Sports Coaching

Commissioning Editor: Claire Wilson
Development Editor: Catherine Jackson
Project Manager: Kiruthiga Kasthuriswamy
Designer/Design Direction: Stewart Larking
Illustration Manager: Bruce Hogarth

Sports Coaching

Professionalisation and Practice

Edited by

Prof. John Lyle EdD and
Dr Chris Cushion PhD

Foreword by

Prof. Patrick Duffy PhD

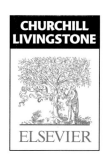

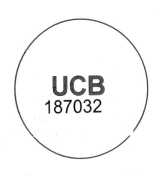
Edinburgh   London   New York   Oxford   Philadelphia   St Louis   Sydney   Toronto   2010

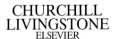

CHURCHILL LIVINGSTONE
ELSEVIER

ISBN 978 0 7020 3054 3
 Reprinted 2011

British Library Cataloguing in Publication Data
A catalogue record for this book is available from the British Library

Library of Congress Cataloging in Publication Data
A catalog record for this book is available from the Library of Congress

Notices
Knowledge and best practice in this field are constantly changing. As new research and experience broaden our understanding, changes in research methods, professional practices, or medical treatment may become necessary.

Practitioners and researchers must always rely on their own experience and knowledge in evaluating and using any information, methods, compounds, or experiments described herein. In using such information or methods they should be mindful of their own safety and the safety of others, including parties for whom they have a professional responsibility.

With respect to any drug or pharmaceutical products identified, readers are advised to check the most current information provided (i) on procedures featured or (ii) by the manufacturer of each product to be administered, to verify the recommended dose or formula, the method and duration of administration, and contraindications. It is the responsibility of practitioners, relying on their own experience and knowledge of their patients, to make diagnoses, to determine dosages and the best treatment for each individual patient, and to take all appropriate safety precautions.

To the fullest extent of the law, neither the Publisher nor the authors, contributors, or editors, assume any liability for any injury and/or damage to persons or property as a matter of products liability, negligence or otherwise, or from any use or operation of any methods, products, instructions, or ideas contained in the material herein.

 ELSEVIER your source for books, journals and multimedia in the health sciences

www.elsevierhealth.com

Working together to grow
libraries in developing countries

www.elsevier.com | www.bookaid.org | www.sabre.org

ELSEVIER   BOOK AID International   Sabre Foundation

The Publisher's policy is to use **paper manufactured from sustainable forests**

Printed in China

Contents

Foreword vii

Preface xi

Acknowledgement xii

Dedication xiii

Chapter summaries xv

Contributor biographies xxi

Chapter 1   Conceptual development in sports coaching 1
            Chris Cushion and John Lyle

Chapter 2   Complex practice in coaching: studying the chaotic nature of
            coach-athlete interactions 15
            Robyn L. Jones, Imornefe Bowes and Kieran Kingston

Chapter 3   Coaches' decision making: a Naturalistic Decision Making analysis 27
            John Lyle

Chapter 4   Coach behaviour 43
            Chris Cushion

Chapter 5   Athlete development and coaching 63
            *Jean Côté, Mark Bruner, Karl Erickson, Leisha Strachan and
            Jessica Fraser-Thomas*

Chapter 6   Planning for team sports 85
            John Lyle

Chapter 7   The professionalisation of sports coaching: definitions, challenges and
            critique 99
            Bill Taylor and Dean Garratt

Chapter 8   Becoming a high-performance coach: pathways and communities 119
            Clifford J. Mallett

Chapter 9   Coach education effectiveness 135
            Pierre Trudel, Wade Gilbert and Penny Werthner

Chapter 10 The learning coach…the learning approach: professional development
            for sports coach professionals 153
            Kathleen M. Armour

Chapter 11 Towards a socio-pedagogy of sports coaching 165
            David Kirk

Chapter 12 Understanding athlete learning and coaching practice:
utilising 'practice theories' and 'theories of practice' 177
Tania Cassidy

Chapter 13 Coaching workforce development 193
Alan Lynn and John Lyle

Chapter 14 Coaching practice and practice ethics 209
Hamish Telfer

Chapter 15 Coaches' expertise 221
Paul G. Schempp and Bryan McCullick

Chapter 16 Coaching philosophy 233
Simon Jenkins

Chapter 17 Narrowing the field: some key questions about sports coaching 243
John Lyle and Chris Cushion

Index 253

Sports coaches are pivotal to the delivery of quality experiences in sport. Millions of paid and unpaid coaches provide children, players and athletes with guidance and support to help them fulfil their goals, follow their dreams and enhance the quality of their lives. Alongside professions such as teaching and medicine, coaching is one of the most ubiquitous services across the globe. Despite this enormous contribution, the value placed on coaching and support for the professional development of coaches is varied. While sport is now a global language, the emergence of connected communities of coaches has been slow to progress both within and outside of national and sport-specific boundaries.

As a consequence, there has neither been the sustained discourse nor the vehicle to advance the position of coaching as a professionally regulated vocation. Until relatively recently, there has been an absence of clarity on terminology relating to coaching roles, systems of qualification and recognition, and the essential elements of effective coaching systems. In this context, it has not been easy to crystallise the key research questions to inform and guide practice and policy.

This publication, edited by John Lyle and Chris Cushion, comes at a critical time as sports coaching takes the early steps in the application of a framework that is gaining international and cross-sport currency. In recent years, there has been increased mobilisation of lead national agencies and federations in coaching; among international federations; within the higher education sector; through Olympic Solidarity and through the efforts of the World Anti-Doping Agency (WADA) and other agencies. This activation has focused on enhancing the education and development of coaches, recognising sport-specific variations, as well as the diversity of need among paid and unpaid coaches in the different nations and continents of the world.

In September 2007, over 20 European agencies adopted the Rio Maior Convention on the recognition of coaching competence and qualifications, named after the Portuguese city in which it was adopted (European Coaching Council, 2007). In addition to leading European agencies in coaching and coach education, the International Council for Coach Education (ICCE) signed the Convention, adding a global dimension to the accord. ICCE has recently signalled its intention to develop a Global Framework for the Recognition of Coaching Competence and Qualifications (ICCE, 2009), building on its support for the Rio Maior Convention.

The Convention stated that 'the framework for the recognition of coaching competence and qualifications as proposed by the European Coaching Council (ECC) in the Review of the 5-level structure is the European recognised reference point for the period 2008–11. During this period, a revised Framework for the Recognition of Coaching Competence and Qualifications will be developed.' (European Coaching Council, 2007: 1). Central to the Review of the 5-level structure was the specification of the core elements of coaching as a professional area within the broader sport sector of the European Union (European Coaching Council, 2007a). This analysis occurred within the context of a wider project that also identified the requirements of the professional areas of health and fitness; physical education and sport management (Petry et al, 2007).

Coaching was defined in the Review as 'the guided improvement, led by a coach, of sports participants and teams in a single sport and at identifiable stages of the athlete/sportsperson pathway' (European Coaching Council, 2007a: 5). As well as providing a sport-specific and participant-centred view of coaching, the EU Review also signalled a revised paradigm that recognised *both* performance-oriented and participation-oriented coaching. Coach of Participant-Oriented Sportspeople and Coach of Performance-Oriented Athletes were identified as the two standard occupations in coaching in paid and unpaid contexts. Participation-oriented coaching includes two sub-roles: Coach of Beginners (child, junior, adult) and Coach of Participation-Oriented Sportspeople (child, junior, adult). Performance-oriented coaching also includes two sub-roles: Coach of Talent Identified/Performance Athletes (child, junior, adult) and Coach of Full-time/High Performance Athletes (European Coaching Council, 2007a: 3).

The emergence of these standard occupations and role descriptors did not occur in isolation. As well as the interaction between leading coaching and coach education agencies in Europe and around the globe since the mid 1990s, research and academic analysis have played an increasing role. One of the editors of this publication was in the frontline of the process to define the broad domains of coaching (Lyle, 2002). This was followed up by a number of studies that aligned the classification of coaching roles and the study of coaching practice with the needs of the participant (for example, Cote et al 2007, Gilbert & Cote 2009).

So, the release of this authoritative publication is timely, in that it clarifies and addresses many research questions in coaching and coach development that have begun to emerge in recent years. The creation of a more solid platform for the further development of coaching as a profession will be significantly advanced by the thoughtful and well-researched contributions that follow. Through the eyes of many of the leading thinkers in the field, the book raises questions, collates evidence and provides a clearer focus on how coaching should move on from here. At a conceptual level, the editors set the scene in Chapter 1, highlighting the complex, dynamic, social, domain and context dependent nature of sport coaching.

In the final Chapter, Lyle and Cushion also provide an overview of emergent themes and issues, recognising that the journey towards conceptual clarity is far from complete. They also suggest that fundamental issues around the definition of sports coaching and its relationship with teaching and instructor roles need to be addressed. This conceptual perspective is augmented by in-depth analyses of the methodological issues associated with the research of coach-athlete interactions through course of action analysis by Jones in Chapter 2 and added to by the insightful perspectives offered by Cushion on coach behaviour in Chapter 4, Kirk on the contribution of pedagogy to coaching in Chapter 11 and Cassidy on practice theories/theories of practice in Chapter 12.

A central theme of the book relates to the long-term development of coaches and the nature of coaching expertise. In Chapter 5, Cote et al elucidate an athlete-centred approach to describe coaching expertise. This important contribution has recently provided the basis for an integrated framework for defining coaching expertise in terms of athletes' outcomes, professional knowledge, inter-

personal knowledge and intra-personal knowledge (Cote & Gilbert, 2009). Drawing on powerful examples from research and practice, Mallet synthesises a number of key themes dealing with the issue of pathways and communities among high-performance coaches in Chapter 8. He cites the need for further research on phased models of coach development, as well as the development by coaches of their own social networks to enhance their craft. In Chapter 15, Schempp and McCullick provide a clear and instructive overview of key findings relating to coaches' expertise, citing a number of key skills demonstrated on a consistent basis by expert coaches: planning; predicting outcomes, intuitive decision-making; communication, automatic coach behaviour; giving attention to the atypical, solving problems; self-monitoring and perceptual skills.

The limitations of looking at coach development purely in terms of coach education are highlighted by Trudel, Gilbert and Werthner in Chapter 9, with a strong emphasis placed on the wider concepts of coach development and lifelong learning. The placement of the development of the coach in a wider, life-long context is also taken up by Armour in Chapter 10. She makes a clear and compelling case for the concept of the 'learning coach'. Armour also emphasises that coaches are likely to take more notice of development opportunities when they see the potential to bring about meaningful learning and progress for the participants with whom they work. Lyle reminds us in Chapter 6 that the development of expertise in team sports brings with it additional challenges, a topic which requires further analysis.

A common theme from these chapters on coach development and expertise is the importance of, as Trudel, Gilbert and Werthner state, 'the responsibility to develop as a coach should stay primarily in the hands of the individual'. The value of situated learning, the ability of the coach to reflect, analyse and adjust their practice; and the creation of communities of practice all emerge as key themes for future development. It is also apparent from these contributions that the creation of formal, informal and non-formal opportunities for coaches should be based on the clear identification of their needs and stage of development and crucially the needs of the participants with whom they work.

The development of coaching as a profession poses many challenges, as highlighted by Taylor and Garrat in Chapter 7. The creation of a professional and regulatory framework will depend on the existence of a distinct knowledge base, organisation and ethics to guide engagement. Notably, Taylor and Garret highlight the absence of an independent body for coaches as a potential limitation in moving the agenda forward. Pragmatically, they highlight 'the considerable problems evident in transforming a mainly voluntary structure and workforce towards one that can provide a sustainable future that serves individual sports, meet government directives and policy and supports a new breed of sports coaching professionals'.

As Armour pointed out in Chapter 10, there are many lessons to be learned from other professions and she draws on the experience of pharmacy to outline three key principles that are of relevance to the professional behaviour of sports coaches: engendering trust, exercising professional judgement and engaging in continuing education. Coaches with a clear sense of their own philosophy, as proposed by Jenkins in Chapter 16, are likely to be in a better position to behave like professionals. He draws on the work of Milton Rokeach to clarify our understanding of beliefs, values and principles – all of which are critical to the development of a profession.

It is evident from many of the contributions in this book, therefore, that the individual responsibility and behaviour of the coach will be the cornerstones of the emergent profession. In this regard, Telfer's illuminative Chapter 14 on coaching practice and coaching ethics draws together a number of essential components that ought to be taken on board in the evolution of coaching towards professional status. He highlights the need for a set of core principles; ethical decision-making, appropriate training, responsibility and accountability for coaches. Telfer states that 'the role and function of the coach is to bring to bear … a degree of judgement about correct or 'right' actions'. He also highlights the need to position the ethical principles associated with coaching as part of a wider set of principles within sport.

The book, therefore, will significantly enhance the discourse and clarity on coaching and the emergent profession. The European and proposed Global Frameworks for the Recognition of Coaching Competence and Qualifications provide important elements of the architecture within which these concepts can be further developed. The creation of momentum in developing coaching as a profession should take full account of the needs of coaches, their sport, their national and cultural contexts and, crucially, their professional choices and decision-making in providing high-quality experiences for sports participants.

The further evolution of the coaching workforce is on-going around the globe and is a critical element in the creation of pathways for coaches and in the supply of quality coaches to participants. Lynn and Lyle in Chapter 13 raise a number of key issues that need to be addressed in the more systematic analysis and development of the coaching workforce. This pragmatic and front-line focus is an essential feature of bringing about change that is needs-led and empirically based. This approach also provides the basis for more effectively supporting coaches in the role that they play. The UK Coaching Framework (sports coach UK, 2008) and The UK Coaching Workforce 2009–15 (North, 2009) are cited as recent examples of how a systems-based approach to workforce development can be built upon participant and coach need, while taking into account government and sport specific objectives.

While the book has not provided all the answers, it has crafted a more coherent architecture for the emergent profession of coaching. It has highlighted that the fledgling profession has made significant strides in recent years and the chapters have combined to plot an exciting and challenging journey ahead. Future developments will be country-, context- and sport-specific, but will increasingly be underpinned by a language, structure and system of training, ethics and accountability that will have a global resonance. Sport coaching must seek to position itself within a wider and more clearly defined profession of sport and physical activity. This wider profession should, in turn, seek to take its place as a valued and effective service area within a globalised world, supporting people of all ages to experience the joy and fulfilment of a life enriched by physical activity.

Prof. Patrick Duffy PhD
Chairman, European Coaching Council,
Vice President (Europe), International Council for
Coach Education, Professor of Sports Coaching,
Leeds Metropolitan University, UK

References

Côté, J., Young, B., North, J., Duffy, P., 2007. Towards a definition of excellence in sport coaching. International Journal of Coaching Science 1, 3–17.

Côté, J., Gilbert, W., 2009. An integrative definition of coaching expertise. International Journal of Sports Science and Coaching 4, 307–323.

European Coaching Council, 2007. Rio Maior Convention on the recognition of coaching competence and qualifications. European Network of Sports Science, Education and Employment: Koln.

European Coaching Council, 2007a. Review of the EU 5-level structure for the recognition of coaching qualifications. European Network of Sports Science, Education and Employment: Koln.

International Council for Coach Education, 2009. Building the coaching profession across the globe. Consultation document. Presented to the ICCE Global Coach Conference, Vancouver.

Lyle, J., 2002. Sports coaching concepts: a framework for coach's behaviour. Routledge, London.

North, J., 2009. The Coaching Workforce 2009–2016. sports coach UK: Leeds.

Petry, K., Froberg, K., Madella, A., Tokarski, W. (eds.), 2008. Higher Education in Sport in Europe. Maidenhead: Meyer & Meyer Sport.

sports coach UK, 2008. The UK Coaching Framework. Leeds.

Sports coaching continues to grow as an academic discipline and, as a vocation, is developing the workforce education, infrastructure, and regulation that will lead to professionalisation. Increasing academic interest and its accompanying research and dissemination are being directed, more and more, to the enhancement of coaching practice through more sophisticated knowledge and understanding. Research has begun to coalesce around the key elements of the coaching process and a number of emerging coaching-related themes. Through the writing of international scholars in the field, *Sports Coaching: Professionalisation and Practice* aims to bring this work together in one volume in such a way that we are able to evaluate the progress made over the past 10–15 years. The overarching purpose is to make a 'position statement' about the nature of coaching, and our understanding of it 'in practice'. In doing so, we provide an overview of coaching research themes that critically considers key research findings, links to practice, and identifies areas for future research and development.

The book opens with a critical appreciation of the theoretical and conceptual 'strength' of sports coaching, and it closes with a polemical stance on a number of issues that impact professionalisation. The authors of the intervening chapters have been encouraged to approach their research themes in a critical and questioning way. This questioning of assumptions is undertaken in the broad interests of coaching and its fate as it moves toward professionalisation. We believe that students of coaching should be aware of the current 'state of play'. However, a further outcome of the book's use is the fostering of discussion and debate. This is needed to enrich the future development of coaching, while ensuring a strengthening link between conceptual development and coaching practice. We believe that the result will be new and important understandings for scholars, coaches and coach educators. The book will become a catalogue of new insights and possibilities, a point of reference that offers, in aggregation, a new analytical framework for coaching research.

Although not formally subdivided into distinct sections, there is a rationale for the ordering of chapters. The opening chapter by the editors serves as an introduction to the book. Chapters 2–6 are concerned with the coach's behaviour and practice. The remainder of the book is rooted in the professionalisation issue. An appraisal of the process of professionalisation (Chapters 7–9) is followed by a detailed exploration of the place of coaching pedagogy as a specialised field of study (Chapters 10–12). The remaining chapters (13–16) examine professional practice in its wider context. The editors conclude the book with a challenging interpretation of some of the themes to emerge across the chapters. All of the chapters draw on theoretical concepts and empirical data, wherever possible all have tangible links to practice and the practitioner.

Acknowledgement

We have worked together, debated furiously and at length, and looked into the future of coaching. Our conclusion was that the time was right to say something about the academic study of sports coaching. We have greatly enjoyed the collaboration that has culminated in this book, and we thank Elsevier for supporting the project. In particular we would like to thank the other authors for taking the time to make meaningful and high quality contributions.

We each benefit hugely from the unconditional support of our families in all our endeavours, and the book is dedicated to them.

John and Chris

Conceptual development in sports coaching

The authors, Chris Cushion and John Lyle, review the emergence of a conceptual understanding and representation of sports coaching and the coaching process. They acknowledge the variety of lens – science of performance, pedagogical, humanistic, sociological – through which coaching can be viewed. However, they point to an emerging consensus that the practice of coaching can be described as a complex, dynamic, social, domain and context-dependent enterprise, with often-contradictory goals and values. Although this appreciation of the complexities of practice may not yet be reflected in coach education, the fact that previous assumptions about coaching are now considered problematic is perceived as a significant step forward. There is a tension between the planned intervention to improve performance and a layer of contingency that requires a continuous process of accommodation, integration and coordination. The authors suggest that research and scholarly activity and its attendant methodologies have not yet addressed the challenges posed by this appreciation of coaching practice and the questions it poses about coaches' expertise.

Complex practice in coaching: Studying the chaotic nature of coach-athlete interactions

The complex interactive nature of coaching is being increasingly recognised. This recognition presents issues around investigative methodologies that are capable of capturing the detail and nuance of coaching practice. The authors, Robyn Jones, Imornefe Bowes and Kieran Kingston develop arguments around the intricacies and complexity of coaching as a social process. They go on to critique current and more traditional methods employed to explore

coaching. Course of action analysis, inclusive of situated action and activity theory is then introduced as an alternative method for exploring the complexity of coaching. This analysis allows particular incidents and interactions to be explored in detail and presents a way to understand why such incidents have meaning for coaches and athletes. This enables a deconstructing of precise actions and reactions within ever-changing contexts, and presents opportunities to theorise practice as a means of explanation and development.

Coaches' decision making: A Naturalistic Decision Making analysis

Decision making in its various forms is argued to be a crucial element of coaches' expertise; ranging from the deliberative decision making in planning to the semi- and non-deliberative decision-making characteristics of coaches' behaviour in managing interventions and competition. Naturalistic Decision Making is proposed as a useful paradigm for understanding how expert coaches make decisions, and cope with the complexity inherent in the coaching context. This theoretical approach stresses the 'reading' of the environment, comparison to stored images of previous coaching situations, and matching to solution that have previously proved effective. John Lyle suggests that adopting this paradigm as a contribution to our understanding of coaches' expertise and coach education will create a new discourse – pattern recognition, situational awareness, mental simulation, forward reflection, and decision choice heuristics. Intuition is explained as a 'speedy' form of mental simulation; an explanation that offers some answers for the seemingly problematic tacit and intuitive decision behaviour of the coach. The chapter ends with some proposals for a more decision-making-friendly approach to coach education.

Coach behaviour

The coach's behaviour is described as a more sophisticated phenomenon than has been adequately captured by research to date. In particular, the nuances of transmission by the coach and reception by the athlete are explored, in addition to the antecedents of behaviour and features of the environment such as gender, age level of expectation and relative status. Indeed, Chris Cushion reminds us that, rather than being thought of as an aggregation of isolated elements of coaching activity, the coach's behaviour can best be understood as multi-dimensional and the outcome of the active engagement of the coach, the athlete and the context – and the effect that each has on the other. Although most often studied in intervention situations, the coach's behaviour is 'all-pervasive', and therefore always contributing to the wider process. The most common 'surface' behaviour, instruction, silence and feedback/reinforcement are reprised but more valuable is the message that the number of context and outcome contingent factors makes the prescription of seemingly generic and effective behaviours almost impossible. Nonetheless, reflecting on discrete behaviours is worthwhile, particularly for novice coaches, and experts develop a 'toolbox' of behaviours that ensure relevance to the athletes' needs and the context.

Athlete development and coaching

Models of coaching and athlete development tend to evolve on parallel paths. The outcome of such research demonstrates that athletes will vary in terms of age, development level and goals, while coaches will work in various contexts with varying resources, equipment and facilities. Jean Côté, Mark Bruner, Karl Erickson and Leisha Strachan argue that while the coach's characteristics and situation will impact coaching, an examination of the development needs of the athletes at different ages and competitive levels should be the driver for a coaching system. The authors review the youth development literature highlighting the 4Cs as outcomes for developing athletes (competence, confidence, connection, character/caring). This conceptual framework is utilised within the developmental model of sport participation to describe a typology of coaching. From this the authors are able to produce four categories of coaching (participation coaches for children, participation coaches for adolescents, performance coaches for young adolescents, performance coaches for late adolescents and adults) aligning each to the athlete's developmental needs and highlighting implications for coaching practice, i.e. what coaching should look like to achieve the goals at each stage and aligned to the athlete's needs. The chapter provides a useful map to help coaches align their knowledge and skills with a specific athlete's developmental needs. In doing so suggests different coach behaviours are necessary along with different types of knowledge skills and training.

Planning for team sports

The evidence provided by the coaches in the study demonstrated that planning was a highly contextual and highly contingent part of the coaching process. The season-long planning framework conforms to a periodised model based on the competition schedule, and is strongly influenced by strength and conditioning needs. Detailed 'operational' planning most often takes the form of 4-week cycles. These are subject to a range of contingencies, the most influential being both the result and the perceived 'form' demonstrated in the most recent games. Session plans are in skeleton form; with implementation relying on the coaches' accumulated expertise. There were clear differences in the planning behaviour of academy, part-time and full-time coaches. John Lyle identifies a sound technical model, regular communication with colleagues, and good information/monitoring systems as mechanisms for coping with the contingent nature of the process. Coaches appear to create a 'vision' (or mental model) of their 'goals in action' and this is used to regulate their decision making. There is a constant tension between the ordered management of contingency, progression and preparation, and the need for a 'reactive flexibility'.

The professionalisation of sports coaching; definitions, challenges and critiques

The professionalisation agenda in sports coaching faces a number of challenges, not least is to give a predominantly volunteer work force, and the governing-body-driven sport landscape a unified and bona fide professional status. Bill Taylor and Dean Garratt critically discuss the drivers behind professionalisation and link this to an imposition of a new managerialist ideology. The discussion surrounding developing sports coaching and a process of professionalisation is used as a mechanism to interrogate the contested discourse of professionalism. The authors consider the issues surrounding the process for coaching, and are critical of the extant literature on this issue in terms of its potency, direction and conceptualisation. The contested terms and definitions discussed highlight the problematic nature of the process. The authors consider some of the theoretical tools for examining professional occupations, and draw on some of their own data highlighting issues pertinent to coaching. The authors demonstrate the lack of meaningful consultation around the process, and question if the envisaged model of the coach will produce a valued and independent intellectual. Instead, arguing that there is a real risk of producing 'docile' technocrat coaches without progressive coach education and development.

Becoming a high-performance coach: pathways and communities

A convincing case is made for the complexity of the high-performance coaching role (not simply the complexity of the complexity process itself), and this reinforces the concept of the high-performance coach as 'performance director', albeit with a variable role in directing coaching interventions. Although not a sole contributor to developing expertise, the evidence on the value of 'time in the role' complemented many previous studies on the extent to which coaches value experience. Nevertheless, our attention is drawn to the preparatory phases of 'development of prior commitment' and occupational socialisation. There is a clear demonstration of 'immersion' in the role, and in the technicalities of the sport. The role is domain-specific, and recruitment takes place from within the sport; coaches generally having had extensive playing experience. Cliff Mallett proposes further research on the 'scaffolding' of high-performance coach development. He questions simplistic interpretations of communities of practice and invites us to

appreciate the full range of social networks from which the coach might receive support.

Coach education effectiveness

A review of the empirical evidence provides no evidence to support the effectiveness of small-scale, university-based, or large-scale national coach education programmes. Receiving any intervention may change behaviour in the short term. However, interventions are rarely measured against coaching practice indicators, and there is limited, if any, evidence of sustained impact. Domain- and role-specificity appear to confound the research. Studies using younger adolescents, university students and high-performance athletes as part of the 'effectiveness' measure provide a confusing array of athlete objectives and outcomes. The study of university-based coach education programmes highlights the issues of realism and embeddedness in education-related practice. The authors, Pierre Trudel, Wade Gilbert and Penny Werthner go on to propose an alternative view of coach education that provides a more realistic set of expectations for coach education. Formal coach education cannot be divorced from other 'spheres' of life and the coach's choices and priorities in relation to development and education should be understood in the context of this personography. This helps to explain the difficulty in measuring the effectiveness of isolated elements of, particularly formal, coach education.

The learning coach ... the learning approach: professional development for sports coach professionals

Continuing professional development (CPD) is proposed as a hallmark of a profession and the chapter considers the ways in which professional learning could be conceptualised, designed and organised. Kathy Armour makes the case for the 'learning coach' with situated professional learning at the heart of coaching as a profession. While acknowledging the enormity and contested nature of 'learning', the author is critical of approaches that are not explicit about assumptions around the learner, knowledge and learning. She warns against the dangers of implicit assumptions and unchallenged beliefs that are not necessarily athlete-centred. Constructivism is proposed as a theory that helps explain how learning is undertaken within communities of practice. The notions of apprenticeship and transformative learning are introduced as concepts to help learning to be engaging and the learner to be engaged. The CPD literature from education is reviewed and highlights salient lessons learned around structure, content and delivery of learning that could be used to inform developments in coaching. These are pulled together to give an overview of the conditions required to create a 'learning coach'.

Towards a socio-pedagogy of sports coaching

Pedagogy is defined as the interdependence and irreducibility of subject matter, learning, instruction and context. The components are interdependent as changes in one will impact the other. David Kirk draws on Mauss' thesis of techniques of the body, and McIntyre's concept of a social practice, including the notion of intrinsic and extrinsic goods, to understand coaching as both a social and embodied practice. The author argues that learning is central to coaching practice, and a socio-pedagogy requires coaches to understand pedagogy, relations among pedagogical settings, and the moral responsibilities surrounding cultural production and reproduction. The importance of subject matter knowledge is highlighted as being vital to coaching and the author urges coaching not to repeat the mistakes of school physical education by abandoning a deep understanding of subject matter and developing content-less pedagogical processes.

Understanding athlete learning and coaching practice: utilising 'practice theories' and 'theories of practice'

'Practice theories' derived from biographical and other descriptive accounts are a rich source of evidence about coaches' pedagogical practices. However, the value of the accounts is diminished by the absence of a conceptual appreciation and vocabulary about pedagogy. 'Theories of practice' are usefully informed by accepting pedagogy as a process of knowledge production that engages the coach, the

athlete, the content, and the context. Coaching knowledge is a 'way of doing something' rather than 'knowledge about something', with implications for building relationships and linkages that should interest coach education designers. Tania Cassidy warns against relying solely on the process knowledge of former performers when making coaching appointments. She goes on to stress the role of the athlete as an active participant in learning strategies, noting that coaches will benefit greatly from reflecting on their implicit assumptions about learning and being exposed to 'theories of practice' about learners. The focus is on the athlete as an active learner and on the process of learning. This poses questions about the tradition hierarchy of coach-athlete relationships.

Coaching workforce development

Workforce development is shown to be much more than coach education. It involves the management of supply and demand (including recruitment and retention), the quality of provision (including upskilling and the regulation of deployment), and the continuing professional development of the workforce. With a dispersed workforce, a limited role as employers, and a traditional role as education and training providers, Governing Bodies of sport have a particular set of challenges in managing the coaching workforce. Alan Lynn and John Lyle identify a number of issues: the largely voluntary nature of the workforce, skills shortages, the absence of a pool of labour, and the limited mobility of the workforce. They draw particular attention to the danger of using 'aspirational' growth targets to set coach education targets, and make the case that much greater understanding of coaches' motives and career development is required. Data management, such as the tracking of coach education throughput and databases of active coaches, is required. The value of a 'licensing scheme' is emphasised, both as a catalyst to better workforce management and as a prerequisite for professional development.

Coaching practice and practice ethics

An argument is presented that emphasises the centrality of moral values in determining the coach's ethical decision making. Individual probity, rather than a reliance on codes of professional conduct, is required and the process of making ethical judgements should be viewed as one of critical interpretation. The process is complex and situationally dependent. Concern is expressed over the minimal role that ethical decision making plays in coach education, and questions are raised about whether the coach can be assumed to have a well-rehearsed sense of appropriate ethical behaviour. Hamish Telfer reviews the guiding principles on which ethics are based. He stresses the values of beneficence, non-malfeasance, autonomy, respect for others, and justice (or fairness). These are challenging to apply in an outcome-based context. Nevertheless, the coaching environment can be argued to create inherent risk since the athlete can be 'situationally vulnerable'. However, being able to justify one's ethical decisions is a mark of the professional, as is an environment in which these decisions are open to scrutiny.

Coaches' expertise

Expert–novice differences are well-documented, and there is a growing body of literature that is helping to identify the characteristics that distinguish the expert coach. Paul Schempp and Bryan McCullick draw on a range of research literature including their own to consider the three elements that consistently emerge as contributing to expertise; experience, knowledge and skills. The authors identify that both experiential learning and learning from experience are crucial to developing expertise. Importantly, in order to be meaningful, experiences need to be reflected upon and deliberate, systematic and continual; that is, experts actively and consistently seek this kind of learning. Superior knowledge is characterised not by volume but by the ability to synthesise and apply. The authors identify strategic knowledge as crucial, enabling the expert coach to distinguish the important from the unimportant. A number of skills are indentified, these include; planning, ability to predict outcomes, decision making, communication, automatic coaching behaviour, paying attention to the atypical, self-monitoring and perceptual skills. The authors argue that these are earned through experience and deliberate practice, suggesting that becoming more expert is a possibility for all coaches motivated to develop the key areas.

Coaching philosophy

Coaching philosophy will impact coaching practice implicitly or explicitly. Developing self-awareness as a coach, and being critically reflective about practice requires that coaches should 'know themselves' and be able to articulate their coaching philosophy. Simon Jenkins attempts to add to the conceptual depth of this exercise by developing the concepts of beliefs, values and principles. Interrogating existing coaching literature the author draws on the work of Milton Rokeach to develop a broader understanding on human values and principles and offers Rokeach's work as a useful framework for coaches clarify their beliefs, values, attitudes and norms. The review of literature highlights that coaches' espoused philosophy, their actual philosophy and their coaching behaviour may not, for a variety of reasons, always align. The author offers the idea of 'story telling' and critical incidents as a means for coaches to develop and articulate their coaching philosophy. In discussing developing a philosophy, the author uses the lens of John Wooden as an example to demonstrate that coaching philosophy evolves over time and to emphasise that the espoused and public philosophy may be at odds with the reality of practice.

Narrowing the field: some key questions about sports coaching

The editors, John Lyle and Chris Cushion, take the opportunity to 'make a statement' about a number of issues that they believe to be at the heart of future challenges to coaching research and researchers. They recognise the situational dependency that pervades much of the literature and attribute this to the distinctive milieux in which coaching communities of practice operate. They describe the domain-specific factors that impact on coaches' practice and argue that it is misguided to assume that a coherent set of processes and practices exist across coaching domains. Sports coaching is attacked as too imprecise a term to be useful; it connotes a family of related roles but the authors suggest that these do not represent a continuum of expertise or roles. It is important to distinguish between coaches, instructors and teachers of sport; and it is argued that professionalisation depends on an appropriate threshold of expertise, experience and education. Mental models are identified as a mechanism for coaches' regulatory practice. These points of references are a focus for investigating the social construction of knowledge, education, experience, and coaches' behaviour. The need for empirically sound models of practice is contrasted with practitioner prescriptions from other fields. The authors counsel against over-ambitious expectations about modelling the coaching process.

Prof. John Lyle EdD
Adjunct Professor of Sports Coaching, School of Human Movement Studies, The University of Queensland, St Lucia, Qld, Australia

Until recently John was Professor of Sports Coaching in the Carnegie Faculty of Leeds Metropolitan University. This appointment followed a long and successful career in higher education, first in physical education and thereafter specialising in sports coaching studies. He established the first professional diploma in sports coaching and the first Masters degree in coaching studies in the UK. He has played a significant role in the development of sports coaching as an academic field of study, and is the author of the influential textbook *Sports Coaching Concepts* (Routledge, 2002). John has contributed widely through publications, conference presentations and professional developments in sports coaching. He is an Adjunct Professor at the University of Queensland, Australia, and sits on the editorial boards of two academic journals. He has recently returned to a role as a full-time research consultant, collaborating with a number of universities and national sports agencies. John's academic experience is complemented by a considerable personal experience as a coach, and engagement in the delivery of coach education and development.

Dr Chris Cushion PhD
Senior Lecturer and MSc Sports Coaching Programme Leader, School of Sport, Exercise and Health Sciences, Loughborough University, Loughborough, UK

Chris Cushion is the programme leader for the MSc Sports Coaching at Loughborough University. He has a wide interest in coaching being involved in the development of the UK Coaching Certificate and a range of coaching-related consultancy projects. He is also actively involved in coaching practice being a UEFA-qualified soccer coach. Chris has a range of research and teaching interests around coaching. These include understanding the coaching process, coach education, learning and professional development, coach behaviour and learning environments. He is involved with a number of research projects in and around these areas. Chris is an

editorial board member and reviewer for a range of peer-reviewed journals including *Physical Education and Sport Pedagogy, International Journal of Sport and Exercise Psychology, Psychology of Sport and Exercise, The Sport Psychologist, Journal of Sport Sciences, European Journal of Sport Psychology* and the *Journal of Applied Sport Psychology*.

Prof. Kathleen M. Armour PhD
Professor of Physical Education & Sport Pedagogy; Director of Research, School of Sport, Exercise & Health Sciences, Loughborough University, Loughborough, UK

Kathleen Armour is Professor of Physical Education & Sport Pedagogy, and Director of Research, in the School of Sport, Exercise & Health Sciences at Loughborough University, UK. Her research interests centre on professional development for teachers and coaches. In particular, Professor Armour is interested in effective, career-long professional development for teachers and coaches, and in PE teachers' learning needs in the areas of health and vulnerable children.

Imornefe Bowes
British Beach Volleyball Womens Coach, Bath, UK

Imornefe Bowes is currently the Head Coach of the Great Britain women's beach volleyball programme, and formerly a Teaching and Coaching Fellow at the University of Bath, where he lectured in coach education and sports psychology. He was also head coach of the University of Bath's high-performance volleyball programme. He is completing a PhD at the University of Wales Institute Cardiff with supervisor Prof Robyn L. Jones where his main research interest is examining the application of complexity theory to sports coaching.

Dr Mark W. Bruner PhD
SSHRC Postdoctoral Research Fellow, School of Kinesiology and Health Studies, Queen's University, Kingston, ON, Canada

Mark Bruner is a SSHRC Postdoctoral Research Fellow in the School of Kinesiology and Health Studies at Queen's University. He received his

Doctorate in Kinesiology (Exercise and Sport Psychology) at the University of Saskatchewan. His externally funded programme of research focuses on examining and understanding how we can utilise group dynamics (e.g., team building, group cohesion, group identity) to enhance physical activity adherence and foster positive youth development.

Dr Tania Cassidy PhD
Senior Lecturer, School of Physical Education,
University of Otago, Dunedin, New Zealand

Tania's research interests focus on the learning process from the perspectives of athletes and coaches. Currently, she serves on the editorial boards of four journals, namely; *International Journal of Sports Science and Coaching, Physical Education and Sport Pedagogy, International Journal of Sport and Exercise Psychology* and the *International Journal of Coaching Science*. Tania is first author of the text *Understanding Sports Coaching: The social, cultural and pedagogical foundations of sports practice* (2004; 2009), which has been translated into Korean and Norwegian, and has had her work published in professional and scholarly journals and books.

Prof. Jean Côté PhD
Professor and Director, School of Kinesiology and Health Studies, Queen's University, Kingston, Ontario, Canada

Dr. Jean Côté is Professor and Director of the School of Kinesiology and Health Studies at Queen's University at Kingston in Canada. His research interests are in the areas of athletes' development, coaching, and sport expertise. He has delivered 24 keynote addresses at major national and international conferences in Europe, Asia, North America, and Australia. In 2009, Dr. Côté was the recipient of the 4th EW Barker Professorship from the Physical Education and Sport Science department at the National Institute of Education in Singapore. Dr. Côté is co-editor of the *International Journal of Sport and Exercise Psychology*.

Karl Erickson
School of Kinesiology & Health Studies, Queen's University, Kingston, ON, Canada

Karl Erickson is a doctoral student at Queen's University, working under the supervision of Dr Jean Côté. Karl's research is currently focused on coach-athlete interactions in youth sport in relation to athletes' psychosocial development. He has also examined the learning and development of sport coaches. Karl's research on coaching at both the masters and PhD level has been externally funded by the Coaching Association of Canada (CAC) and the Social Sciences and Humanities Research Council (SSHRC) of Canada. More practically, Karl is heavily involved in coaching both basketball and rugby at a number of different levels.

Dr Jessica Fraser-Thomas PhD
Assistant Professor, York University, Toronto, Ontario, Canada

Jessica Fraser-Thomas is an Assistant Professor in the School of Kinesiology and Health Science at York University, Toronto, Canada. Her research interests are in youth sport with a specific focus on sport pedagogy, psychosocial influences, life skills development, mental skills training, and how youth sport contexts can be better designed to facilitate children and adolescents' healthy physical and psychosocial development. Jessica is a former physical education teacher, national team athlete, and coach of youth, varsity, and master athletes. In her leisure time Jessica enjoys competing in triathlons, coaching and consulting athletes in her community, and spending time with her family.

Dr Dean Garratt PhD
Senior Lecturer in Education Studies, Faculty of Education, Community and Leisure, Liverpool John Moores University, Liverpool, UK

Dr Dean Garratt is a senior lecturer in Education Studies and postgraduate programme leader at Liverpool John Moores University. His research interests span a broad and eclectic range of themes, but have tended to focus upon the critique of citizenship education, analysis of education policy and theme of professionalism in the context of sports coaching. These are complemented by a long-standing fascination and curiosity of social theory and towards the philosophy of qualitative research, in particular aspects of phenomenology, hermeneutics and post-structural theorising.

Dr Wade D. Gilbert PhD
Associate Professor, Department of Kinesiology, California State University, Fresno, CA, USA

Wade Gilbert is an Associate Professor in the Department of Kinesiology at California State University, Fresno. He directs the Sport & Exercise Psychology Lab and is the project coordinator for

SHAPE (School-based Healthy Activities Program for Exercise). Dr. Gilbert is the editor of a special issue of the *Sport Psychologist on Coach Education*. His work has been published in a wide array of scientific outlets including *Research Quarterly for Exercise and Sport*, *The Sport Psychologist*, and the *Journal of Teaching Physical Education*.

Dr Simon Jenkins PhD

Principal Lecturer in Sports Coaching, Leeds Metropolitan University, Leeds, UK

Simon Jenkins is a Principal Lecturer in the Carnegie Faculty of Sport and Education at Leeds Metropolitan University. He is the Founder and Editor-in-Chief of the *International Journal of Sports Science and Coaching, Annual Review of Golf Coaching* and *Annual Review of High Performance Coaching and Consulting*. Simon is also the author of *Sports Science Handbook: The Essential Guide to Kinesology, Sport & Exercise Science*. He was an Associate Coach with the English Golf Union (1996–2001), providing education and training on the mental, physical and technical sides of the game for talented boy golfers in the South Region of England.

Prof. Robyn L. Jones PhD

Professor of Sport and Social Theory, University of Wales Institute – Cardiff (UWIC), Cardiff, UK

Robyn L. Jones is a Professor at the Cardiff School of Sport, University of Wales Institute, Cardiff (UWIC), UK and a Visiting Professor at the Norwegian School of Sport Sciences, Oslo, Norway. His research area comprises a critical sociology of coaching in respect of examining the complexity of the interactive coaching context and how practitioners manage the power-ridden dilemmas that arise. He has published several books and articles on coaching and pedagogy, and serves on the editorial boards of *Sport, Education and Society*, *Physical Education and Sport Pedagogy* and the *International Journal of Sports Science and Coaching*.

Dr Kieran Kingston PhD

Senior Lecturer in Sport Psychology (Sport Psychology). Cardiff School of Sport, University of Wales Institute Cardiff, Cardiff, UK

Kieran Kingston is a Senior Lecturer and Discipline Director of Sport Psychology at the University of Wales Institute Cardiff (UWIC). He completed his PhD (University of Wales) in 1999 under the supervision of Professor Lew Hardy. Kieran is an active

researcher primarily in the area of sport motivation, particularly focussing on the areas of: goals, self-determination, goal climate, and self-confidence; he also continues to work in the area of golf psychology. Kieran has worked as a sport psychology consultant in a variety of elite individual and team sport environments (including rugby, track and field and snooker), although the majority of his work has been in professional and elite amateur golf.

Prof. David Kirk PhD

Alexander Chair in Physical Education and Sport, University of Bedfordshire, Bedford, UK

David Kirk is currently Alexander Chair in Physical Education and Sport at the University of Bedfordshire. Between 2005 and 2009 he was Dean of the Carnegie Faculty of Sport and Education at Leeds Metropolitan University. Professor Kirk has also held academic appointments at the University of Ghent, Loughborough University, the University of Queensland and Deakin University. He is Editor of *Physical Education and Sport Pedagogy* and is a former European Editor of the *Journal of Curriculum Studies*. Professor Kirk's latest book, *Physical Education Futures*, was published by Routledge in 2009.

Alan Lynn

Course Director, MSc Sports Coaching at the University of Stirling, Stirling, UK

Alan Lynn is an experienced swimming coach and coach educator. He has coached Olympic Games finalists and world-class swimmers in his 25-year coaching career and was Technical Director for Scottish Swimming before his move into Higher Education. Currently the Course Director for the MSc Sports Coaching at Stirling University, he has research interests in personal construct psychology, particularly as it relates to the analysis of elite sports coaches and is presently completing his PhD on this topic. Still an active coach with age group swimmers, he also mentors young coaches across several sports. He has authored three successful books on performance swimming with a fourth book in press.

Dr Cliff Mallett PhD

Senior Lecturer & Coordinator Postgraduate Programs in Sports Coaching, School of Human Movement Studies, The University of Queensland, St Lucia, Qld, Australia

Dr Mallett teaches and researches in sport psychology and coaching, and manages the postgraduate programmes in sports coaching at The University of

Queensland. A former national and Olympic team athletics coach, Cliff has coached many sprinters and relay teams to international success. He is a leading coach educator and sport psychologist consulting to several organisations, including the IAAF, Sport Knowledge Australia, Australian Sports Commission, professional and Olympic sporting bodies, and elite athletes. Cliff is an active researcher in high-performance coaching and sport performance, and a member of the International Council for Coach Education. He is on the Editorial Boards of several international sport psychology and coaching science journals.

Dr Bryan A. McCullick PhD
Associate Professor, Sport Instruction Research Laboratory, The University of Georgia, Athens, GA, USA

Bryan McCullick is an Associate Professor in the Department of Kinesiology at the University of Georgia. His research interests are focused on studying expert teachers and coaches, and the participants in and assessment of coach education programs (CEPs). Bryan's work provided the first examination of expert sport instructors' working memory and the implications for instruction. A key theoretical article applying Berliner's framework of teaching expertise to coaching 'greats' is often cited in contemporary publications. His work has generated invitations to speak at meetings of learned societies in the United States, Germany, Turkey, and Taiwan. Dr McCullick held a visiting scholar post at University College, Cork in 2008, and has received external funding on CEPs from the LPGA and GOLF Magazine.

Prof. Paul G. Schempp PhD
Professor, Sport Instruction Research Laboratory, University of Georgia, Athens, GA, USA

Dr. Paul G. Schempp is a Professor at the University of Georgia where he serves as the Director of the Sport Instruction Research Laboratory. He has taught at Kent State University and University of Oregon. In 1990, he was appointed a Senior Fulbright Research Scholar at the University of Frankfurt, Germany and was a visiting professor at the National Institute of Education in Singapore in 2001. The author of six books, and over 100 articles, Paul's research focuses on teaching and coaching expertise.

Dr Leisha Strachan PhD
Assistant Professor, Faculty of Kinesiology and Recreation Management, University of Manitoba, Winnipeg, Canada

Leisha Strachan is an Assistant Professor in the Faculty of Kinesiology and Recreation Management at the University of Manitoba in Winnipeg, Canada. As a coach and judge in the sport of baton twirling, she has a keen interest in the growth of children and youth in highly competitive sport contexts. With help from the Social Sciences and Humanities Research Council (SSHRC) and in collaborations with Dr. Jean Côté and Dr. Janice Deakin, she has examined outcomes and experiences in youth sport programs. She plans to examine further recreational and elite sport programmes for children and youth and delve more deeply into their sport experiences.

Bill Taylor
Senior Lecturer in Coaching Studies, Department of Exercise and Sport Science, Manchester Metropolitan University, Manchester, UK

Bill Taylor is a senior lecturer in Coaching Studies and postgraduate programme leader at the Department of Exercise and Sport Science of Manchester Metropolitan University. His research interests centre around the conceptualisation and critical deconstruction of notions of professionalism in sports coaching and sports medicine. He has undertaken projects and research for a number of National Governing Bodies and government agencies on this subject. As a coach he has worked with a number of athletes at international level as well as being employed as a consultant within the UK and USA in coach education within paddle sports.

Dr Hamish Telfer PhD
Senior Lecturer in Sports Pedagogy, University of Cumbria, Lancaster Campus, Lancaste, UK

Having trained as a teacher of physical education at the Scottish School of Physical Education in Glasgow, Hamish followed a brief spell of school teaching with a full-time post as Great Britain National Coach and Technical Officer in Life Saving. This was followed by lecturing posts at the Universities of Liverpool and Lancaster and then St Martins College, Lancaster (now University of Cumbria). He established six undergraduate degrees and one Masters degree course whilst at Cumbria, as well as fulfilling the role of Great Britain National Team Coach for cross country running for British Universities. He specialises in coaching practice, practice ethics, reflective practice and child protection issues.

Prof. Pierre Trudel PhD

Professor, Faculty of Health Sciences, School of Human Kinetics, University of Ottawa, Ottawa, Canada

Pierre Trudel is a Professor in the School of Human Kinetics, University of Ottawa, Canada. In the last 15 years his research group has been funded by the Social Sciences and Humanities Research Council of Canada and the Coaching Association of Canada (CAC) to conduct research on coaching and coach education. He has published 90 articles in a variety of journals and books and supervised many graduate students at the master and doctorate levels. Dr. Trudel has been a consultant for many sport organisations, developing programmes and supervising coaches. He is the current Chair of the CAC Coaching Research Committee.

Dr Penny Werthner PhD

Assistant Professor, Faculty of Health Sciences, School of Human Kinetics, University of Ottawa, Ottawa, Canada

Penny Werthner is an Assistant Professor in the School of Human Kinetics, University of Ottawa, Canada. She is part of the research group at University of Ottawa conducting research on coaching and coach education. Other areas of research include women and coaching, and the use of bioneurofeedback for Olympic coaches and athletes (the latter research funded by Own The Podium, the agency responsible for high-performance sport in Canada). Dr Werthner has been published in *The Sport Psychologist*, *The International Journal of Sports Science and Coaching*, and the *International Journal of Coaching Science*. She has also been a sport psychology consultant to Olympic coaches, athletes, and teams over numerous Olympic Games. Dr. Werthner is currently a member of the Review Committee for the Canadian Sport Psychology Association.

Conceptual development in sports coaching

Chris Cushion and John Lyle

Introduction

In approaching this book, we begin by asking our-selves how much progress has been made since the publication of the early attempts to conceptualise the field (Lyle 1996, Cross & Lyle 1999). This research attempted to explore the coaching process and coaching practice and move the focus from sports performance and the purely 'technical' aspects of coaching delivery onto the search for a conceptual framework that represented coaching sufficiently well to underpin coach education. Indeed, publications such as those above (see also Abraham & Collins 1998) were stimulated by the realisation that research and academic writing had made little if any impact on coach education.

Therefore, we have posed the question, 'what progress has been made in "filling out" a conceptual framework for coaching?', and it is this question that we asked our fellow authors to address in their approach to each chapter. Thus, we were driven by issues such as: has a theory of coaching begun to emerge?, is there a consensual position within aca-demic writing?, how has conceptualisation dealt with the clearly distinctive domains within which coaching is practised?, what is the relationship between coaches' practice and our concept of coaching?, and what has been the impact of a devel-oping conceptualisation on coaching research? In this introductory chapter we have adopted the same challenging approach that we encouraged in our fel-low authors.

In their recent review of coaching research Gilbert and Trudel (2004a) identified in excess of 1000 coaching-related publications. An examination of this considerable landscape of coaching research reveals a bewildering range of theoretical and empir-ical perspectives and insights into coaching. Despite this seeming depth of empirical work and the recog-nition within it for two decades (Lyle 1984) of the existence of a coaching process, we conclude that an in-depth understanding of coaching and a con-ceptual underpinning with which to inform practice is absent (Cushion et al 2006, Cushion 2007a). Regardless of our research efforts we seem as far removed from consensus or clarity about the nature of coaching as ever (Cushion 2007a) and hence have no clear conceptual framework to inform practice or the development of practice.

More broadly, the test of the utility and value of research to a community is the extent to which its findings are (a) used as recommended practices in the preparation of practitioners and (b) incorpor-ated by practitioners in everyday practice (Ward & Barrett 2002). Research tends to suggest that many coaches work without any reference to a coaching process model, but we have to distinguish between our knowledge of how coaches operate and our capacity to describe this, or indeed how we educate and develop coaches. In reality, the research find-ings suggest that coaches base their coaching on feelings, intuitions, events and previous experience that trigger actions (Lyle 1992, Cross 1995a, 1995b, Gilbert & Trudel 2001, Cushion et al 2003, 2006). Furthermore, despite some positive research examples (e.g. Smoll & Smith 2006) there is no evidence for the systematic application of these, or any other findings, in the development of coaching practice or coach education (Abraham & Collins 1998, Abraham et al 2006, Lyle 2007a) in terms of either methodology or results (Cushion 2007b). As both Gilbert (2007) and Cushion (2007b) remark they are yet to 'meet a coach that referenced a coaching model when describing what they do'. Indeed, a somewhat disheartening picture of the 'effectiveness' of coaching research to impact practice can be drawn particularly considering the pragmatic nature of coaching practitioners; models or theories that do not work are quickly discarded or ignored (Brewer 2007).

In passing, however, we must note that the criticism of existing 'models' needs to be placed in context, and we must be careful not to criticise models for what they were never intended to do. It would be strange indeed if a coach described practice in terms of a coaching process model, given the complex environment and the contingencies and exigencies within which they operate. On the other hand, coaches might be expected to be exposed to models as a means of helping them to reflect on their practice. Conceptualisations of the coaching process are not necessarily there to be 'drawn upon' directly and overtly by practitioners. They should, however, inform coach education and development, in addition to underpinning research. Prescriptions for practice that coaches can relate to are likely to be much more focused, simply presented, and couched in appropriate technical language; albeit underpinned by sound theoretical concepts.

These limitations notwithstanding, the literature has broadly come to acknowledge that coaching is a social activity built on a web of complex, context-dependent and interdependent activities that come together to form a holistic process (Lyle 2002, Jones et al 2004, Cushion et al 2006). It is a remarkably complex, intricate yet coherent process incorporating myriad individual variations that each coach, player and environment adds to the blend (Cushion et al 2006, Cushion 2007a). Perhaps it is this very complexity that has resulted in a dearth of 'research that has explored the conceptual development of the coaching process', possibly because it is too complex to research neatly or about which to draw straightforward conclusions (Lyle 1999 p 13, Cushion et al 2006).

At the same time, we have to acknowledge that this is an interpretation, and the view may differ depending on perspectives and underlying assumptions about coaching. However, much of the writing in this book will demonstrate that the sociocultural

and pedagogical aspect of coaching has been given insufficient attention, both in coach education and in our conceptualisation of the process. In addition, coaching is also a cognitive activity (Abraham & Collins 1998, Lyle 2002, Abraham et al 2006). The apparent reliance on intuition, the everyday 'management' of interventions, and the capacity to take non-deliberative decisions in the 'heat' of practice suggests a cognitive expertise that is certainly not well understood, and is also not a commonplace feature of coach education and training.

With increased research attention devoted to coaching and yet little apparent impact on coaching practice or coach education, this chapter attempts to give an overview and critical evaluation of 'what we currently know' about coaching. It is of course beyond the scope of this chapter to 'review' coaching research in its entirety, but drilling into key issues and linking these arguments with others presented throughout the book has the potential to provide a broad and comprehensive analysis of the substantive nature of inquiry into coaching. We suggest that a critical examination of the state of the field in terms of conceptual development, research direction and research evidence provides a framework to understand and bridge the 'theory–practice' gap (Abraham & Collins 1998). Indeed, Gilbert and Trudel (2004a) argue that utilising such guiding frameworks has the potential to allow a number of things to be achieved; first, researchers to set research agendas, and second, coaches to access and realise the potential of coaching research and finally, to allow the full scope of research findings to be integrated into coach development programmes.

Conceptual development

The conceptual features of the coaching process are wide-ranging and multifaceted, and there remains a need to clarify this process so that effective coaching methods can be established (Mathers 1997, Lyle 2002). Conceptualisation creates a mechanism for representing the coaching process, without which there is no adequate basis of understanding, analysis or modelling. Such a representation is required to underpin research and education, and to appreciate the impact of interpersonal and environmental factors. Conceptual schema will address questions about terminology, purpose, variability in practice, meaning, genericism versus specificity, and domain distinctions; and these understandings form the basis of subsequent assumptions about effectiveness, expertise, and good practice prescriptions (Lyle 2002).

Note, however, that conceptualisation is not value-free. Any particular interpretation of sports coaching has the potential to influence coach education [a current example would be the linkage between Long-Term Coach Development and Long-Term Player Development (Stafford 2005)], research validity, and accountability measures. For example a sociological perspective (Jones 2000), a pedagogical perspective (Armour 2004), instructional perspective (Sherman 1997), humanistic perspective (Kidman 2005), or science of performance perspective (Johns & Johns, 2000) each makes assumptions that lead to practical consequences. Naturally there are barriers to conceptualisation that derive from coaching itself. The most obvious is the vast range of coaching contexts in which coaching is said to take place. The challenge of linking in a meaningful way domains characterised by school sport, children's activities, recreational sport, elite Olympic competition, highly commercialised professional sport, and so on, is considerable, and made even more so by considerations of team and individual sports, environmental differences, and the role of the coach in competition. Would or should a conceptualisation imply that a generic coaching process exists, or should the conceptualisation embrace more than one concept of coaching?

One particular issue has been the difficulty in dealing with the complexity of the coaching process: coaching practice exists within such a variable and dynamic environment of conflicting goals, socio-pedagogical delivery, sports specificity, non-consensual values, coaching traditions, and mores. This complexity has implications for researchers and the validity and utility of their research. Indeed, a number of researchers have argued that without studies specifically directed toward describing the complexity inherent in coaching, knowledge informing the coaching process is likely to largely remain ambiguous and a matter of conjecture (Saury & Durand 1998, Jones et al 2004, Cushion et al 2006). The danger is that attempts to simplify the complexity appear not to represent adequately the complexity of the environment or coaching practice. Indeed, it could be argued that to date research approaches have taken an overly simplistic approach to coaching resulting in a dearth of useful research into the conceptual development of the coaching process (Jones et al 2002, Cushion et al

2006). As Lyle (1999, 2002) points out, a fragmented or episodic approach to coaching knowledge tends to underestimate the complexity of the coaching process, and because coaching can be represented as 'episodes' and therefore parts of the process described in individual terms, it is easy to overlook the degree to which the inter-relatedness and interconnectedness of coaching sustains the process (Cushion et al 2006, Cushion 2007a, Jones 2007). Consequently, it becomes (and has become) easy to take an asocial, linear view of coaching. This, in turn, leads to immature or limited understanding that hides meaning but gives the illusion of a more complete understanding (Cushion 2007a). It could be argued therefore that this hinders genuine conceptual development and growth.

As Jones and Wallace (2005) suggest, we do not understand the phenomenon of coaching sufficiently in-depth as a precursor to proscribing coaching practice. As a result, the complexity has not been acknowledged or sufficiently understood before attempting to produce models. Consequently, 'oversimplification of the phenomenon and over-precision of prescriptions is the unfortunate price paid' (Jones & Wallace 2005 p 123). The outcome has been an approach that fails to fully encompass coaching practice (Lyle 2002, Cushion et al 2006); hence the contribution of such an approach to coaching has been useful but limited. It was for this reason that Lyle (2007b) argues that we should distinguish the intent from the practice – or at least attempt to appreciate the latter in terms of the former. It might, for example, be argued that the coaching intervention is an instrumental, managed process that can be planned in a more or less systematic fashion. Implementation of those intentions, and the on-going process of negotiation and accommodation, becomes susceptible to the complex dynamic environment within which it is delivered.

Although the conceptual development and understanding of the coaching process has been somewhat limited, a promising and growing body of work that explores coaching practice, and the debate that it has stimulated, has begun to emerge. This line of enquiry has been worthwhile in recognising more explicitly the complexity inherent in coaching. This body of work demonstrates that coaching is not something that is merely 'delivered' but is a dynamic social activity that engages coach and athlete in an active way (Cushion et al 2006, Jones 2006). The conceptual inference that could be drawn from this is that the coaching process is evident at two levels. On one level is the social context/meaning and flow of delivery created by coach and performer (at all levels and stages of sport), but at the same time, there is the planned intention/direction/delivery from the coach (and potentially influenced or designed with the performer). An interesting conjecture is whether the nature of such 'levels' changes with sports domains.

Coaching then is a practical, social activity that has as its characteristics 'multidimensionality, simultaneity, uncertainty, publicity and historicity' (Côté et al 1995 p 255). Echoing these sentiments, Saury and Durand (1998) argue that coaching can be characterised as complex, uncertain, dynamic, singular, and with conflicting values. Indeed, Saury and Durand (1998) suggested that the 'actions of coaches were full of context based, opportunist improvisations and extensive management of uncertainty and contradictions' (p 268). Increasingly, research is suggesting that each coaching situation carries some degree of novelty, thus practice is characterised in terms of 'structured improvisation' that is neither entirely reason-based or planned, and is far from systematic but highly problematic and individual; a set of reciprocal relations between athlete, coach and context (Saury & Durand 1998, Sève & Durand 1999, d'Arripe-Longueville et al 2001, Cushion 2001, Poczwardowski et al 2002, Jones et al 2003, 2004).

However, Lyle (2007b) has argued that the novelty element can be misunderstood, and to some extent could be dependent on the sport. There is no doubt that the coach's intervention requires active 'application' and the management of the activities/drills/exercises involves a continuous process of adjustment (or not). This management of the situation, embracing the evolving history of the processes and people involved, may be described as the developed expertise of the coach. When perceived this way, the 'improvisation' looks much more like a skilful application of more or less anticipated decisions about progression. This is not novelty as such, particularly for the experienced coach, but perhaps a better description is the 'degrees of freedom' that might be expected in sports preparation and performance, given the complexity involved.

Accounts of coaching practice such as those mentioned earlier tend to be sport-specific, although the research is from a range of sports, both team and individual. The coaches involved in the research were all operating in the 'performance domain' (Lyle 2002) and thus fully engaged with the coaching process. The degree to which the cumulative findings of this body of work can be generalised to coaching in all domains is a matter for debate; but there is arguably enough in the findings to challenge the more 'traditional' conceptions of coaching (we take to mean an unproblematic, acontextual, linear assumption, within a performance science framework). Indeed, the utility of the work perhaps lies in its use as a gateway to a more sophisticated and rich view of coaching practice. It is able to identify in coaching what Wenger (1998) identifies as the explicit: language, roles, tools, documents; and also the implicit: relationships, tacit conventions, subtle cues, untold rules of thumb, recognisable intuitions, specific perceptions, well-tuned sensitivities, embodied understandings, underlying assumptions and shared world views. While most of these can never be articulated, they are unmistakable signs of coaching practice and arguably crucial to its effectiveness (Cushion 2007a).

The tacit, uncertain and contradictory nature of coaching has been conceptually well developed by Robyn Jones (e.g. Jones & Wallace 2005, Jones 2007) who highlights both the pathos and ambiguity *of* and *in* coaching. His work attempts to reach beyond the problems of capturing the complexity of coaching arguing that coaching is in fact largely uncontrollable, incomprehensible and imbued with contradictory values (Jones & Wallace 2005, Jones 2007). This work draws on some empirical research to support it, and while interesting and indeed appealing, the concepts that Jones develops need further empirical exploration and scrutiny. Empirical research might demonstrate that this 'uncontrollability' is overstated and perhaps significantly environment-dependent, while the contradictory values are no more evident than in other similar enterprises. However, perhaps the greatest benefit of Jones' work has been to highlight and problematise many underlying assumptions made about coaching practice. Indeed, the work has highlighted the challenge in identifying the coach's expertise when the links between intentions and practice are often compromised or blurred. Indeed, the ability to orchestrate and maximise (perhaps, optimise) detailed technical analysis, planning and performance, in the context of the various social, psychological, and organisation milieus, may be the emerging mark of coaching expertise.

Immersion in, and engagement with, the detail of coaching practice reveals much about the construction and complexity evident within it (Cushion 2007a). We detect a movement towards some clearer and coherent concepts around, ironically, understanding ambiguity and inconsistencies in practice. Structured improvisation (managing the degrees of freedom), or the interaction of order and chaos, suggests that continuity in coaching in fact may not come from stability but from adaptability (Cushion 2007a). The notion of structured improvisation and the degrees of freedom therein, themselves require some considerable elaboration. The terms are useful, however, because they imply that coaching practice is not without an intentional framework, but identifies the continual process of application that appears to characterise the coach's actions. As we have already argued, the term improvisation may suggest compromise, and an absence of pre-determination that may also not adequately capture the coach's practice. However, what has become clear is that the ever-changing nature of coaching practice means that we must focus on the totality of that practice and the practitioner, and not simply on 'episodes' that occur in the process.

Coaching domains

It is difficult to conceptualise coaching without mention of coaching domains, particularly if recognising these specific contexts helps both to understand the complexity, and perhaps ameliorate some of it. We would argue that coaching domains are distinctive sporting milieus in which the environmental demands lead to more or less coherent coaching practice, and a community of coaches recognisable within it. These coaching domains place specific demands on the coach's expertise and behaviours, and require domain-specific knowledge and understanding to operate within them. The environmental demands refer to the meeting place of agent and structure, that is, an accommodation of the tensions between the performers' aspirations, abilities and developmental stage, the consequent development and preparation provision, the coach, and the organisational and social context. In a sense, coaching domains are simply a conceptual device; each domain can be thought of as constituted by an aggregation of countless coaching contexts, processes and episodes that exhibit a similar characteristic pattern. The very complexity of the domain practice is recognisable in those elements that are likely to differ: for example, intensity of

participation, complexity of performance, coach recruitment, interpersonal skills, value systems, competition emphasis, and the strength of the community of practice.

The result of these differences is differential demands on the coach in terms of knowledge, behaviour, practice and expertise. For example, the coaching process that emerges from each set of circumstances will require different planning skills, tactical preparation, decision making, refining/teaching skills, resource management, interpersonal skills and so on. In addition, the knowledge base and associated skills will differ across domains. It is difficult to avoid suggesting that the higher the levels of athlete performance the greater the sophistication required of the coaches' knowledge and skills. However, this should be avoided. The coaching processes in each domain should be thought of as different, and presenting their distinctive challenges. Nevertheless, when thought of in these terms, the arguments for distinctive perspectives on coaching are persuasive. Perhaps most persuasive is the notion that coaches will learn to 'frame' their roles and expectations within a particular set of personal, educational, and experiential circumstances.

Furthermore, the idea of domains is important as Trudel and Gilbert (2006) argue that a single typology of coaching contexts/domains is required to facilitate research within a meaningful framework, and to assist with the design of coach education. The authors reviewed a number of coaching context classifications, characterised by terms such as community, instruction, competition, professional, volunteer and school. Following the review, Trudel and Gilbert (2006) decided upon a typology of recreational sport, developmental sport and elite sport. This they acknowledge is most analogous to Lyle's (2002) typology, which they describe as the most thoroughly described, grounded in concepts of the coaching process, and consistent with empirical research on stages of performance development. It may also be the case that the incorporation of developmental strategies such as the Long-Term Athlete Development model (Stafford 2005) will, de facto, create coaching domains.

Understanding coaches and coaching practice across domains remains the cornerstone to conceptual development and engaging practitioners (Cushion 2007b). For example, how coaching impacts the subjectivities of those involved and how coaching is experienced as both a social space and a social structure offers fertile ground for further conceptualising coaching (Cushion 2007b). Against this backdrop, as Cushion (2007b) argues, any consideration of interaction and discourse within the coaching process, and of the coaching process itself that is devoid of context is both flawed and limited. Nevertheless, we reinforce this change in emphasis in the knowledge that the central purpose of sport coaching (improvement of sports performance) and how that can be achieved is sufficiently well understood in its domains to provide a core process against which the social construction of practice can be understood. Our thinking then should not be focused on the production of all-embracing definitions, but about enquiring with greater breadth, depth and detail in order that we increase our understanding about practice. As a consequence, the search for an adequate conceptualisation of sports coaching has implications for how we research sports coaching. For this reason we now turn to a commentary on coaching research.

Research

Despite the growing body of work to which we have already alluded, coaching unfortunately remains relatively speaking, largely under-researched. The existing research tends to be 'sparse, unfocussed and subjective' (LeUnes 2007 p 403). We might argue that there are two key reasons for this. First the coaching research agenda is too often driven by personal research interest, with coaches and coaching a convenient data set for some other issue. Second, despite a seemingly compelling argument for a 'paradigm shift' in coaching research (Cushion et al 2006, Jones 2007), perhaps reflecting the wider sport science research field, there remains a predominantly narrow, reductionist, rationalistic and bio-scientific approach to coaching research (Jones et al 2002, 2004, Cushion et al 2003, 2006).

This is despite the significant changes taking place in the methods employed. Gilbert and Trudel (2004) found that the balance of qualitative to quantitative research had moved from 11%/81% to 28%/70% between 1990–93 and 1998–2004. Gilbert and Trudel (2004) note that there had been marked changes into interview-based and observation-based research away from questionnaire studies. This methodological shift perhaps reflected the change away from 'characteristics' and 'career development' research (emanating from North America) to coach behaviour and cognitive organisation.

Despite this shift, the research remains largely positivistic.

However, we have to be careful about generalising across all coaching research, and about criticising research for not being something that it didn't set out to be. Therefore, we might be critical of the research community for paying less attention to the complexity of the coaching milieu, but we also need to address the methodological challenges that this brings. The criticism that positivism is reductionist and attempts to reduce 'interference' (for example, systematic observation of coaching behaviours) is apt; more interpretive methodologies are able to identify the complex interweaving of personal, performance, and environmental factors, but may not, as yet, have contributed substantively to theory building or practice prescriptions.

Coaching research itself may be a misnomer, and we ourselves may be guilty of perpetuating the concept of a unified field or consensual purpose that we will later argue does not exist. Without wishing at this stage to offer a taxonomy of research fields, we can point to coaching practice, both environment and career (e.g. Mallett & Côté 2006, Jones 2007), coaches' behaviours, both intervention/delivery and interpersonal (e.g. Smith & Cushion 2006, Jowett & Poczwardowski 2007), coaches' cognitions, both decision policies and decision making (e.g. Vergeer & Lyle 2007), coaches' expertise (Schempp et al 2006), and coach education and training (e.g. Gilbert & Trudel, 2006, Nelson et al 2006). This catalogue of emerging coaching research fields does not, of course, absolve us from reflecting in their methods the generally 'messy' nature of coaching for which we have argued.

Coaching research is not yet at a stage of development in which the influence of funding agencies or publishing policies has impacted on the 'weight of focused research'. With such a diverse research community, 'schools' have developed that reflect personal agendas. Personal research agendas are seldom coaching specific, but tend to be driven by disciplinary or sub-disciplinary outcomes. This may be understandable in an under-theorised field, but recourse to models and theories from other fields has limited value in building a coherent conceptual or theoretical body of knowledge (Cushion 2007b). Too often, this means that the 'coaching' within the research is superficial or secondary. Again, it is understandable that the core purpose of coaching – improved performance – should be an obvious driver. This may have focused attention on the 'what to do' rather than the 'how or why' and understandably under those circumstances the driver is the promotion of athletic achievement, with a dominant focus on performance enhancement. Nevertheless, coaching practice and its process has received considerably less attention than the 'performance' outcomes. Note, however, that this should not imply that such research is automatically useful. Our review of coaching research finds few if any links between coaching practice and performance outcomes, limited attention to intervention research (Gilbert & Trudel 2004), and performance outcomes are rarely the dependent variables in such research.

In these circumstances, 'coaching' research becomes characterised by distinct and fragmented categories and coaching itself is reduced in scale and scope, often viewed as unproblematic with coaching portrayed as a matter of simplistic technical 'transfer'. Even in circumstances in which there has been an attempt to investigate the 'how' of delivery, for example, motivational climate (e.g. Pensgaard & Roberts 2002, Mageau & Vallerand 2003), feedback (e.g. Hodges & Franks 2002), communication (e.g. LaVoi 2007), there is a danger that its singular focus does not have the capacity to capture sufficiently the dynamic and complex nature of coaching. Furthermore, research topics such as the coach–athlete relationships (e.g. Jowett & Cockerill 2002) and decision making (Vergeer & Lyle 2007) are self-evidently important to coaching but the most-often used methodologies are limited in the extent to which they are able to embrace the wider coaching context. In addition, although an integral part of coaching practice, they alone do not account sufficiently in their resultant prescriptions for the breadth of coaching expertise. From a practitioner's perspective, the impact of this 'competition of importances' has been confusion and, not unsurprisingly, a perception of much the majority of research as being irrelevant, of not being linked to the real world (Jones et al 2004, Cushion et al 2006).

Why then do we engage in this type of research and treat the coach as the 'other' to be studied (Gilbert 2007)? This question requires further elaboration. The answer is linked to wider epistemological issues associated with scientific enquiry in sport generally and coaching specifically. The questions coaching research has posed to date have by and large been shaped by the methods and assumptions of the positivist paradigm (Lyle 1999, Cushion et al 2006). This is important as 'paradigmatic allegiances can determine the theories, perspectives, or operationally, the theoretical frameworks that shape the research process' (MacDonald et al 2002 p 134). A core concept of the positivistic paradigm is reductionism, which is an attempt to understand the functioning of the whole through an analysis of its individual parts (Brustad 1997). By its nature, this approach provides a 'mechanistic' guide to understanding; viewing human behaviour as measurable, causally derived and thus predictable and controllable (Smith 1989). In addition, the positivist paradigm structures the types of questions asked (Brustad 1997), with the main goal when applied to coaching to establish causal relationships in a quest for generalisable theories (Cushion 2007a).

This nomothetic approach has resulted in the complexity of coaching practice and the coaching process being greatly reduced by the simplifying nature of 'efficient' research design, thus stifling a more holistic understanding. Indeed, according to Kahan (1999) 'it would seem that due to its nomothetic pursuit', a positivist approach is 'incongruous with, and insensitive to, the peculiarities of coaching and the unique conditions under which coaches act' (p 42). Furthermore, content focus stems from the perceived methodological possibilities; thus, 'too many studies have adopted a quantitative survey approach (where) the need for the control of variables and reliable operationalisation of constructs has militated against a more insightful and interpretive investigation of values, behaviours and context' (Lyle 1999 p 30).

The outcome is a body of work that is in some part useful, but ultimately limited, in developing our understanding of aspects of coaching. This type of research consistently, and frustratingly, reduces the complexity of practice by presenting coaching in overly systematic and unproblematic ways (Jones 2007). More seriously perhaps, there persists a fundamentally flawed assumption that a positivist science, with a sub-disciplinary focus, inevitably reducing coaching to episodes of neat dependent and independent variables, can account fully for what coaching practice actually entails (Cushion 2007a). Indeed, the process of separating and specialising components of real life coaching and feeding them back to coaches in order to enhance understanding or prescribe practice, results in abstractions that clearly fail to substitute for real life-derived intuitions about coaching (Cushion 2007a, Jones 2007). Viewed from this perspective, coaches are considered to be solely motivated by a narrow reductionist logic (Jones 2007), and this reinforces the concept of coaching as efficient technical transfer. It is important to stress that these arguments are not designed to claim superiority of one method or paradigm over another, but suggest that making a reductionist approach central to understanding practice is problematic in that it serves only to define coaching both narrowly and unilaterally (Cushion 2007a). What Schön (1983) would characterise as 'technocratic rationality' has thus far produced dominant, but at the same time, weak notions of theory–practice relations, and as such has impoverished practice (Cushion 2007a). As Cushion (2007a) argues, it is these representations that produce on one hand, the illusion of a 'complete' understanding but in reality are weak and limited; while on the other hand, are viewed with irony and even cynicism by practitioners and hence fail to impact the practice realm to the disadvantage of coaching and its professional standing.

Our critical appraisal of the positivist paradigm is neither new nor exclusive to coaching. Nevertheless, we suggest that it contributes very significantly to the failure of coach research to impact on coach education (Abraham & Collins 1998). Indeed, this raises the issue of how much coaching research is 'used' by coaches, performers, or coach educators. Although we point to the link between the dominant research paradigm and a narrow concept of coaching, we also suggest that the problem lies as much with the absence of other competing paradigms rather than the overstated claims of positivist research. We are also careful to acknowledge that some practitioner cynicism is attributable to both a residual 'anti-intellectualism' and a disregard for any non-self-experiential research, rather than the limitations of particular paradigms.

To a large extent, coaching research is dependent on, and characterised by, design, and ultimately our research designs are hostage to our understanding, perspectives, and theories (Cushion 2007b). As Cushion (2007b) argues, it is important that debate and discussion should not become an end in itself, and 'waving theory from the balcony' (McDonald et al 2002 p 149), will result in the development and perpetuation of 'knowers' of theory, and perhaps more significantly, the establishment and firming of a theory–practice binary.

Coaching research has its own history and character. The early systematic observation studies (e.g. Lacy & Darst 1985) and leadership model (Chelladurai & Saleh 1980) were influential in the devising of behaviour frameworks. These gave way to the interview and observation approaches of Salmela (1995), Gould (1990), Gilbert (Gilbert & Trudel 2004b), and Côté (Côté et al 1995). In the last 10–15 years, the acknowledgement of a coaching *process* has spawned a search for the most appropriate means to represent and understand it (Lyle 2002, Jones & Wallace 2006, Cushion et al 2006). It is interesting to observe the ebb and flow that characterises the development of the coaching research base. There are, as we have discussed here, pockets of empirical research that are contributing to the conceptual and intellectual development of coaching; these force us to go back and question earlier perspectives and help us form new understandings of coaching practice. This research, and the debate it engenders, has great potential to develop coaching's conceptual base and add meaningfully to coach education and development. Moreover, as our understanding of coaching becomes more sophisticated and a shift in the nature of coaching research occurs we should not disregard existing accumulated knowledge, but rather, consider ways to integrate new knowledge with what is already known (Cushion 2007b). It is not in the interests of coaching and its development to block or delay integrating existing contributions or ideas in establishing a more sophisticated knowledge base (Rink 1993, Cushion 2007b). The challenge, therefore, lies in not only looking for new ways to understand coaching but also to build on existing work.

A close examination of the existing body of research, however, also reveals that amongst the insightful empirical work there is arguably also a large amount of 'theory waving'. Coaching *is* ill-defined and under-theorized (Jones 2006) and needs to take both a critical and a reflexive stance for which theory provides the necessary 'thinking tools'. Indeed, the utilisation of theories from other fields need to be considered as threshold concepts (Toole & Seashore-Lewis 2002, Jones 2006) that act as signposts to new ways of seeing and understanding (Jones 2006), rather than convenient scaffolding for isolated and unintegrated enquiry. However, too many researchers are guilty of speaking seemingly authoritatively about coach education and coaching practice based solely on the production of a well-argued, but ultimately arbitrary theory (perhaps derived from their own research agenda, or through 'spotting a perceived gap', rather than driven by the needs of coaching). As Bourdieu reminds us 'research without theory is blind, and theory without research is empty' (Bourdieu & Wacquant 1992 p 160). We should be cautious therefore of being indoctrinated into 'seeing' coaching through the eyes of empty theory or being drawn to 'theoretical tinsel' (Cushion 2007b).

Often these theories, tinsel and all, come from outside the coaching field. There is of course a utility in drawing on relevant theoretical resources and learning from other perhaps 'similar' fields. However, the world is transformed by transforming its representation (Bourdieu & Wacquant 1992) and pre-constructed theories with limited empirical evidence or basis in coaching can produce a representation that is a fiction obscuring true meaning and understanding (Nash 1990, Cushion 2007b). Empirical objects appear to 'emerge' from coaching and become the focus of research. Yet they are ultimately arbitrary. Somehow the discourse of the moment becomes deemed important by researchers and research agendas, but not always of interest or value to the coaching field. There is a danger that coaching research pays inadequate attention to the issues of importance to coaching and coaching practice. Clearly to establish coaching as an autonomous field, we need to do more than uncritically accept and apply theories from other disciplines; there is an overwhelming need for our own evidence-based theories and concepts. Indeed, regardless of the method or approach adopted to engage with coaching and coaching practice, conceptual development and understanding needs to be grounded in coaching practice and empirically supported. In the meantime as the research grows and we attempt to fill the theoretical and conceptual void and establish the relevance of our work to practitioners, we should be mindful of the real threat of being overly influenced or colonised from other fields (Cushion 2007b).

A research agenda

Constructing a research agenda forces us to consider the limitations of existing research, but also to recognise the barriers to more ecologically valid research. The very factors that we identify as necessary to an appropriate description of coaching are those that present considerable challenges to future research. Perhaps we might ask if this is the reason for more writing *about* the shortcomings of current research than remedial contributions. We certainly hope that the chapters that follow will in

aggregation form a research agenda. One of the most obvious first steps is to bridge the gap between relevance and feasibility, to site coaching research within practice and the practice community. Coaching practice, however, is not a construct that is in someway subordinate to the needs of empirical work (Cushion 2007b). The relationship between research and practice, and researchers and practitioners therefore needs to be better established and further developed. We need to strike up a dialogue with practitioners and demonstrate an engagement and collaboration with coaching practice (Cushion 2007b). This may seem self-evident but so far has proven elusive. There is a need to ensure that research questions arise from practice, are seen to be relevant to the problems and challenges of the day-to-day work of the coach, and of course, have an appropriate level of utility for coach education and development, improved practice and more effective coaching. At the same time this, of course, should not stifle innovation and alternative conceptualisations.

In doing so, coaching researchers and research must face up to and grasp the dual character of coaching practice with its subjective and objective aspects (Cushion 2007b). An overly polarized research field can lead to a reductionist and misleading (or perhaps simply 'less helpful' and 'less useful') portrayal of practice and research approaches. Of course the objective/subjective dichotomy is an enduring metatheoretical dilemma (Swartz 1997) and as this chapter has argued is a considerable obstacle to the development of a meaningful portrayal of coaching practice (Cushion 2007b).

Focusing on explicit features of the coaching process and at the same time arguing for engagement with practice that is neither episodic nor reductionist may seem somewhat paradoxical or even contradictory (Cushion 2007b). A focus on episodes as evidenced by existing research, has tended to develop and promote an impersonal, reductionist, and decontextualised view of practice. The episodic concept may result in a profile of behaviour and expertise that negates, or at best fails to capture, the very coordination and management of the coaching process that the emerging complexity, interrelatedness, and inter-dependence imply. Alternatively, a focus on the social and contextual aspects of coaching practice may provide a perspective that can appear relativist and unable, and indeed unwilling, to capture any 'generic' (there have to be generic features of coaching practice to enable us to recognise coaching as coaching, as has been argued elsewhere, there is a 'sameness' about our uniqueness; not all coaching practice is the same, but it is nonetheless coaching practice; the continuous adjustment inherent in practice captures the meeting place of object and subject and forces a consideration of the degree of predictability and control within practice, the *how* and *why*, rather than the *what)* features of practice (i.e., the structure of 'structured improvisation'). Framing an analysis to focus on coaching practice in the social world will provide a conceptualisation with the potential to capture specific practice in specific circumstances, thus doing justice to the multiple relations through which practice is defined (Lave & Wenger 1996), and which seems so necessary for sport-specific analysis. Such an approach perhaps offers the potential to transcend some of the 'oppositions' outlined in this chapter, while integrating them into a broader knowledge framework (Cushion 2007b).

Summary

We have attempted throughout to focus on higher-order matters that are relevant to conceptualising sport coaching, and we conclude with some selective remarks about the 'current state of play'. As we have shown throughout the chapter, there is a body of literature that has contributed to the debate on conceptualising coaching and a consensus seems to be emerging around its complexity, social and dynamic context, and competing goals and values. The measure of control and adherence to planned interventions across sports and domains has yet to be established empirically.

As is often the case, it is easier to identify shortcomings, particularly in an ill-defined field of study, than to take the next step of building the framework that can account for the headline description, useful analytical 'chunks', and detailed and immediate behaviours. We have stressed throughout that there is a very significant challenge in marrying subject and object, of reconciling intention and practice, of layering social and organisational context with personal and inter-personal histories. It is easier to identify the need for management, accommodation and coordination than to describe and explain *how* the coach copes with this. There seems no doubt that coaches are faced with a dynamic set of interdependent circumstances, and

we might assume that expert coaches, even in the demanding arena of intensive elite-level sport, are able to cope with the demands. It does not seem too presumptive a leap to imagine that these demands are perceived, organised, and solved within a set of capacities that we might term cognitive expertise. This produces two layers of expertise: the 'how and why' that connotes coping strategies and decision-making, and the craft-based 'how' that expresses itself in communication, feedback, planning and so on. The obvious corollary to this concept of coaches' expertise is that it provides difficult methodological challenges to the researcher. Thus we might suggest that research should not be reductionist, but going beyond overt behaviours to cognitive processes in the context of the conceptualisations described earlier leads us to other paradigms that are not without their own limitations.

We would appear to be moving to an agreement that the social and environmental context provides a layer of contingency that requires a continuous process of accommodation, integration and coordination between goals and actuality. We have been careful to stress that the image of coaching as a 'transfer of technical knowledge' does not do justice to the coaching role. Nevertheless, it should not be forgotten that there is a technical and knowledge element to the role that circumscribes practice as *sports* coaching. The expertise of the coach not only depends on this technical knowledge, but the effectiveness of the coach depends on a capacity to achieve performance improvement while navigating and understanding the given context.

We have attempted to demonstrate that conceptualisations about coaching are related to coaching research. Lyle (2002) characterised coaching research as failing to adequately describe coaching practice, of failing to deal with coaching effectiveness, of relying on satisfaction studies in lieu of sport performance outcomes, of being a diverse community of practice, of failing to impact on coach education, and of being unable to devise appropriate intervention studies. There was also a criticism that coaching domains were not recognised for their specificity. However, this is less evident, although not yet theorised. We have argued that a paradigm shift is required both to reflect the complexity of the role and practice and adequately to enquire into it. In addition, the bulk of the criticisms above remain pertinent. Academic writing about sports coaching is increasing in scale and the 'coverage' is spreading. At present, however, this does not seems to be the result of conceptual agreement and a consequent consensual or coordinated agenda. Research is characterised by personal agendas and methodological comfort, rather than practitioner problems and application. At this stage of the development of the field, we need to be concept and theory building, but not losing sight of the danger of isolation from the practitioner community.

Coaches deal with ill-defined problems and practice is subject to high levels of variability and uncertainty. Indeed, the constraints of practice may be context-specific or common to all coaches, but we know little about them and how they operate (Saury & Durand 1998, Cushion 2007b). As coaching scholars there remains a real danger that isolated paradigm debate and a forced retreat to disciplinarity (Kirk & McDonald 2000) will lead to a

polarisation of the field and marginalise coaching research and its conceptual development further from practice (Cushion 2007b). If we are to stay close to its social, dynamic and complex nature a more sophisticated understanding of coaching practice needs to be developed. As Marx argued, '…all social life is essentially practical. All the mysteries that lead theory toward mysticism find their rational solution in human practice and in the comprehension of this practice' (cited in Bottomore & Rubel 1963 p 84). Indeed, as Cushion (2007b) argues, authentic analysis of coaching practice in situ (in collaboration with coaches), not driven by arbitrary theory or personal research agendas, has the potential to provide the empirical tools to understand and connect with coaches' and athletes' individual and collective work.

References

Abraham, A., Collins, D., 1998. Examining and extending research in coach development. Quest 50, 59–79.

Abraham, A., Collins, D., Martindale, R., 2006. The coaching schematic: validation through expert coach consensus. J. Sports Sci. 24, 549–564.

Armour, K., 2004. Coaching pedagogy. In: Jones, R.L., Armour, K., Potrac, P. (Eds.), Sports coaching cultures: from practice to theory. Routledge, London, pp. 94–115.

Bottomore, T.B., Rubel, M. (Eds.), 1963. Karl Marx: selected writings in sociology and social philosophy. Pelican, Harmondsworth.

Bourdieu, P., Wacquant, L.J.D (Eds.), 1992. An invitation to reflexive sociology. Chicago University Press, Chicago.

Brewer, B., 2007. Modelling the complexity of the coaching process: a commentary. International Journal of Sport Science and Coaching 2 (4), 411–413.

Brustad, R.J., 1997. A critical-postmodern perspective on knowledge development in human movement. In: Fernandez-Balboa, J.M. (Ed.), Critical postmodernism in human movement, physical education, and sport. State University of New York, Albany, pp. 87–98.

Chelladurai, P., Saleh, S.D., 1980. Dimensions of leader behavior in sports: development of a leadership scale. Journal of Sport Psychology 2, 34–45.

Côté, J., Salmela, J.H., Trudel, P., et al., 1995. The coaching model: a grounded assessment of expert gymnastic coaches knowledge. Journal of Sport and Exercise Psychology 17 (1), 1–17.

Cross, N., Lyle, J. (Eds.), 1999. The coaching process: principles and practice for sport. Butterworth-Heinemann, Oxford.

Cross, N., 1995a. Coaching effectiveness in hockey: a Scottish perspective. Scottish Journal of Physical Education 23 (1), 27–39.

Cross, N., 1995b. Coaching effectiveness and the coaching process. Swimming Times 72 (3), 23–25.

Cushion, C.J., 2001. The coaching process in professional youth football: an ethnography of practice. Unpublished Ph.D. thesis, Brunel University, UK .

Cushion, C.J., 2006. Mentoring: harnessing the power of experience. In: Jones, R.L. (Ed.), The sports coach as educator: re-conceptualising sports coaching. Routledge, London, pp. 128–144.

Cushion, C.J., 2007a. Modelling the complexity of the coaching process. International Journal of Sport Science and Coaching 2 (4), 395–401.

Cushion, C.J., 2007b. Modelling the complexity of the coaching process: a response to commentaries. International Journal of Sport Science and Coaching 2 (4), 427–433.

Cushion, C.J., Armour, K.M., Jones, R.L., 2003. Coach education and continuing professional development: experience and learning to coach. Quest 55, 215–230.

Cushion, C.J., Armour, K.M., Jones, R.L., 2006. Locating the coaching process in practice models: models 'for' and 'of' coaching. Physical Education and Sport Pedagogy 11, 83–99.

d'Arripe-Longueville, F., Saury, D., Fournier, J., et al., 2001. Coach–athlete interaction during elite archery competitions: and application of methodological framework used in ergonomics research to sport psychology. Journal of Applied Sport Psychology 13, 275–299.

Gilbert, W., 2007. Modelling the complexity of the coaching process: a commentary. International Journal of Sport Science and Coaching 2 (4), 427–433.

Gilbert, W., Trudel, P., 2001. Learning to coach through experience: reflection in model youth sport coaches. Journal of Teaching in Physical Education 21, 16–34.

Gilbert, W., Trudel, P., 2004a. Analysis of coaching science research published from 1970–2001. Res. Q. Exerc. Sport 75, 388–399.

Gilbert, W., Trudel, P., 2004b. Role of the coach: how model youth team coaches frame their roles. The Sport Psychologist 18, 21–43.

Gould, D., Giannini, J., Krane, K., et al., 1990. Educational needs of elite US national team, Pan American and Olympic coaches. Journal of Teaching Physical Education 9, 332–334.

Hodges, N.J., Franks, I.M., 2002. Modelling coaching practice: The role of instruction and demonstration. J. Sports Sci. 20, 793–811.

Johns, D.P., Johns, J., 2000. Surveillance, subjectivism and technologies of power: an analysis of the discursive practice of high-performance sport. International Review for the Sociology of Sport 35, 219–234.

Jones, R.L., 2000. Towards a sociology of coaching. In: Jones, R.L., Armour, K.M. (Eds.), The sociology of sport: theory and practice. Addison Wesley Longman, London, pp. 33–43.

Jones, R.L., 2007. Coaching redefined: an everyday pedagogical encounter. Sport, Education and Society 12 (2), 159–174.

Jones, R.L., Wallace, M., 2005. Another bad day at the training ground: coping with ambiguity in the coaching context. Sport, Education & Society 10, 119–134.

Jones, R.L., Wallace, M., 2006. The coach as 'orchestrator. In: Jones, R.J. (Ed.), The sports coach as educator: re-conceptualising sports coaching. Routledge, London, pp. 51–64.

Jones, R.L., Armour, K.M., Potrac, P., 2002. Understanding the coaching process: a framework for social analysis. Quest 54, 34–48.

Jones, R.L., Armour, K., Potrac, P., 2004. Sports coaching cultures: from practice to theory. Routledge, London.

Jones, R.L., 2006. How can educational concepts inform sports coaching? In:

Jones, R.L. (Ed.), The sports coach as educator: re-conceptualising sports coaching. Routledge, London, pp. 4–13.

Jowett, S., Cockerill, I., 2002. Incompatibility in the coach-athlete relationship. In: Cockerill, I.M. (Ed.), Solutions in sport psychology. Thomson, London, pp. 16–31.

Jowett, S., Poczwardowski, A., 2007. Understanding the coach–athlete relationship. In: Jowett, S., Lavallee, D. (Eds.), Social psychology in sport. Human Kinetics, Champaign IL, pp. 3–13.

Kahan, D., 1999. Coaching behaviour: a review of the systematic observation research literature. Applied Research in Coaching and Athletics Annual 14, 17–58.

Kidman, L., 2005. Athlete-centred coaching: developing inspired and inspiring people. Innovative Communications, Christchurch, NZ.

Kirk, D., McDonald, D., 2001. The social construction of PETE in Higher Education: towards a research agenda. Quest 53, 440–456.

Lacy, A.C., Darst, P.W., 1985. Systematic observation of behaviours of winning high school head football coaches. Journal of Teaching in Physical Education 4, 256–270.

Lave, J., Wenger, E., 1991. Situated learning: legitimate peripheral participation. Cambridge University Press, Cambridge.

LaVoi, N.M., 2007. Interpersonal communication and conflict in the coach-athlete relationship. In: Jowett, D., Lavallee, D. (Eds.), Social psychology in sport. Human Kinetics, Champaign, IL, pp. 75–90.

LeUnes, A., 2007. Modelling the complexity of the coaching process: a commentary. International Journal of Sport Science and Coaching 2 (4), 403–406.

Lyle, J., 1984. Towards a concept of coaching. Scottish Journal of Physical Education 12 (1), 27–31.

Lyle, J., 1992. Systematic coaching behaviour: an investigation into the coaching process and the implications of the findings for coach education. In: Williams, T., Almond, A., Sparkes, A. (Eds.), Sport and physical activity: moving towards excellence. E & FN Spon, London, pp. 463–469.

Lyle, J., 1996. A conceptual appreciation of the sports coaching process. Research Papers in Sport, Leisure and Physical Education 1 (1), 15–37.

Lyle, J., 1999. The Coaching process: an overview. In: Cross, N., Lyle, J. (Eds.), The coaching process: principles and practice for sport. Butterworth-Heinemann, Oxford, pp. 3–24.

Lyle, J., 2002. Sports coaching concepts: a framework for coaches' behaviour. Routledge, London.

Lyle, J., 2007a. A review of the research evidence for the impact of coach education. International Journal of Coaching Science 1 (1), 17–34.

Lyle, J., 2007b. Modelling the complexity of the coaching process: a commentary. International Journal of Sports Science & Coaching 2 (4), 407–409.

MacDonald, D., Kirk, D., Metzler, M., et al., 2002. It's all very well in theory: theoretical perspectives and their applications in contemporary pedagogical research. Quest 54, 133–156.

Mageau, G.A., Vallerand, R.J., 2003. The coach–athlete relationship: A motivational model. Journal of Sport Sciences 21, 883–904.

Mallett, C., Côté, J., 2006. Beyond winning and losing: guidelines for evaluating high performance coaches. The Sport Psychologist 20, 213–218.

Mathers, J.F., 1997. Professional coaching in golf: is there an appreciation of the coaching process? Scottish Journal of Physical Education 25 (1), 23–35.

Nash, R., 1990. Bourdieu on education and cultural reproduction. British Journal of Sociology of Education 11 (4), 431–447.

Nelson, L.J., Cushion, C.J., Potrac, P., 2006. Formal, nonformal and informal coach learning. International Journal of Sport Science and Coaching 1 (3), 247–259.

Pensgaard, A.M., Roberts, G.C., 2002. Elite athletes' experiences of the motivational climate: the coach matters. Scand. J. Med. Sci. Sports 12 (1), 54–59.

Poczwardowski, A., Barott, J.E., Henschen, K.P., 2002. The athlete and coach: their relationship and its meaning. Results of an interpretive study. International Journal of Sport Psychology 33, 116–140.

Rink, J.E., 1993. Teacher education: a focus on action. Quest 45, 308–320.

Salmela, J.H., 1995. Learning from the development of expert coaches. Coaching and Sports Science Journal 2 (2), 3–13.

Saury, J., Durand, M., 1998. Practical knowledge in expert coaches: on-site study of coaches in sailing. Research Quarterly in Exercise and Sport 69, 254–266.

Schempp, P., McCullick, B., Mason, I., 2006. The development of expert coaching. In: Jones, R.L. (Ed.), The sports coach as educator: reconceptualising sports coaching. Routledge, London, pp. 145–161.

Schön, D.A., 1983. The reflective practitioner: how professionals think in action. Basic Books, New York.

Sève, C., Durand, M., 1999. The action of a table tennis coach as situated action. Avante 5, 69–86.

Sherman, C., Crassini, B., Maschette, W., et al., 1997. Instructional sport psychology:

a reconceptualisation of sports coaching as sports instruction. International Journal of Sport Psychology 28 (2), 103–125.

Smith, J.K., 1989. The nature of social and educational inquiry: empiricism versus interpretation. Ablex, Norwood NJ.

Smith, M., Cushion, C.J., 2006. An investigation of the in-game behaviours of professional, top-level youth soccer coaches. Journal of Sport Sciences 24 (4), 355–366.

Smoll, F.L., Smith, R.E., 2006. Development and implementation of coach-training programs: cognitive-behavioral principles and techniques. In: Williams, J.M. (Ed.), Applied sport psychology: personal growth to peak performance. fifth ed. McGraw-Hill, Boston, pp. 458–480.

Stafford, I., 2005. Coaching for Long Term Athlete Development. Coachwise, Leeds.

Swartz, D., 1997. Culture & power: the sociology of Pierre Bourdieu. The University of Chicago Press, Chicago.

Toole, J.C., Seashore, L.K., 2002. The role of professional learning communities in international education. In: Leithwood, K., Hallinger, P. (Eds.), Second international handbook of education leadership and administration. Kluwer Academic, Dordrecht, pp. 245–279.

Trudel, P., Gilbert, W., 2006. Coaching and coach education. In: Kirk, D., O'sullivan, M., McDonald, M. (Eds.), Handbook of research in physical education. Sage, London, pp. 516–539.

Vergeer, I., Lyle, J., 2007. Mixing methods in assessing coaches' decision making. Research Quarterly for Exercise and Science 78 (3), 225–235.

Ward, P., Barrett, T., 2002. A review of behavior analysis research in physical education. Journal of Teaching in Physical Education 21, 242–266.

Wenger, E., 1998. Communities of practice: learning meaning and identity. Cambridge University Press, Cambridge.

Complex practice in coaching: studying the chaotic nature of coach–athlete interactions

2

Robyn L. Jones, Imornefe Bowes and Kieran Kingston

Introduction

Increasingly, researchers have recognised the complex interactive nature of coaching, highlighting its multifaceted, integrated and dynamic character (e.g. Saury & Durand 1998, d'Arripe-Longueville et al 2001, Jones & Wallace 2005). It is a portrayal of coaching, whilst not totally dismissing its developmental disposition, gives growing credence to the non-processual social pressures to which it is also subject (Puddifoot 2000). Hence, the assumptions of unambiguous linearity and sequence associated with traditional processual conceptualisations of coaching are questioned, with the coach being seen not only as a 'mountain guide' through athletic peaks and troughs, but also someone capable of changing the landscape itself (Mayer-Kress 2001).

Although such an appreciation is welcome, accompanying investigative methodologies have not been forthcoming. Indeed, the growing acknowledgement of the co-operative complexity of coaching, containing elements of initiation, reaction and exchange within a temporal process, means that traditional research methods often miss the details and nuances on which much of coaching actually rests. Consequently, if Jones and colleagues' belief (Jones et al 2002, Jones & Wallace 2006) that coaching is not just delivered through a series of given, linked episodes but is a dynamic unfolding social activity is taken as conceptually sound, research methodologies permitting an effective in-depth exploration of it must be sought. The aim of this chapter is to provide a rationale for, and description of, a method that takes into account the social complexities of

coaching, by scrutinising the meaning and interpretation that an individual gives to a task before deciding on an appropriate course of action. The objective is to discuss and illustrate a means to record and subsequently interrogate coaches' understanding of their actions in relation to why they coach as they do within their collective contexts.

The value of the chapter is two-fold. Firstly, it builds upon Puddifoot's (2000) critique of what counts as a 'social process', arguing that a more intricate and complex appreciation of the concept would be advantageous for a further insightful conceptualisation of coaching. Far from being some underlying regular activity over an unspecified period of time where a predicted linage or causal connection takes place (Puddifoot 2000), the act of coaching is alternatively posited to be founded on the interaction or negotiation between coach and athlete in context (Cushion & Jones 2006). In this respect, coaching is reconceptualised as a 'dynamic social process', de-emphasising considerations of unproblematic chronology and the assumption that an identified linkage in one context would ever be repeated in another (Puddifoot 2000). It is a view gaining increasing credence within the field of pedagogy in general (e.g. Sonsino & Moore 2001) as well as sports coaching (d'Arripe-Longueville et al 2001, Bowes & Jones 2006, Hauw & Durand 2007). Here, it has been claimed that optimum learning occurs at or near the so-called 'edge of chaos'; a state which lies neither in a zone of complete stability nor total flux (Sonsino & Moore 2001). The trick for coaches then, is to keep the coaching context hovering in this ever-evolving zone of dynamism through managing the micro-interactions among the agents who comprise it (Bowes & Jones 2006).

Our claim to originality here is tempered, as we are, to a considerable extent, following in the footsteps of others (e.g. d'Arripe-Longueville et al 2001, Hauw & Durand 2005, 2007). Consequently, the second and principal significance of this chapter lies not so much in breaking virgin ground, but in developing and more firmly locating complexity-related studies, and the methodologies they employ, within the field of coaching research. In doing so, we hope to bring an innovative means of investigation to a wider audience in order to stimulate further study and understanding of coaches' immediate and temporal actions, strategies and responses. In terms of structure, we firstly present a brief critique of traditional methods employed to explore coaching, thus making the case that more sensitive means are required for a greater nuanced understanding of the activity. The method we put forward, course of action analysis, inclusive of both situated action (Suchman 1987) and activity theory (Leont'ev 1978), is then defined and discussed as one example through which this can be achieved. Finally, a conclusion summarises the main points made whilst further outlining the implications of course of action analysis for future coach education programmes and coaching practice.

Exploring and conceptualising coaching: Why a more sensitive approach is needed

Without re-presenting the case made in earlier work, suffice to say that traditional methods used in coaching research have largely followed a positivistic approach, with reductionism and generalisability at its heart (e.g. Jones & Turner 2006). This agenda has been reflected in the use of methods such as questionnaires, systemic observation and structured interviewing, giving rise to a conceptualisation of coaching through particular constructs (e.g. Jowett & Ntoumanis 2004) and various models (e.g. Côté et al 1995). In many ways, this approach represents an attempt to identify 'effective' practice from 'good' coaches; to extract knowledge and actions considered tried, tested and, therefore, repeatable by others. It is a conceptualisation of coaching as a knowable sequence of decisions over

which coaches have command, and reflects the assumption that the coaching process is primarily governed by a set of measurable, achievable goals with resources being freely available to realise those goals.

Recently, Jones and Wallace (2005) argued that a fundamental problem with this approach, and the subsequently espoused coaching knowledge, is that the phenomenon of coaching itself is insufficiently understood to effectively prescribe a model of 'best practice'. They go on to discuss that, in utilising a reductionist perspective, behaviour is explained in a mechanistic manner and, hence, is viewed as causal and predictable; the price paid being over-precision in guiding coaching practice. Furthermore, Cushion (2007), in his critique of Lyle (2002), argues that plotting a series of hierarchical relationships and proposed interactions in a model of coaching does little to illuminate the complex actions and their precursors, which actually underpin the activity (Jones et al. 2006). This is because such an approach takes little account of social, moral and cultural influences on individual behaviour, thus disenfranchising the person (McFee 2005). The problem, therefore, with adopting a positivistic approach, which still holds considerable sway in some quarters (e.g. Voight 2007), is that it leaves many coaches frustrated because of the extent to which its representations are divorced from reality. As Jones and Wallace (2005) alluded, the direction given in coaching models is not viewed as applicable as it ignores the tensions and social dilemmas that characterise coaching practice. What we are often left with then is an unbridgeable gap between the best intentions and goals that drive and inspire coaches, and their capacity to attain them – a situation which Jones and Wallace (2005, 2006) described as a 'pathos' within the coaching theory to practice domain.

Coaching has also come to be recognised as a personal venture, negotiated between various stakeholders within a specific context (Jones et al 2004, Purdy et al in press). Such a position further problematises many of the processual assumptions and discourses that underpin our understanding of coaching and how we go about researching it. In depicting the activity as being reliant on patterns of interactions between individuals, this evolving conceptualisation has placed coaching close to the tenets of complexity theory inclusive of both predictable and random results, and where small differences in initial conditions can result in large changes in outcomes (Puddifoot 2000, Mayer-Kress 2001, Bowes & Jones 2006). To date, however, a definitive framework to adequately explore this complexity in coaching has proved elusive.

While we have outlined the principal limitations of the positivistic approach, the works of Côté et al (1995) and Lyle (2002) in particular have provided an impetus for recognising coaching as a sophisticated interpersonal process. Hence, although criticised for oversimplifying a complex practice (e.g. Cushion 2007, Jones 2007), it could be argued that such work has served as a necessary precursor for a subsequent more discerning approach (Lyle 2006). If the initial signposts were there for us to read, much of the credit for leading us in this critical, complex direction goes to the work of Saury and Durand (1998), Sève and Durand (1999), and d'Arripe-Longueville et al (2001). It is to this body of work that we now turn to further make the case for a more sensitive methodological approach to study the phenomena of sports coaching.

One of the first studies that began to shed some light on the complexity of the coaching process in situ was that of Saury and Durand (1998). Having critiqued Côté et al's (1995) model for portraying coaching tasks as being specifiable in advance, Saury and Durand (1998) adopted a cognitive ergonomic (i.e. designed along human need) perspective where the task was presented as a set of constraints facing individuals (e.g. the varying abilities of athletes, the facilities at hand, and/or the immediate objectives of particular actors). The interaction of these constraints generated a set of complex, contradictory, and ill-defined problems. Given this unpredictability, the approach embraced by the coaches studied by Saury and Durand (1998) was based on past experience and was characterised by negotiation and (to varying degrees) shared responsibility with athletes. The study also demonstrated that elite coaches draw upon knowledge far beyond the procedural, rule-based information conveyed in training manuals. Rather, it extended to practical and personal knowledge tied to experience; highly context-dependent knowledge which, because it is often characterised by automation, is difficult to articulate (Saury & Durand 1998). Similarly, Sève and Durand (1999) in their investigation of the temporal and contextual organisation of the working behaviours of three elite coaches, found that such practitioners' activities were not planned in advance but were reactive and heavily typified by flexibility in response to ever-changing, unforeseeable situational characteristics (Bowes & Jones 2006).

Applying this conceptualisation of coaching to the context of competition, d'Arripe-Longueville et al (2001) explored coach–athlete interaction during elite archery contests. Defining situated actions as actions taken in the context of specific, concrete circumstances where cognition is seen as inherently linked to experience and ecological constraints, they identified coaching per se as being collectively constructed. This was particularly so in relation to the shared control that was evident between the actors present. Here, they suggested that so-called 'common' goals were not entirely predetermined, but were collectively constructed through interaction between the agents. Coordination between team members was considered as emerging from mutual constraints, a process which did not follow a general procedure or pre-defined plan. Saury and Durand (1998) similarly proposed coaching as a set of interacting constraints: that coaching tasks comprise a series of routines and cognitive anticipation in relation to flexible plans, whilst works by Sève et al (2003), and Hauw and Durand (2005, 2007) amongst others, have also positioned coaching along such complex lines. Therefore, although grounded in experience, coaches' practice is increasingly being viewed as very flexible and responsive to unforeseeable situational characteristics (Bowes & Jones 2006, Sève & Durand 1999). Coaches' subsequent planning then, is not considered as being related to pre-set applied goals, but rather is dependent on 'continuous step-by-step tuning to the context' (Saury & Durand 1998 p 264).

Such a conceptualisation of coaching echoes that of Jones and Wallace (2005, 2006), who recently posited that the quantifiable processual goals often set by coaches are doomed to failure given the need for variable and constant adaptation to context; where physical, social and personal factors militate against any sequential, unproblematic progression. The implications of such work are that coaching expertise requires constant adjustment to evolving constraints (albeit within certain parameters) imposed by the situation, the actors, and the broad pedagogical objectives. In this respect, coaching becomes a contested, negotiated practice between those involved within the social setting (Cassidy et al 2004, Jones 2007). Although many of the studies we have considered here utilised small samples, which preclude their findings' general application, we believe that the uncovered evidence points to potential commonalities and, hence, to a very fruit-ful area of investigation.

In an attempt to accommodate this increased appreciation of complexity as an important facet in explaining coaching interaction, Bowes and Jones (2006) utilised the notion of relational schemas and complexity theory. Here, relational schemas pro-vided a coherent explanation for coaches' possession of an experience-based, constantly evolving frame-work for expected patterns of interaction (which regulate their behaviours). Complexity theory meanwhile was used to depict the coaching environ-ment as problematic and non-linear, therefore aligning it with propositions of coaching theorists (e.g. Sève & Durand 1999). Within this framework, the pedagogical process is viewed as complex and dynamic, with controlled yet chaotic interaction being the catalyst for learning (Sonsino & Moore 2001). Teaching moments are derived rather than pre-ordained, with the coach's role being essentially to manage the various agendas and goals held by those present for the greater good within a context characterised by continuous transformation (Sonsino & Moore 2001, Jones & Wallace 2005). Conse-quently, studying coach–athlete interaction as a dynamic process involving measured reflection within flexible plans necessitates an exploration and understanding of situated action, the meanings of such action, and the constructed cognition underpin-ning such actions within a given social (coaching) sys-tem. It is to a considered discussion of course of action analysis as a means through which we can real-ise this goal that we now turn.

Course of action analysis: What's it all about?

To fully understand an activity, its history and growth should be taken into consideration. In study-ing development, Thelen and Smith (1996) argued that although descriptions of events are useful if not essential to understanding, they also hold the potential of being flawed explanations. This is because the move from description to explanation requires only a subtle shift. As evidence of this, descriptions of coaching have tended to become 'how to' models leading to a superficial acceptance or adoption of causality (Jones & Wallace 2005). This has resulted in some neophyte coaches unpro-blematically replicating the behaviours of their more experienced counterparts with little appreciation of

social or individual factors that may have affected the original development, resulting in an often inef-fective interaction and confusion for the coach (Jones et al 2003).

An alternative position argued by Thelen and Smith (1996) is that of viewing development as a process that possesses non-linear flexibility while still acknowledging a (target) goal state. This con-ceptualisation of a self-modifying process moves away from the proposed division between cognition and behaviour, where the boundary between action and response is difficult to define (Varela et al 1991). Instead, such a stance contends that it is impossible to separate the products from the pro-cesses because the processes used change the user (Minsky 1986). Research involving reflection (e.g. Schön 1983, Kolb 1984) supports the impact of this evaluative or self-modifying process, where the implications for the act of coaching look more like the complex picture given elsewhere, and less like a knowable coaching process (Bowes & Jones 2006). Anecdotally, this also seems to match the reality of coaching, where athletes' perceived need is gleaned through exposure to various competi-tion-related situations as opposed to repetitive coach instruction. It is a position which suggests the importance of participation in less controlled activity in order to develop the skills needed to negotiate the complexities of (game and social) interaction, thus questioning the assumed causal link between prescribed coaching acts and defined outcomes.

Course of action analysis (Theureau 1992) is sug-gested as a means to better engage with the com-plexity of non-linear phenomena such as coaching as it seeks to describe and analyse the action of agents from their point of view in relation to the characteristics of the situation. Epistemologically then, without wishing to apply definitive and, hence, restrictive labels, course of action analysis lies within the interpretive realm, inclusive of inter-active and subjective methods.

Grounded in both activity theory (Leont'ev 1978) and situated action (Suchman 1987), course of action analysis acknowledges three dimensions of the 'human system'; the task, individual differ-ences and, importantly, the timescale of behavioural acts. It is a perspective that increases the focus or the unit of analysis to include more than just the individual actor or the environment, to the interac-tion that occurs between these elements over time. Underlying the notion of course of action is the premise that cognition utilises many sources including the social, cultural and material characteristics of the context in which it occurs. It is a sentiment that echoes that of Simon (1977), whose work highlighted the dynamic and indistinct quality of real life problems, which are both impacted upon by current knowledge and generated from interaction with the environment.

Course of action analysis fundamentally argues for the importance of participation in structuring thought (Varela et al 1991). Here, it emphasises the dynamic quality of experience, suggesting agents' interactions with their environment are developed in line with particular contexts and are not predefined (Varela et al 1991). Such experiences are not solely individually enacted but collectively manufactured, meaning that individual events are interwoven with culturally bound artefacts, symbols or actions.

It is a position that draws heavily from three key ideas of situated approaches. Firstly, that cognition is inseparable from the activity where it is produced, thus actors can mobilise and build their own knowledge from the emergent coupling of activity and situation (Guillou & Durny 2007). Secondly, that activity is a construction of meaning which does not pre-exist activity but emerges with it (Theureau 1992). Finally, that activity is a dynamic totality, with no distinction between action and interpretation (Varela et al 1991). Such a perspective holds the potential to examine what recent research has termed the seemingly intuitive, unplanned actions of coaches; actions which accommodate the 'unforeseeable contingencies of particular situations' (d'Arrippe-Longueville et al 2001 p 277). This last notion, that activity is a dynamic totality, is rooted in Simon's (Newell & Simon 1972) concept of 'satisficing', where problem-solving and decision-making rest not on a painstaking search for optimal idealistic solutions as the dynamic context does not allow such opportunity. Rather, they rely on a judgement regarding what is good enough, that satisfies the needs of the complex real world. Consequently, a course of action constitutes a dynamic entity comprising actions, communication, interpretations and feelings that are meaningful for the actor in situ. Furthermore, the action (described from the actor's point of view) is presented and analysed in relation to the overall extrinsic characteristics of the situation (d'Arripe-Longueville et al 2001).

The remainder of this section is devoted to a further examination of course of action analysis, paying particular attention to activity theory (Leont'ev 1978) and situated action (Suchman 1987), from which it largely derives.

Activity theory

Broadly defined, activity theory is a philosophical and cross-disciplinary framework that can be used to study forms of human practice where both individual and social processes are interlinked (Kuutti 1996). The core aspects of activity theory centre on situational 'goings-on', and include subject, object, actions, and operations, which are taken as creating a flexible dynamic picture of actors at a specific task in a particular situation (Leont'ev 1978). Activity then is defined as the dynamic reactor to changing circumstance, with an individual's action being perceived as a response to a task. Activity theory discusses the *subject* as a person engaged in an activity, an *object* as something that motivates the subject's activity in a specific direction, and an *action* as a conscious goal-directed process that is carried out to achieve the object (Nardi 1995). For example, in a coaching context, the subject could be the athlete, the object a ball, and the action a deliberate movement to gain possession of the ball. However, emphasising the in-built allowance for complexity, it is acknowledged that objects and actions need not be seemingly coherent. For example, in an invasion game, creating space by *moving away* from the ball (action) might be the best method of getting possession or receiving the ball (object). Similarly, the appropriateness of action will be dependent on the immediate context. Such contextualisation is important as it follows the change present during activity, recognising it neither as a static entity nor as something that develops in a linear fashion (Kuutti 1996).

Actions can, according to Nardi (1995), become unconscious over time. This is as a result of practice when conscious cognitive action ceases to exist (Leont'ev 1978). Consequently, it can become difficult to gain insight from an actor about specific differences and developments as related to achievements. This feature has been highlighted as a weakness in self-report studies questioning the validity and reliability of the data gathered (Lyle 2003). Within course of actions analysis, the participants are actively engaged to make such actions explicit. This feature reflects the capability of activity theory to capture the shifting nature of actors in situ

(Nardi 1995). Specifically, it encourages them to reflect upon and disclose motives for their behaviours that are crucial to understanding how they make sense of, and subsequently navigate, social spaces. Allowance is also made for the mediating influence of artefacts such as instruments, signs, procedures or laws created and transformed during any activity. Such artefacts also carry a historical and cultural residue (Kuutti 1996) and have been identified within coaching research, albeit in numerous guises; for example habitus (Bourdieu & Passeron 1977, Cushion & Jones 2006), relational schema (Bowes & Jones 2006), and self-presentation (Jones 2006a). Such work has highlighted the crucial role that culture and personal biography have on action, which is often only manifested when actions break down, or alter dramatically.

The interpretative nature of activity theory can be seen in its explanation of context, as something not divorced from the observer. An acknowledgement exists, therefore, that context can be generated through activity, allowing actors to reframe their actions as they engage with that activity (Leont'ev 1978). Context is thus both created by and acts upon individuals, rather than simply existing as the canvas upon which coaching is painted. The relevance of activity theory here is that it permits analyses of social phenomena at the levels of both social systems and individual behaviour. This allows differentiation between and among motives, goals and conditions, and for unpredictable behaviour due to changing circumstances (Kaptelinin 1996). Taken as such, activity theory appears well positioned to explore the context of coaching, which was recently depicted by Cushion and Jones (2006) among others (e.g. Purdy et al in press) as both constructing and constructed by the actions of those who comprise it.

Situated action

Situated action is concerned with how individuals achieve integrated action from unique experience. According to Suchman (1987 p 50), it reflects a view whereby 'every course of action depends in essential ways upon its material and social circumstances'. In contrast to the reductionist perspective where each element is considered in isolation, situated action theorists propose the unit of analysis to be the unfolding real activity occurring in a setting which is defined as 'a relation between acting persons and the arenas in which they act' (Nardi 1995 p 36). Hence, it emphasises the emergent, contingent nature of human activity, focusing on the in situ rather than the constituent parts (Suchman 1987). As opposed to the linear link assumed between intentions and desired outcomes in traditional approaches, the situated action perspective recognises that there is a difference between what we say we will do and knowing exactly how that action will unfold (Suchman 1987). In dynamic social settings (such as coaching), where the sequence of actions cannot be known in advance, the effectiveness of 'plans' and 'goals' as the only source of intent becomes questionable (Jones & Wallace 2005). For example, although coaches are encouraged to plan sessions detailing practices, learning outcomes and methods of provision, the actual delivery of the session relies more on instinctive, contextual skills. Consequently, the plan becomes only a loose guide to orientate coaches in such a way as to make best use of those in situ abilities (Suchman 1987). Plans, therefore, become approximations, requiring constant recourse to the physical environment for confirmation and adaptation: at best, they can only be considered a weak resource, insofar as they must be able to allow for the unpredictable incidents and eventualities of particular situations (d'Arripe-Longueville et al 2001). Such a conclusion echoes the empirical findings of Jones et al (2003), whose subject, Steve Harrison, emphasised the importance of being flexible and of reacting to changing circumstances, particularly when issues of maintaining players' respect were at stake. Within situated action, the importance of contextually adhered action is accentuated. This practical objectivity, the necessity of everyday actions in creating meaning, becomes the essence of understanding activity.

Central to situated action is the 'research programme' that focuses on how individuals use their circumstances to achieve meaningful action (Suchman 1987); that is, how people find evidence for plans in what they do. Intent is thus borne out of two aspects; the first contends that cognitive experience has an essential relationship to a 'publicly available, collaboratively organised world of artefacts and actions'; that is, to a surrounding culture (Suchman 1987 p 50). The second meanwhile argues that 'the significance of artefacts and actions, and the methods by which their significance is conveyed, have an essential relationship to their particular, concrete circumstances' (Suchman 1987 p 50).

Such a position renders the claim for objective pre- or post-action intent a little meaningless and, instead, posits action as dynamic, situated and enacted. It is a perspective that eliminates the need to explain intuition as stored knowledge; rather it can be seen as something that emerges, being present within any situation. Both activity theory and situated action reflect the nature of the individual editing or constantly refining as he or she negotiates their respective environments. This is not so much in physical terms, but by constantly adjusting the focus of their activity towards a desired outcome. In this way, the experience is made unique and equally improvisatory based on their minute-to-minute preferences (Nardi 1995). Jones and Wallace (2005) recently conceived of coaches as involved in such orchestrating actions; endlessly evaluating and fine-tuning actions to bring sought-after developments back 'on-track'.

According to course of action analysis, what informs these micro decisions is not only cognition which generates awareness of experience (Theureau 2003), but also experience through social interaction, and the construction of that experience at any given moment. Such a proposition takes inspiration from Pierce's 'thought-sign' model (1931), which stated that to understand experience is not to describe the physical processes but to develop an awareness and appreciation of how the culture, immediate situation and the individual all join the physical environment to initiate action (Theureau & Jeffory 1994). Given that such a position would seem an appropriate location from which to view coaching (Cushion & Jones 2006), the following section attempts to articulate a method through which it can be effectively researched.

Course of action: An alternative method to investigate coaching

Based on the assumption that a particular event carries meaning for the parties involved, it can be viewed as a sign. That is, it represents something for an individual and generates an equivalent sign in the mind of that person. It is this meaningful use of signs, which is at the heart of semiotics, reflecting the on-going quest to categorise complex social processes. According to Pierce's (1931) foundational work, a sign comprises three aspects; the *Representamen*, the *Object* and the *Interpretant* which, in turn, combine to create an elementary unit of meaning (EUM) (Theureau 1992). The Representamen is the contextual element to which the actor gives meaning (i.e., the particular contextual event or experience), and can be internal or existing within the external environment. Based on this, the Object is the consciousness or the intentional state of the individual as related to the possible range of actions available to him or her. Consistent with situated action's stance, the chosen action or behaviour does not need to be defined prior to the task but becomes apparent based on the Representamen. The mediator of this relationship is the Interpretant, which consists of previous knowledge brought to bear by the person who impacts on the current situation (Hauw & Durand 2007). This triangular or triadic form combines to give the eventual EUM, which also contains or acknowledges the temporal qualities or sequences (in terms of the collective interaction) often missing from previous analyses (Theureau 1992). It is a position based on the inference that static, discrete and well-defined problems do not exist in real-life. Rather, problems are endlessly altering, being modified on the basis of agents' recall of past experiences, which, in turn, are founded on changing perceptions of their environment (Simon 1977). Such a perspective, of course, is equally applicable to any coaching 'domain', be it working with elite athletes or 7- and 8-year-old beginner-level children. This is because the fundamental objective here, giving weight to Jones' (2006b) critique of a perceived artificial dichotomy between performance and participation coaching, relates to social communication and action in context, and how, as communal beings, we make sense of the messages we send to and receive from each other. The importance of such interaction was illustrated in Purdy's (2006) recent study, where the uncovered dysfunctionalities in a coach–athlete relationship were attributed to misunderstandings and mis-readings of social 'signs'.

In relation to positioning course of action theory as a particular analytical framework, participants (or researched subjects) are interviewed while reviewing a video recording of themselves coaching (or being coached), which they break down into personally meaningful semiological units of experience (i.e. the EUMs) (Guillou & Durny 2007). The basic methods employed within course of action theory then, are observation, video recording and self-confrontation interviews in relation to those recordings (von Cranach & Harré 1982).

The primary purpose of these interviews is to assess on-going thoughts and feelings, and consist of a procedure where participants are faced with their actions soon after the events in question (von Cranach & Harré 1982). In doing so, participants are encouraged to reconstruct past experience and behaviour 'in all its complexity' (Therueau 1992, d'Arippe-Longueville et al 2001 p 279). The resulting segments of experience may be physical actions, communications, interpretations or feelings and can be connected through either sequential or serial coherence (d'Arripe-Longueville et al 2001, Sève et al 2003). Although d'Arripe-Longueville et al (2001) constructed their EUMs according to the pre-determined categories above (i.e., 'physical actions', 'communications', 'interpretations' or 'feelings'; with the addition of 'focalizations'), we see no reason why a more preliminary inductive analysis of videoed data could not yield other categories still related to addressing the fundamental questions of 'what is happening?', 'why is it happening?' and 'what are its consequences?'

Relating to the temporal or processual nature of coaching, it is acknowledged that EUMs create a sequential chain when in close succession, and where the previous in some way determines the following. However, due to the unpredictable nature of action, sequences can be discontinued or interrupted at any time often by an EUM from another sequence. On the other hand, serial coherence relates to repeated preoccupations and resultant actions of an individual that do not form part of a sequential relation (d'Arripe-Longueville et al 2001). Through such coherences, the partial predictability of such systems is acknowledged while the emphasis remains on their basic chaotic, non-linear state (Jacobsen 2000, Puddifoot 2000). Additionally, through further analysis, archetypal structures or regularities can also be deduced from the data where the sequences and series of particular courses of actions are compared and contrasted (d'Arripe-Longueville et al 2001).

The whole process echoes that of grounded theory (Glaser & Strauss 1967) where data are organised and moderated into meaning units which, in turn, are subjected to a fine-grained search for commonalities and uniqueness (Tesch 1990). The relevance to coaching thus becomes increasingly obvious, as each coaching context is an exceptional, novel system housing a network of social agents (i.e. coaches, athletes and others) comprising constant action and reaction between and among them, albeit within given boundaries which themselves are often in flux (Bowes & Jones 2006).

To make this task workable, d'Arrippe-Longueville et al (2001) selected a number of differing interactive situations from earlier recorded coaching sessions from which EUMs could be deducted. Although this naturally involved an element of construction, one could argue that a degree of theoretical sampling and preliminary review is unavoidable. In d'Arrippe-Longueville et al's study (2001) these situations or events were firstly identified by the researchers and confirmed by the coaches as being significant interactions or moments between themselves and athletes. The temporal events or related EUMs prior to and following from the principal incidents were also taped and discussed, so that the latter could be more properly contextualised. In this way, each EUM was 'chronologically chained' to others, with condensed narratives being developed for each situation (d'Arrippe-Longueville et al 2001). Such narratives, stemming from the interviews, focused on the participants' actions, feelings, communications, motivations and interpretations (Theureu & Jeffroy 1994, d'Arrippe-Longueville et al 2001). Indeed, this is where such a data collection method principally differs from embedded ethnographic approaches. In focusing on discrete events with participants through recourse to video evidence, a detailed investigation of the context in terms of its creation and consequence in relation to future interactions can be explored.

The purpose of such a method is to collect detailed contextually rich data from a living, bounded and connected social system; a system like coaching which is grounded in a collective (albeit porous) understanding of social signs and grammar, yet possesses the potential for individuals to follow and occupy differing locations within it. Through probing and provoking verbalisations from those under study (be they athletes or coaches) during the analysis of their activity, course of action analysis allows for the observation of knowledge creation; that is, through unveiling the evolving interpretation and subsequent construction of each EUM and how, if at all, they are related (Theureau 2003). These individual and chained constructions comprise data from the observer's viewpoint, from the subject's position, from the diverse components of variable situations (e.g., the prescribed task and organisational roles, the existing interfaces, the workspaces, the organisation of training, etc.), and from both the micro and macro culture within which the interaction is taking place (Theureau 2003). In this way, we can observe the development of knowledge about coaching as it is formed (Theureau 2003). It is a recognition of cognition as being experienced, embodied and dynamically situated, whilst also being indissolubly individual, collective and cultural (Theureau et al 2001). Course of action analysis then is a framework that allows us to develop lines of inquiry based on individuals' personal criteria of relevance in relation to the real-time coaching situation encountered. It provides an opportunity to explore coach and athlete cognitions in greater depth than previously possible in that it illuminates the impetus for particular actions, what the consequences of such actions are for all concerned, and how such complex and often intersecting sequences construct what we define as coaching.

Conclusion

In this chapter we have tried to present an alternative conceptualisation of coaching, one that is gaining increasing recognition within the literature (e.g. Bowes & Jones 2006, Hauw & Durand 2007). The acknowledgment of coaching's complex nature within this body of work is a welcome development from previous portrayals of a largely unproblematic, sequential activity. This is not to deny the processual nature of coaching per se, but rather to qualify such claims in light of non-processual social pressures (Puddifoot 2000). With the exception of work by Durand and colleagues (e.g d'Arippe-Longueville et al 2001, Hauw & Durand 2005,

2007), increasingly nuanced methods to explore this complexity have not generally been forthcoming. Within this chapter, we have presented course of action analysis, a position based on situated action and activity theory, as one such means to realise this goal. By exploring the nature of particular incidents and interactions and why they have meaning for coaches and athletes, in addition to where these then lead the coach–athlete relationship, we can extend and enrich the comments and claims we make on behalf of our findings (Theureau et al 2001). Course of action assists in this quest by allowing us to thoughtfully consider and deconstruct the meaningful, lively, everyday contextual moments and sequences which comprise social interaction within coaching.

Viewing and researching coaching as a series of noteworthy, although often non-linear, events has obvious ramifications for how we teach and facilitate the activity. Indeed, the principal significance of the approach, and the value of this chapter, lies in its potential to inform more credible coach education programmes, grounded in the messy reality of everyday practice. For example, through engaging coaches in deconstructing their precise actions and reactions to ever-changing contexts, whilst maintaining a focus on athlete learning and improvement. Subsequently, appropriate theory can be introduced into the conversations both to explain and further explore practice. Doing so could give coaches more definitive, realistic pegs on which to hang their contextually laden reflections and thoughts about why they coach as they do and how they can do so better.

References

Bourdieu, P., Passeron, J., 1977. Reproduction in education, society and culture. Sage, London.

Bowes, I., Jones, R.L., 2006. Working at the edge of chaos: understanding coaching as a complex interpersonal system. The Sport Psychologist 20, 235–245.

Cassidy, T., Jones, R.L., Potrac, P., 2004. Understanding sports coaching: the social, cultural and pedagogical foundations of coaching practice. Routledge, London.

Côte, J., Salmela, J., Trudel, P., et al., 1995. The coaching model: a

grounded assessment of expert gymnastic coaches knowledge. Journal of Sport and Exercise Psychology 17 (1), 1–17.

Cushion, C., 2007. Modelling the complexity of the coaching process. International Journal of Sports Science & Coaching 2 (4), 395–401.

Cushion, C., Jones, R.L., 2006. Power, discourse and symbolic violence in professional youth soccer: The case of Albion F.C. Sociology of Sport Journal 23 (2), 142–161.

d'Arripe-Longueville, F., Saury, J., Fournier, J., et al., 2001.

Coach–athlete interaction during elite archery competitions: an application of methodological frameworks used in ergonomics research to sport psychology. Journal of Applied Sport Psychology 13, 275–299.

Glaser, B.G., Strauss, A.L., 1967. Discovery of grounded theory: strategies for qualitative research. Aldine, Chicago, IL.

Guillou, J., Durny, A., 2007. Students' situated action in physical education: analysis of typical concerns and their relations with mobilized knowledge in table tennis. Physical Education and Sport Pedagogy 1, 1–17.

Hauw, D., Durand, M., 2005. How do elite athletes interact with the environment in competition? A situated analysis of trampolinists' activity. European Review of Applied Psychology 55 (3), 207–215.

Hauw, D., Durand, M., 2007. Situated analysis of elite trampolinists' problems in competition using retrospective interviews. J. Sports Sci. 25 (2), 73–183.

Jacobson, M.J., 2000. Butterflies, traffic jams and cheetahs: Problem solving and complex systems. In: Paper presented at the American Educational Research Association, April 21st, New Orleans, Louisiana.

Jones, R.L., 2006a. Dilemmas, maintaining 'face' and paranoia: An average coaching life. Qualitative Inquiry 12 (5), 1012–1021.

Jones, R.L., 2006b. How can educational concepts inform sports coaching? In: Jones, R.L. (Ed.), The sports coach as educator: re-conceptualising sports coaching. Routledge, London, pp. 3–13.

Jones, R.L., 2007. Coaching redefined: An everyday pedagogical endeavour. Sport, Education and Society 12 (2), 159–174.

Jones, R.L., Turner, P., 2006. Teaching coaches to coach holistically: the case for a Problem-Based Learning (PBL) approach. Physical Education and Sport Pedagogy 11 (2), 181–202.

Jones, R.L., Wallace, M., 2006. The coach as orchestrator. In: Jones, R.L. (Ed.), The sports coach as educator: re-conceptualising sports coaching. Routledge, London, pp. 51–64.

Jones, R.L., Wallace, M., 2005. Another bad day at the training ground: Coping with ambiguity in the coaching context. Sport, Education and Society 10 (1), 119–134.

Jones, R.L., Armour, K.M., Potrac, P., 2002. Understanding the coaching process: a framework for social analysis. Quest 54, 34–48.

Jones, R.L., Armour, K.M., Potrac, P., 2003. Constructing expert knowledge: a case study of a top-level professional soccer coach. Sport, Education and Society 8 (2), 213–229.

Jones, R.L., Armour, K., Potrac, P., 2004. Sports coaching cultures: from practice to theory. Routledge, London.

Jones, R.L., Potrac, P., Hussain, H., et al., 2006. Exposure by association: maintaining anonymity in autoethnographical research. In: Fleming, F., Jordan, F. (Eds.), Ethical issues in leisure research. Leisure Studies Association, Eastbourne, pp. 45–62.

Jowett, S., Ntoumanis, N., 2004. The coach–athlete relationship questionnaire (CART-Q): development and initial validation. Scand. J. Med. Sci. Sports 14, 245–257.

Kaptelinin, V., 1996. Activity theory: Implications for human–computer interaction. In: Nardi, B.A. (Ed.), Context and consciousness: activity theory and human–computer interaction. The MIT Press, Cambridge MA, pp. 103–116.

Kolb, D., 1984. Experiential learning: experience as the source of learning and development. Prentice-Hall, Englewood Cliffs.

Kuutti, K., 1996. Activity theory as a potential framework for human–computer interaction research. In: Nardi, B.A. (Ed.), Context and consciousness: activity theory and human–computer interaction. The MIT Press, Cambridge MA, pp. 17–44.

Leont'ev, A., 1978. Activity, consciousness, and personality. Prentice-Hall, Englewood Cliffs NJ.

Lyle, J., 2002. Sports coaching concepts: a framework for coaches' behaviour. Routledge, London.

Lyle, J., 2003. Stimulated recall: a report on its use in naturalistic research. British Educational Research Journal 29 (6), 861–878.

Lyle, J., 2006. Sports coaching: Pedagogy, professionalisation, and precedent. Inaugural professorial lecture, Leeds Metropolitan University, 28th November.

McFee, G., 2005. Why doesn't sport psychology consider Freud? In: McNamee, M. (Ed.), Philosophy and the sciences of exercise, health and sport: critical perspectives on research methods. Routledge, London, pp. 85–116.

Mayer-Kress, G.J., 2001. Complex systems as foundational theory of sports coaching. In: Keynote presentation to the 2001 International Sports Coaching Symposium of the Chinese Taipei University Sports Federation, Taichung, Taiwan. November 16th–18th.

Minsky, M., 1986. The society of mind. Simon and Schuster, New York.

Navrdi, B.A., 1995. Context and consciousness: activity theory and human computer interaction. MIT, Cambridge MA.

Newell, A., Simon, H.A., 1972. Human problem solving. Englewood Cliffs, Prentice Hall.

Pierce, C., 1931. Collected papers of Charles Sanders Pierce (Vols. 1–6, C & P Weiss, Eds.). Harvard University Press, Cambridge, MA.

Puddifoot, J., 2000. Some problems and possibilities in the study of dynamical social processes. Journal for the Theory of Social Behaviour 30 (1), 79–97.

Purdy, L., 2006. Coaching in the 'current': Capturing the climate in elite rowing training camps. University of Otago, Dunedin, New Zealand.

Purdy, L., Jones, R.L., Cassidy, T., in press. Negotiation and capital: athletes' use of power in an elite men's rowing programme. Sport, Education and Society.

Saury, J., Durand, M., 1998. Practical knowledge in expert coaches: on-site study of coaching in sailing. Res Q Exerc Sport 69 (3), 254–266.

Schön, D.A., 1983. The reflective practitioner: how professionals think in action. Basic Books, New York.

Sève, C., Durand, M., 1999. L'action de l'entraîneur de tennis de table comme action située [The action of a table tennis coach as situated action]. Avante 5, 69–86.

Sève, C., Saury, J., Ria, L., et al., 2003. Structure of expert players' activity during competitive interaction in table tennis. Res. Q. Exerc. Sport 74 (1), 71–83.

Simon, H.A., 1977. Models of discovery. Reidel, Dordrecht.

Sonsino, S., Moore, J., 2001. Only connect: teaching and learning at the edge of chaos. In: Paper presented at the ITP Conference, NYU, New York.

Suchman, L., 1987. Plans and situated actions: the problem of the human/machine communication. University Press, Cambridge.

Tesch, R., 1990. Qualitative research: analysis types and software tools. Falmer Press, New York.

Thelen, E., Smith, L.B., 1996. A dynamic systems approach to the development of cognition and action. MIT Press, Cambridge MA.

Theureau, J., 1992. Le cours d'action: analyse sémiologique. Essai d'une anthropologie cognitive située [The course of action: Semiological analysis. Essay in situated cognitive anthropology]. Peter Lang, Berne.

Theureau, J., 2003. Course of action analysis and course of action centred design. In: Hollnagel, E. (Ed.), Handbook of cognitive task design. Lawrence Erlbaum, Hillsdale NJ, pp. 55–81.

Theureau, J., Jeffory, F., 1994. Ergonomie des situations informatisées [Ergonomics of computerised situations]. Octares, Toulouse.

Theureau, J., Filippi, G., Saliou, G., et al., 2001. A methodology for analysing the dynamic collective organisation of nuclear power plant operators in simulated accidental situations. In: Paper presented at the Conference in Cognitive Science Approaches to Process Control CSAPC'01, 23–26 September, Munich, Germany. Available: http://www.coursdaction.net/06-English/2001-JTal-C82.pdf.

Varela, F., Thomson, E., Rosch, E., 1991. The embodied mind: cognitive science and human experience. MIT Press, London.

Voight, M., 2007. Modelling the complexity of the coaching process: a commentary. International Journal of Sports Science & Coaching 2 (4), 415–416.

von Cranach, M., Harré, R. (Eds.), 1982. The analysis of action: recent theoretical and empirical advances. University Press, Cambridge.

Coaches' decision making: a Naturalistic Decision Making analysis

3

John Lyle

Introduction

There seems little doubt that decision making plays an important part in coaches' everyday practice and is a significant component of coaching expertise. It might be argued, however, that coach education has yet to pay sufficient attention to this aspect of the coach's skills set. This chapter makes the case for the centrality of decision making in coaches' practice and offers the Naturalistic Decision Making (NDM) paradigm (Lipshitz et al 2001) as an appropriate mechanism for describing and explaining how coaches make decisions. As subsequent sections will demonstrate, NDM is a (relatively) recent research paradigm in psychology that focuses on the decision making of proficient and experienced practitioners. The more traditional Judgement/Decision Making (J/DM), based on the rational assessment of alternatives (Teigen 1996), did not appear to offer an adequate mechanism for describing and understanding the apparently intuitive decision making of these practitioners. NDM (Cannon-Bowers et al 1996, Flin et al 1997, Zsambok & Klein 1997, Lipshitz et al 2001, Montgomery et al 2004) offers a number of alternative models of decision making, the best known of which is Klein's (1998) Recognition Primed Decision model. This model illustrates the central theme of NDM, which is that for proficient practitioners the decision to act 'emerges' from a largely sub-conscious process in which the decision is generated from previous experience and is based on a reading and recognition of the situation.

Although the literature referred to will confirm the recognition of decision making as an element of sports coaches' expertise, it will also demonstrate that there has been very limited exploration, in theory or concept, of the mechanisms through which the coaches' cognitions enable this decision making. Therefore, this chapter offers a research agenda, and provides an account of how the NDM paradigm could provide insights that resonate with coaching practice.

Practising coaches will have no problem with an assumption that much of their functioning as coaches involves taking decisions. Indeed, if we conceive of the coach's behaviour, in all but its most instinctive or reactive forms, as being the result of an 'action decision', it might be argued that decision making assumes a pre-eminent place in the coach's expertise. Of course, conceptions are never as straightforward as this, and it is necessary to distinguish between deliberative and non-deliberative decision making. Deliberative decisions involve those aspects of practice in which the coach has time and space to consider options and weigh the relevant evidence to decide upon the most appropriate course of action. This will characterise much of forward planning, but also aspects of team selection, reflecting on progress, considering tactical options, or dealing with some relationship issues. On the other hand, non-deliberative decision making is perhaps most evident in game or competition situations in which the coach has to take decisions under considerable time pressure (perhaps thought of as 'reactive'). This may be too 'black and white' for the messiness of coaching practice, in which much of the coach's decision taking can be categorised as semi-deliberative; that is, there is an element of time pressure, but no suggestion that the coach's behaviour is (or should be!) completely without conscious deliberation. It is not too much of a jump to characterise the greater part of the coach's management of interventions (the training session), competition, and interpersonal interactions as semi-deliberative.

The reason for introducing these distinctions at this early stage is that NDM will be shown to contribute most to the coach's decision taking in semi-deliberative and non-deliberative circumstances. It will also be obvious to students of sports coaching that the literature will show, or at least conceive, that much of the coach's action decision taking appears intuitive and draws upon personal knowledge in ways that are described as tacit or implicit. It will be necessary, therefore, to demonstrate throughout this chapter that NDM offers insights into such behaviour, and can make a contribution to both research and coach education.

The chapter begins with a brief account of the decision-making circumstances in which NDM provides the most apt explanation for decision-making behaviour, and demonstrates why this is particularly appropriate for sports coaching. This is followed by a more in-depth examination of NDM, which illustrates how some of its findings resonate with semi-deliberative decision making in coaching practice. There are two focused sections. The first provides an example of 'story telling' as an exemplar of NDM-related analysis of coaches' narratives; the second examines intuition and the role that this plays in NDM accounts of decision making. The chapter concludes with an identification of the implications for understanding sports coaching expertise and designing coach education.

Sports coaching and decision making

An acknowledgement that the sports coaching practice of expert coaches is a predominantly cognitive activity is relatively recent (Côté 1998, Vergeer & Lyle 2007), although research into coaches' cognitive organisation is clearly not yet a coherent field (Gilbert & Trudel 2004). Studies have focused on general decision processes (e.g. Jones et al 1995, 1997) or specific coaching problems (e.g. Vergeer & Hogg 1999). This latter study is an example of a policy-capturing approach in which the focus is on identifying the 'rules' used by coaches to make decisions in given circumstances. There have been notable attempts to study coaches' knowledge structures in relation to coaches' practice (e.g. Saury & Durand 1998) but coaches' decision making has received limited attention. To some extent this is surprising given that recent literature identifies decision making as the core of coaches' expertise. For example, Abraham et al (2006) suggest that coaching is 'fundamentally a decision-making process' (p 549), although they fail to elaborate on what this means for coaching expertise. Nash and Collins (2006) reinforce the point, stating that decision making is 'one of the key functions that define a coach' (p 466), adding that knowledge gained from everyday (practice) is 'tacit' and often 'unarticulated' by the coach.

A simple and workable definition of decision making is provided from within the NDM paradigm: a decision is 'committing oneself to a course of action' (Lipshitz et al 2001). It may therefore be more profitable if we work on the assumption that coaching requires decision making, and as with other professions it constitutes the mark of the professional (Beckett 1996). At the same time, it is necessary to keep in mind that the range of decisions will stretch from the automatic and unconscious; the routine, repetitive decisions about which there is no conflict; decisions with a choice of alternatives (with impact on achieving goals); to fluid, real-life decisions in which there is no clarity about the alternatives or the basis on which the decision might be taken – perhaps better thought of as problem solving (Svenson 1996). It does not take too much imagination to visualise this as part of coaching practice. The useful categorisation of deliberative, semi-deliberative, and non-deliberative helps to bring some order to the mix of routine training interventions, coach–performer interactions, planning and management activities, crisis interventions, competition management, and so on. The 'pressured' action in response to a performer's reaction to the coach and the control of the competition situation with key momentum-turning decision points are often visible manifestations of the coach's skills (or lack of skills!). Nevertheless, the cumulative, and perhaps more reflective, decisions about managing the progress of the training interventions may be even more crucial to achieving success.

Lyle (2002) suggests that the aim of the coach is to 'manage uncertainty and retain control' (p 137), while acknowledging the factors that make this difficult. However, there is limited value in identifying the uncertainty that undoubtedly characterises coaching practice without working towards an explanation for how the coach copes with this. It is also worth pointing out that 'control' does not refer to performer behaviour but to maintaining focus on the individual and group targets and goals that have been agreed. Lyle (2002 p137) offers some hypotheses about decisions taken. These high-light the balance between impact and certainty in making decisions, the ability to reduce option choices, the influence of personal biases and prefer-ences, and the use of heuristics that optimise rather than maximise outcomes. He cites Lipshitz and Bar-Ilan (1996) who suggest that we should diagnose (recognise the need for action) as early as possible, delay decision taking, and select actions that do not completely restrict our 'room for subsequent manoeuvre'. For coaches reading this text this advice is likely to resonate with their experience and practice.

The purpose of the chapter is to draw attention to the extent to which NDM offers a plausible explana-tion for coaches' decision making. Teigen (1996) dis-tinguishes between the traditional experimental, laboratory-based Judgement/Decision Making (J/DM) research with structured, contrived problems, and NDM, which is ill-structured, 'messy' and untidy, and with fewer 'givens'. The question there-fore, is whether sports coaching offers the sort of decision-making environment within which NDM analyses and explanations might be profitably applied. Randel et al (1996 p 579) describe the con-trast between NDM and more traditional research problems. They characterise NDM contexts as: deal-ing with ill-structured problems; suited to uncertain dynamic environments; operating best with shifting, ill-defined or competing goals; process-orientated; time-constrained problems; having outcomes with high stakes; and having multiple actors involved. The 'high stakes' element is derived from the kind of outcome consequences that accompany military fire control officers, firefighters and air traffic con-trollers. Although there may be personal, economic and career consequences from coaches' decisions, the day-to-day practice of the sports coach does not satisfy this criterion. However, recent descriptions of the coaching environment (e.g. Bowes & Jones 2006, Cushion 2007) match extremely well with all of the other characteristics.

Sports coaching involves decision making, partic-ularly in semi-deliberative practice, but this is not of the 'choice of options' type. Not only is it rare to be able to demonstrate that an action decision was 'correct', but practice generally consists of a series of inter-dependent decisions. Therefore, decision taking is not about option choices (in the language of Judgement/Decision Making psychology) but about coming to the most appropriate decision on an on-going basis. The decision making of interven-tion and progression by coaches should not be thought of as necessarily problematic (although the literature speaks of problem-solution linkages), but merely as the minute-by-minute job of the coach in managing intervention, interaction and pro-gression in complex circumstances.

Naturalistic Decision Making

Naturalistic Decision Making (NDM) has estab-lished itself as a 'force' within psychological research over a period of 10 or 15 years (Cannon-Bowers et al 1996, Flin et al 1997, Zsambok & Klein 1997, Lipshitz et al 2001, Montgomery et al 2004). NDM 'is an attempt to understand how people make deci-sions in real world contexts that are meaningful and familiar to them' (Lipshitz et al 2001 p 332). NDM emerged in response to an awareness that decision makers who could be described as proficient, that is, had considerable knowledge and experience in a professional domain, appeared not to use a process that considered alternative options, and also appeared to operate at a tacit or sub-conscious level. This decision-making process is most useful in cir-cumstances characterised by complexity, uncer-tainty, goal conflict, and time constraints. NDM describes decision making where there is a dynamic interplay of experience/knowledge, a high level of complexity, and the environment, and where the generalisability of laboratory-based research would be questionable (Currey & Botti 2003). In these cir-cumstances, the limitations of human cognition become evident, and resultant actions emerge as appropriate rather than being measured by their dis-tance from the 'correct' solution (Meso et al 2002).

Lipshitz et al (2001) in their overview of NDM point to several differences from the traditional J/DM. NDM is about matching rather than choosing, is process-orientated rather than output-driven, and is context-bound rather than context-free (p 334). The centre of focus is the experienced decision maker. However, the field setting is important because its constraints and affordances shape the decisions taken. NDM was a response to the realisation that expert decision makers who cope with complex, novel and dynamic situations do not employ a (fully) rational choice approach to their decision making. An important feature of NDM is the emphasis on the process of taking decisions, rather than the action selected. In general, NDM models are variants of 'situation-action matching'. In other words, proficient decision makers take action because it is appropriate for the situation, not because it is better than the alternatives. Appropriate actions 'emerge' because of their compatibility to situational needs. The process is based on an expert knowledge structure that is domain- and context-specific, and in which attention is paid to the semantic content (meaning) inherent in the situation.

There are a number of descriptive models within NDM. The best known of these is the Recognition-Primed Decision making (RPD) model (Klein 1998). This model in essence describes pattern recognition of a situation leading to a known course of action. More elaborate versions deal with enhanced diagnosis and a reconsideration of action decisions. Klein's (1993, 1998) Recognition-Primed Decision model is a development of the immediate reaction to the perception of the problem space. Klein stresses the situational assessment that allows the experienced worker to immediately generate the most appropriate response based on previous experience. The individual adopts the solution or action associated with the 'recognition', which obviates the need for consideration of multiple alternatives. This reinforces the 'recipe-led' executive command response to recognised patterns.

Time pressure is a common feature of decision contexts in which NDM has been used to explain behaviour. One element of this is the opportunity–cost equation. This contrasts the limitations of 'deciding too soon' (but not being sure of the situation) and delaying choice (which gives a lower return). Payne et al (1996) suggest three ways to react to time pressure: accelerate the processing (spend less time deciding), become more selective, or change one's decision strategies. This is made easier by using simple and fast rules of thumb (heuristics). For example, Payne and colleagues suggest that when under time pressure the decision taker should identify and use the important attributes in the first instance, and consider options only on those attributes. These speedy search heuristics allow the decision maker to recognise common domain-specific patterns (Devine & Kozlowski 1995). In other words, experts can 'decompose' complex and ill-structured situations and convert to more recognisable and manageable attributes. This is the 'is able to read situations and people' that we may recognise in those who cope well with the need to deconstruct unusual circumstances and events.

Many of the NDM explanations deal with the issue of risk or threat (firefighting, nursing care, command and control, air traffic control). This implies that physical harm may follow, or the consequences of an inappropriate decision may lead to serious consequences. For the sports coach the consequences are much less dire, and may involve a threat to performance objectives or personal relationships. The 'reading' of threat is one of the learned abilities for which NDM offers an explanation. This 'reading' may be problematised by uncertainty or time pressures. In such circumstances a default option or weak solution may be employed (Orasanu 1997). In practice, this often means that coaches respond with a generalised action that has wide coverage (address many circumstances), but only attends to the issue when that default response does not appear to 'work'. An example might be a coach who makes a substitution because of a lack of momentum, but considers more specific tactical changes once the problem persists. One of the hypotheses that deserves attention is that novice coaches interpret 'threat' too soon (do not allow variation, and respond to too many issues), whereas the more expert coach may be willing to allow the circumstances to settle down or accept less 'smooth' progress. This hints at the education and training process within which Lipshitz and Strauss (1997) suggest that 'programmes should aim at teaching novices and medical performers the strategies and tactics that are used by experienced decision makers in the same domain' (p 160).

Randel et al (1996) used situational awareness to examine the differences between expert and novice coaches. Their findings were that experts put greater emphasis on the situational analysis rather than the decision taking. This may be explained by the expert having had more opportunities to benefit from feedback and therefore a more extensive repertoire of 'solutions'. As a result, the solution or required action becomes 'obvious', providing the reading of the situation has been accurate. Randel and colleagues also found that experts had the ability to recall patterns visually, although these had to be meaningful and domain-specific. Their conclusions were that experts would spend time on understanding and assessing the situation, rather than evaluating the best course of action. The distinctions between novices and experts were reflective of the experts' integration of cues, knowledge and imagery, rather than each individual element. In relation to the heuristics or mechanisms for prioritising options, they suggest that 'experts do not have more or different rules of thumb than novices but they do show a better knowledge of how to apply the rules' (1996 p 594). Randal et al also reinforce the concept of modelling, 'expertise appears to take the form of a complex model of potential situations. For experts, rules of thumb are a short-lived expression for the cause and effect relations of a complex model that they have internalised' (1996 p 595).

Kaempf et al (1996) also emphasised situational awareness. Individuals used 'feature matching' to recognise or categorise events that matched ones they had experienced previously. These 'key attractors' or cues in the display will be domain-specific, and perhaps even difficult to verbalise. If the situation or event is novel or complex, the decision maker will 'story build'. Story building refers to a process of analysis and interpretation based on previous experiences. Another hypothesis is that the expert coach can identify the most appropriate 'cues' and ignore the irrelevant.

Before moving to a couple of NDM-related themes, it is important to emphasise the level of cognitive organisation required, and perhaps why NDM is a mark of the domain expert. The NDM explanation for decision-making behaviour is predicated on accessing 'organised' knowledge. The knowledge is stored in a mixture of knowledge 'about' and knowledge 'how to'. It is also worth pointing out that the expert's ability to 'mentally simulate a course of action and anticipate how it will play out' (Lipshitz et al 2001 p 336) is a form of 'propositional' knowledge; in other words, 'if I do this … that will happen'. This form of knowledge is not necessarily based on having previously taken this action in exactly similar circumstances, but the expert is able to generalise (forward reason) from previous examples, and apply the mental simulation to the newly experienced context. What emerges is a family of terms (mental simulation, reflective anticipation) that suggest a 'feedforwardness'. The sports coach who introduces a new drill, who has to deliver selection decisions, or who loses a player to injury during a competition has experienced a similar situation previously and is able to 'image' or predict what might happen and has already generated an appropriate solution. Beckett (1996) p 140 suggests that 'an anticipative conversation with our practices'

is a good descriptor of this aspect of the professional's ability to cope with dynamic ill-structured contexts. The expert is constantly thinking ahead about the potential consequences of actions taken, and this is continuously monitored as the circumstances unfold and the reactions and responses of the other actors become clearer. This is largely conducted in a selective fashion and at a subconscious level, acting as a form of 'hypothesis narrowing'; the coach becoming gradually more certain that the situation is being understood. Of course, coaching practice is made up of a myriad of interpersonal interactions, performance-related decisions, changing contexts, and so on. These are happening in a continuous stream of sub-episodes that are at different stages of certainty and outcome. It is hardly surprising, therefore, that coaching is described using the terms messy, complex, dynamic, and so on.

From the literature we can point to a series of hypotheses that might populate a coaching research agenda. We might reasonably speculate that expert coaches will be better able to 'model the future' because of more accurate predictions. The coach's behaviour will continue to seem 'intuitive' – the actions taken have already been weighed and judged (albeit rapidly and often sub-consciously) to be appropriate; actions follow as the need to respond becomes pressing. It is worth recalling that not all decisions are non-deliberative. For the most part there will be an element of deliberation about the coach's behaviour, although the sheer scale of the potential interactions and decisions may help us to appreciate why the 'rational analysis' approach seems implausible. The need to 'cope' with the potential range of action decisions also explains why experts use heuristics – rules of thumb that help to simplify the problem of option choices. Identifying the use of heuristics by our best coaches is another task for the researcher.

The apparently intuitive, often sub-conscious, reasoning of the expert is dependent on accessing context-referenced frames of knowledge; that is, the knowledge is domain- and context-specific. It is developed from and through experience, and is meaningful to the individual (for example the coach) only in that context. This specificity of knowledge frames is very significant for the construction of learning programmes in coach education, and questions the genericism of problem-solving capabilities. The speedy form of expert decision making is contrasted with the more deliberative, analytical and explicit behaviour of the novice (Boreham 1994).

The expert's cognitive style is largely 'routinised' and under schematic frame-recognition control. Evans (1989) describes a schema as a 'knowledge structure which is induced or learned from experience, contains a cluster of related declarative and procedural knowledge, and is sensitive to the domain and context of the current focus of cognitive activity' (p 84). These schemata are the frameworks through which we represent the world to ourselves. A good deal of work has been done on clinical decision making by experts. For example, Schmidt et al (1990) describe how doctors move from memory-based knowledge structures to memories of specific illnesses and then to memories of specific patients as they become more expert. This reinforces the move to implicit behaviour by stressing the use of 'scripts' based on particular instances. Scripts are a particular kind of knowledge structure that predicts sequences of events, including likely solutions to problems. Experts recognise the similarity of cases to previous examples and apply highly idiosyncratic 'recipe' solutions.

The reader will be able to recognise the parallels in the coach's practice. The recognition of instances of interaction with performers, training-ground problems, and competition patterns in relation to previous typical cases or specific cases is one way that the coach can enhance situation awareness and reduce the need for deliberation and 'trawling through options'. We can hypothesise that the coach will apply actions that address the case, and perhaps 'attend' to the peculiarities of the situation only if it becomes apparent that the action is inappropriate. Once again the need for experience and a repertoire of 'cases' is highlighted.

In the introduction to this chapter it was suggested that the novelty inherent in the application of the NDM paradigm to sports coaching would have the effect of creating a potential research agenda, and opportunities have been taken throughout to suggest appropriate questions. Vergeer and Lyle (2009) illustrate the insights that might be obtained from such research. In a study of the decision-making policies and practices of more and less-experienced gymnastics coaches, there were differences in both the amount and value of information attended to by coaches with differing levels of experience. Experienced coaches showed evidence of an extensive knowledge and a capacity to weigh a greater range of factors, although they reduced uncertainty by taking earlier decisions about injured gymnasts' participation. The coaches' greater experience appeared to allow them to frame the problem in a broader context. The less-experienced coaches appeared to have less cognitive complexity and more 'surface', rather than performance-related, considerations, perhaps suggesting that they attended to a different set of cues. Another obvious focus of attention for researchers is the nature of the 'mental models' that are becoming acknowledged as an essential part of the coach's cognitive organisation. Mental models were recognised by Côté et al (1995) and Lyle's (2002) simulation model fulfils the descriptor of the mental simulation of future action and how it might unfold given by Lipshitz et al (2001).

There is clearly substantial benefit from applying NDM methodologies and themes to the coaching context, and perhaps reinforcing the relevance of the paradigm for understanding coaches' behaviour. However, the coaching context also offers something to NDM research. In addition to a serial multi-decision context, the contested aspect of sport creates circumstances in which competition-coaching behaviour, for example, is being actively opposed by another coach. The 'winning and losing' element of sport participation, performers' reactions to their (often publicly evaluated) progress and performance, the coaches (in many instances) familiarity with the performers, and the physical and psychological competition between athletes create a working context in which emotion and emotional responses play a significant role. It seems likely that decision making will be impacted by the emotion and personal meaning attached to actions.

Story telling as an example of Naturalistic Decision Making

A study into non-deliberative decision making by expert coaches (reported in Lyle 1999) identified a Slow Interactive Script model as the predominant cognitive mechanism. This suggests that coaches were using a strategy of continual refinement of action and potential action against 'scripts', that is, images or models of the situation, its determinants, and likely future outcomes. These scripts are likely to have been very strongly influenced by an accumulation of previous experiences. From these experiences expectations and appropriate behaviours have been shaped into mental models. These in turn, help coaches to recognise what is happening, situate it within existing experience, and choose appropriate actions. These Slow Interactive Scripts are mediated by the coach's objectives, and the combination of situation, actors, and goals creates a very dynamic and challenging atmosphere. The research was carried out on volleyball coaches during competitive matches and the non-deliberative (time-pressured) nature of the decision making will have exaggerated the fast-moving nature of the context. Coaches in this case appeared to attempt to control uncertainty and the contested nature of the activity through anticipatory modelling of the action.

It was proposed that Naturalistic Decision Making (NDM) offered the most appropriate means for describing and explaining dynamic decisions in this context. The narratives generated by expert coaches were re-examined to investigate the extent to which they demonstrated characteristics of NDM (Lipshitz et al 2001), more particularly story telling and mental simulation. In the language of the field, it was anticipated that retrospective narratives would focus on explanatory links, emphasising single-path reasoning, and demonstrate delaying-impact strategies.

Story building is particularly important in novel and complex situations in which the coach is seeking to understand 'what is happening'. Simple or isolated incidents may be recognised from previous experience, but coaching often involves a serial or 'unfolding' set of circumstances in training, in competition, or in interpersonal interaction. Part of the coach's expertise is to build up a picture, to 'scenario build'. As we now recognise from much of the literature, this may well be a subconscious, tacit process. In more deliberative decision making this may involve mental simulation, including anticipating or predicting future activity. Story telling, therefore, is like a diagnosis, leading to hypothesis testing, and resulting in an emerging solution. Clearly, this has implications for coaching, since coaches need to be educated to recognise and analyse performance- and athlete-related situations, in addition to expanding their range of potential solutions or most effective options. It is worth reiterating, however, that much of the coach's analysis and decision making is likely to be relatively routine and even subconscious (otherwise the practice of coaching would be extremely challenging). Not all coaching action decisions should be thought of as crises or stretching the coach's technical expertise. The element of 'typicality' will be high for much of the coach's practice.

Where the circumstances are less clear, 'the skilled decision maker will often rely on a story building strategy to mentally simulate the events leading up to the observed features of the situation' (Lipshitz et al 2001 p 336). In this context, the coach needs to have the expertise and experience to construct the mental models from which one explanation will emerge as the most plausible.

Narrative accounts of expert volleyball coaches' action decisions during regular competition games were generated. Using stimulated recall of videotaped coach behaviour, immediately following the games, 12 coaches were each asked to select six incidents from the final two sets of a game and to elaborate on their decisions. Seventy incidents were identified, related in the main to substitutions, time outs, and tactical changes. The 70 narratives were coded using an adaptation of Klein's (1998) story-telling and mental simulation characteristics.

Klein's (1998) story-telling elements can be portrayed in this fashion: the agents (recognition of those involved, accountability acknowledged); the predicament (the problem the agents are trying to solve); the intention (the goal); the action chain (description of decisions and behaviours); the causality linkage (recognition of the 'why' of actions, 'this happened or will happen because of …'); the context (catalysts for action recognised); the uncertainty (element of lack of control acknowledged); the future (forward-looking process); the alternatives (what would have happened with different actions); the restatement of objectives (goals restated as a result of ongoing outcomes); the conditions (reference to principles of action, 'I will do this if that…'); the scenarios (alternative interpretations), and the history (reference to previous cases or instances). In the research carried out, meaning units within the narratives were attributed to one of these categories. The final step was to interpret the findings in a model of story-telling elements. These are presented in Figure 3.1 (the numbers refer to the percentage of responses for each element).

The coaches' narratives demonstrated the characteristics of story telling. The narratives were post hoc accounts in deliberative form of decisions taken in a semi-deliberative fashion, although, given that the coaches were asked to give an account of the decision, it is not surprising that they resembled 'stories'. In addition, they will be subject to a number of personal biases (Lyle 2003). Nevertheless, the coaches' narratives identified a hierarchy of decision elements that could be valuable in understanding how coaches came to those decisions.

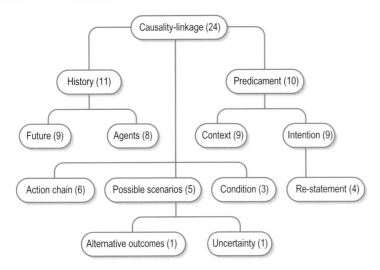

Figure 3.1 • A model of story-telling elements

The predominant meaning units were those related to causality linkage. In other words, coaches were able to build an account of how the situation had arisen and the factors that had 'caused' it to happen. The coaches' 'reasons' assumed that they could 'frame the problem', and, in particular, how this related to previous instances. They were able to frame this set of circumstances in relation to similar instances with the same players, or from their more general experiences as a coach. Significantly, the coaches could verbalise the 'predicament', and why this was a threat to the team goals (or was a positive reinforcement of the team goals). This reinforced a working hypothesis that the coach 'images' the situation or event, creates a mental model of how the circumstances emerged, and compares this to existing models. More interestingly, the coach also simulates the possible future courses of action and evaluates the likely outcomes.

In simple terms, the attributions to the story-telling elements demonstrated that the decision making involved, first, a complementarity to the NDN accounts of decision taking, and second, that the breakdown of the process had an analytical power for subsequent development. It was immediately obvious that coaches had a capacity for (very) informed situational awareness, recognised patterns in the action before them, and could 'narrow the hypotheses' that explained the situation and prompted the solution. In the context of the NDM paradigm, there was no consideration of alternatives.

Intuition

Part of the emerging consensus is that coaches appear to act in an intuitive fashion when making decisions (Schempp et al 2006, Cushion 2007), although the terminology applied to this is often imprecise. Terms such as instinctive, intuitive, automatic, tacit, unconscious, and gut feeling are used to describe the experiential reality that coaches' everyday practice is characterised by a continuous flow of apparently sub-conscious and difficult-to-access action decisions, rather than by rational analysis and consideration of all options. It would be encouraging to think that these conceptions about practice were considered accounts of how coaches went about their business (as with many other professionals), as we have attempted to do in this chapter, rather than merely the absence of a suitable explanation. Nevertheless, we need to give some attention to the concept of intuition, which is so often invoked to account for coaches' tacit decision making.

Sadler-Smith (2008) develops an excellent account of intuition, both theoretically and in its practical realisation. Although he describes intuition as part of the cognitive unconscious, he acknowledges that, when judiciously mixed with rational analysis, it is part of successful decision making (p 10), and is relied upon by everyone at some stage in his or her day-to-day practice (p 9). Most importantly, he situates intuition in expert and learned practice, 'effective use of intuition is one factor that distinguishes expert practitioners from novice practitioners. Developing informed intuitive judgement through intense, focused practice is an important step in the acquisition of expertise and professional development' (2008 p 10).

Sadler-Smith presents an argument that links intuition with the complex, contested, and 'messy' (Jones & Wallace 2005, Bowes & Jones 2006, Cushion 2007) dynamic, which describes much of coaching practice, and with Schön's (1983) 'swampy lowlands' in which professionals operate. Schön refers to this confusion of interacting elements as being 'incapable of being solved by purely rational means' (1983 p 89). From the perspective of coaches' decision making and the extent to which it can be developed or trained, Sadler-Smith's conclusion that intuition forms a learned part of professional expertise provides a prompt that it should form part of coaches' education. A working understanding of intuition is that it is a mental simulation, emerging from existing knowledge in an almost instantaneous way through 'holistic association', and without conscious deliberation. This mechanism is what Lyle (2002) terms a 'cognitive shortcut'. The coach becomes aware of a situation requiring action and this prompts a series of associations at the level of the 'intelligent unconscious' (Claxton 1998). This 'speedy association' (Wierzbicki 1997) enables the coach to operate effectively and efficiently in the context of the routine, repetitive and operational decision making that characterises coaching practice.

One of the corollaries of this interpretation of intuition and decision making is that the action outcome can be described as 'satisficing' (Simon 1990), that is, it is the most appropriate action that emerges from the limited data, confusion of factors, or time pressure under which the professional operates. The availability of data, the uncertainty of outcomes, the time available and the limits of our computational capacity mean that the action decisions are not arising from a completely rational, analytical and considered process. This takes Sadler-Smith to Naturalistic Decision Making as one of his explanations for how intuition becomes part of decision making. He finds an obvious correlation with Klein's (1998, 2003) expert decision makers, who size up the situation, assess its typicality, and enact a course of action that matches previously successful action decisions. Just as we have described, the individual has a capacity to evaluate the feasibility of a course of action by simulating its implementation, with some adjustment if this does not prove to be the most appropriate solution. NDM becomes a plausible explanation for how experienced decision makers are able to operate, and provides a more detailed account of the 'speedy association' that characterises intuition.

Intuition is not best described as instinctive, and it is not inherently creative, although this form of intuition is described separately by Sadler-Smith. Rather it is part of what Schön calls 'professional artistry' (1983 p 49) – a considered judgement, albeit carried out largely sub-consciously. Perhaps more importantly, a number of features of intuitive decision making have emerged that have implications for coach development: (a) it is learned capacity; (b) it can be improved through practice; (c) the pattern recognition on which it depends is context-specific; (d) professionals can operate from 'thin slices of evidence'; and (e) reflection is required to actively develop this expertise. The cognitive knowledge structures that enable the links to be made between events and appropriate actions depend on aggregated experience in the domain and the reinforcement of appropriate practice. The decision taking may be routine and sub-conscious but the capacity is built up from deliberate acquisition of knowledge, experience and reflection on previous practice. The action of the expert professional is not all intuition and not all rationality. Perhaps Saddler-Smith's (2008 p 121) assertion that 'for experts, theory and practice and informed intuition and rational analysis co-exist seamlessly in a harmonious integration', is somewhat idealistic, but a helpful image.

We end this section with a reminder of two of the aspects of decision making that should influence our research and education. The first is the nature of the shortcuts that we use to speed up our decision taking, and second, the importance of mental models in the decision-making process. As to the former, there are a number of biases or heuristics that are used to help us to make choices. These might refer to the representativeness of the event to our preconceptions of 'how it should be', the availability of one solution over another, or a number of decision 'tactics' based on conservatism or risk. This is a research agenda that has not been addressed in coaching. Saddler-Smith (2008) refers to Kahneman and Tversky's (1982) simulation heuristic, 'in order to simulate events in ways that will support good judgement and problem solving, decision makers need to have a robust mental model of how the system, or process under consideration actually works' (2008 p 182). Again we might ask whether this refers to existing coach development.

Implications for coach development

Throughout the text, attention has been drawn to the complementarity and relevance of NDM to the coach's decision-making practice. NDM is a means of describing and providing explanations for the taking of action decisions by experts in domains with which they are familiar. Particular attention was paid to the similarity between typical NDM decision contexts and those of the expert sports coach. Readinger et al (2005) draw links between NDM and sport, 'it attempts to describe what people actually do under conditions of time pressure, ambiguous information, ill-defined goals, and changing conditions. It is therefore, on the surface, very appropriate for application in sport and coaching domains'. In an interesting statement, Readinger et al (2005) suggest that the goal of training 'is to create intuitive decision making'. The implications are straightforward. How are we to help coaches to make better decisions, and more generally to cope with the complex multi-decision context that is characteristic of many coaches' practice.

In the context of the NDM paradigm, we need to (a) give coaches the tools (this refers to specific capacities of situational awareness, pattern recognition, hypothesis narrowing, story telling, and so on); (b) give them the ammunition (this refers to the knowledge and experience (cases) from which they can build their schemata and scripts); and (c) give them the opportunity to reflect on and interpret their decision making (this refers to structured opportunities to learn from their own experiences and those of experienced others). Coach development is a generic term for the growth in the coach's expertise that results from a combination of formal and informal learning over (often extended) periods of time.

Expertise in the context described in this chapter depends on knowledge being accumulated, stored and accessed by coaches. As Abraham et al (2006) propose, coaches develop procedural knowledge (knowing how to do something) as the basis of their operational competence. In relation to two key aspects of action decision making for which this

knowledge becomes operationalised, that is, selecting appropriate actions and dealing with dynamic and evolving circumstances, the expert decision maker's cognitive behaviour is understood best within the NDM paradigm. As we have seen, knowledge is crucial to this model of decision making. The coach builds a mental repository of schemata (linked 'chunks' of knowledge) and scripts (instances, both real and simulated, of how relevant situations unfold). Part of the expertise, indeed the crucial part, is linking the situation being experienced with this knowledge. The difficulties (and by implication the coach development agenda) can be highlighted in the challenges faced by the novice coach. The novice may not recognise the patterns being presented, may not have the awareness and background to interpret (read) this, may fail to 'match up' the need for action with an appropriate solution, and may not have a range of decision strategies or heuristics with which to simplify the options (or may employ an inappropriate heuristic). These are skills that need to be developed in the not-yet-expert coach.

The novice coach will take decisions but his or her actions may need greater deliberation, and the decision-making 'power' will be limited by the potential shortcomings identified above. The process described above also provides a template for action decision making. Each of the elements – knowledge building, imaging, recognition, analysis, option selection, and so on – are learned capacities. This means that they should form part of coach education and training. Although coaches will develop this expertise over time in supportive and appropriate circumstances, the purposeful development of this expertise is yet to be incorporated into formal coach education.

The RPD model described earlier emphasises the 'sense of typicality' that emerges from pattern recognition and leads to easier 'matching'. However, the decision-making contexts for coaches are challenging to 'read', and may even be described as unique because of their complexity. It might be argued that this leads to a pervasive sense of 'uncertainty' that coaches have to cope with. The uncertainty is manifest in a lack of adequate information, having to anticipate the actions of others, conflicting options, and the sheer volume of potential actions. It seems equally clear that coaches are able to live with this uncertainty, so how do we teach coaches to cope with it? The NDM approach is to: (a) reduce the uncertainty by gathering information (which takes time); (b) use assumption-based reasoning to 'fill in the gaps'; (c) weigh the pros and cons; (d) forestall (put the decision off); or (e) simply suppress the uncertainty (Lipshitz & Strauss 1997). Lyle (2002) draws attention to the need to operate with 'thresholds' and 'selective attention' that limit the number of matters about which coaches might feel they need to act.

Were the NDM to offer a plausible explanation of coaches' decision making, a new vocabulary of expertise would need to be developed (albeit one with a recognisable complementarity to existing skills and abilities). From what we have already learned about NDM, coaches would need to develop situational assessment (pattern recognition); recognition of key attractors (features of the environment or event that best account for the variations encountered, for example, what aspects of performers' behaviour best reflect their mood); diagnostic hypothesising; mental simulation, assumption-based reasoning (filling in the gaps when complete evidence is not available); knowledge frames or schemata; development of threshold triggers for action; impact forestalling tactics; and meta-recognition capacities (judgement of threat and advantage). Many of these skills can be recognised in expert coaches' behaviour. What we have yet to do is incorporate these explicitly in coach education and development.

Klein (1998) cites a list of competences: intuition (pattern recognition, taking the big picture, situation awareness), mental simulation (seeing the past and the future), using key features/cues of the environment to understand ill-defined problems; seeing the invisible (perceptual discrimination); story telling; and analogue reasoning. It is worth noting that Klein also adds rational analysis, and working as a team. This is a very different set of skills from the competences normally adduced in coach education. Many of these have their roots in cognitive psychology but are expressed in practitioner language.

The description of NDM clearly places significant emphasis on situational assessment (Kushniruk et al 1995, Randal et al 1996). Thus the attention of the expert decision maker is focused on reading and understanding the situation rather than being concerned about best options. The appropriate action will follow if the circumstances have been read properly. Therefore coaches should be concerned to understand their performers in the training environment or game/competition, rather than constantly thinking – what should I be doing? (which we might hypothesise the novice coach would do) (Hall & Smith 2006). Central to assessing the situation is the capacity to 'frame the problem', which is an ability that could be developed in the not-yet-expert coach. Thus the coach might be advised to wait, let circumstances unfold, and then intervene if necessary. These are similar to Lipshitz and Bar-Ilan's (1996) heuristics of not rushing into action, diagnosing as early as possible before taking action, and choosing solutions with a broad impact.

Inevitably we have to turn our attention to what might be done to develop this catalogue of skills and abilities in coaches. The discourse of NDM is not familiar to most coaches and the capacities identified above are certainly not part of formal coach education. Nevertheless, there seems to be prima facie evidence that expert coaches operate in ways for which the NDM paradigm is an apt descriptor. We might further argue that this expertise was developed through time, experience, and informal learning. The role of coach development is to accelerate this learning process. Inevitably the suggestions that follow are speculative in the sense that the implications of the NDM approach have been applied to coach education and training but there is no supporting evidence that they would succeed. Once again, a research agenda related to the development of decision-making expertise (or perhaps better expressed simply as coping with the day-to-day challenges of coaching intervention) should follow.

Readinger et al (2005) refer to Decision Skills Training, which has been used in a number of occupational settings. They suggest the repetition of decision taking in less-challenging, time-constrained simulations, which are followed by deliberate and reflective practice. Over time the simulations are increased in intensity to mirror the professional environment (more complexity, less time and greater accountability). However, this type of training may be more relevant to the 'event' decision context, than the continuous multi-decision coaching environment. We need to find ways to simplify and simulate the coaching environment, and to do so in ways that allow expertise to develop over time and through 'professional levels'. The list of suggestions that follows is just that – suggestions. The intention is to offer a number of options that might enhance coach education and training, and would be worthy of attention by researchers and coach developers.

- It would be appropriate to begin to use some of the language associated with NDM, for example, situational assessment, pattern recognition, mental simulation, recognition-primed decisions, and so on. This need not be 'jargonised'. However, it would be a useful contribution to expert competences, and might in time replace 'intuition' as a 'catch all' for processes that we do not fully understand.

- All training-related experience should be 'situated'. It is clear that usable knowledge is domain- and context-specific. It is important therefore to ensure that not all training is simulated, and that training is carried out in role-specific situations.

- Problem-based learning is a valuable mechanism for linking in situ experiences and knowledge (Jones & Turner 2006). There are also numerous opportunities for identifying cues and practical heuristics. However, there are two aspects of problem-based learning that need to be emphasised. First, problems need to be derived from the coach's domain. Second, they need to be meaningful. This is not just about the role context, but also about the coach's level of accountability for the decision, and the impact that the decision will have on other aspects of the role.

- Directed and purposeful reflection and peer–expert interaction are essential aspects of learning. It is important that coaches are given the opportunity to reflect on behaviour, but in a way that focuses on some of the skills identified earlier. It is also important that coaches take part in the reflection of experts. Expert coaches should be prompted to reflect on their behaviour, and decisions taken or action followed, in order that the coach's knowledge frames are expanded.

- A sizeable repertoire of case studies and structured scenarios is required for coach education and training at this level. These need to be reflective of many aspects of coaching practice and should be 'worked through', including responses of expert coaches, perspectives from performers, and with 'options' built into the scenarios.

- There are a number of 'basic rules' that emerge from the NDM paradigm, not all of which are new. For example, there is consensus that experts spent time on situational awareness (or reading and understanding the situation) before

acting. Although the individual coach will create a personalised set of meanings, heuristics, threshold values, important cues, and so on, sports should be able to draw together some 'rules of practice' from which the individual can fashion personal expertise.

- A process of introspection is required at this professional stage. This perhaps goes beyond reflection, and might better be described as critical appraisal. What is suggested is an individualised profiling that probes the coach's knowledge, previous experience, and critical instances in which outcomes are examined in the light of decisions taken. This improves the likelihood of understanding better the coach's detailed capacity for existing and improved practice. In NDM language, the coach's capacity for 'feature matching', mental simulation, reflective anticipation, narrowing options, and responding to crises should be examined via case studies and critical incident analysis. This can only be done with the help of others, and a willingness to be open to development-related criticism.

- The necessity for experience as a building block should be acknowledged by insisting on periods of coaching experience in an appropriate role before, and certainly during, learning programmes. This is not simply a generalisation about the value of experience. Coaches need to have a growing repertoire of cases from which 'typicality' can be recognised, and some generic rules established. The coach's capacity for rapidly deconstructing situations, recognising key features, situating the need for action alongside a broad range of other factors, feeding forward the possible outcomes, and narrowing options is derived from previous cases. The coach becomes able to construct usable 'scripts' – courses of action – that can be employed in almost routinised ways. It is difficult to see how this can be accomplished without the necessary experience (although their experiences as athletes in similar situations may give them a 'head start').

- In the context of what has been presented in the chapter about the development of expertise, it may be appropriate to 'drip feed' knowledge, rather than present it in a typical 'programme' fashion. The steady accumulation of knowledge may prove more effective in building the practical competences evident in schemata and scripts. In addition, knowledge should always be presented in 'competence fields', to reflect the domain and context specificity. There are implications here for the structure of coach education (embracing the formal and the less-formal) and continuing professional development.

At the risk of repeating what may seem like tried and trusted principles, a number of crucial guidelines can be seen to emerge: (a) It is essential to educate the process of decision making, of deciding upon a course of action, and not the preferred or most appropriate outcomes of those decisions. Coaches need to learn the process of 'coping', rather than learn the solutions to common problems; (b) There is no substitute for knowledge. It is important to realise that this is not simply the accumulation of declarative knowledge, but the development of personal frameworks of knowledge upon which the coach's decision-making expertise is based; (c) Learning and practice are based on active engagement. The coaches' continued development, but also the everyday expression of their expertise, depends upon purposeful activity, analysis, reflection, responsibility and experimentation. While 'experimentation' may not be the most appropriate term, the coach needs continually to build the repertoire, make new linkages, and incorporate new knowledge and experience through a process of refinement. Perhaps 'use it or lose it' might be appropriate!

Conclusions

The purpose of the chapter was to contribute to our understanding of sports coaching by testing the plausibility of the NDM paradigm for understanding better the decision making of expert coaches and how this aspect of expertise can be further developed. Decision making was understood to be 'deciding on a course of action' rather than a set-piece decision event, and a case was made that the circumstances under which the NDM paradigm was most useful mirrored the emerging consensus on coaching practice.

In the NDM paradigm, individuals do not engage in an elimination of rational alternatives, rather the action decision emerges as the most suitable and plausible option. We need to remember that this conceptualisation of decision making describes the behaviour of 'experts'. The relevance of this is that the actors have an accumulation of knowledge and experience from which 'recognition primed decision

making' (or other NDM models) is able to take place. In non-deliberative and semi-deliberative contexts (dynamic action), the coach is able to match up the demands of the situation (through pattern recognition) with the most appropriate action. These 'solutions', or optimum responses, have been learned from a variety of contexts – formal education and training, experience, watching significant others, reflection and discussion – and then refined through constant use.

Perhaps the most important feature of this account of decision making is that the process is not limited to the matching of situations to existing solutions. The coach's constant engagement in the practice of coaching intervention allows a form of 'propositional knowledge' to be created. This can be represented as 'if I do this, the following will probably happen'. When coaches recognise a set of circumstances that requires action (or non-action) they do not have recourse to an existing 'script' unless the problem demands an exactly similar response to a case that has been experienced before. The coach recognises the key elements in the situation and weighs these very quickly. What emerges is an action decision that can be refined later if it does not have the desired effect; alternatively, in circumstances that are uncertain, the coach may adopt a 'safe' action, a conservative action that can be reinforced later. It is worth remembering that the terms problem and solution in this description of coaching behaviour are not referring to crises, but to everyday decisions about intervening, feeding back, adapting drills, relaying instructions, coping with athlete behaviour and so on. This account helps us to understand the minute-by-minute action decisions taken by coaches in what is often a dynamic and highly charged atmosphere.

The complexity and pace of coaching intervention result in much of the coach's practice being dependent upon semi-deliberative decision making. In this context, it was important to establish that intuition was simply a speedy professional short cut, and not an untestable mechanism for coping with a situation that belies rational analysis and action. The thrust of the argument is that there is a plausible explanation for decision taking in such circumstances and NDM research on experts in their domains demonstrates (largely through comparison to novices or less-experienced practitioners) that it is a learned capacity. It is also very important to remember that coaching practice will demand a combination of decisions/actions based on rational analysis and those that are more sub-conscious.

The more recognition-response-based decisions are a mechanism for coping with complexity and limited information, particularly by allowing a mental simulation of several courses of action.

Attention was given to story building because it is part of the NDM repertoire of skills, but also because the investigation reported in this chapter seemed to confirm that coaches demonstrated the key elements of story building. The coaches could identify causality linkages, and were able to verbalise both historicity and potential scenarios when reflecting on their decision making. An interesting feature was that coaches attempted to minimise their (possible) lack of control (conceptualised as reducing uncertainty), perhaps in order to maintain an expectation of demonstrable expertise.

Perhaps the key message is that a different discourse, and a different set of expectations, is required for describing and developing coaches' decision-making capacities. The NDM-derived terminology used in this chapter appears to provide a coherent framework for describing coaches' decision-making behaviour, and the NDM paradigm itself has the potential to make a contribution to the development of coaches' expertise. Coaching research does not have a good record of impacting on coach education and training, and there is considerable scope for contributing to the development of our best coaches. Naturalistic Decision Making could provide a research paradigm and agenda from which coaching practice and coach education could become better informed.

References

Abraham, A., Collins, D., Martindale, R., 2006. The coaching schematic: validation through expert coach consensus. J. Sports Sci. 24, 549–564.

Beckett, D., 1996. Critical judgement and professional practice. Educational Theory 46, 135–149.

Boreham, N.C., 1994. The dangerous practice of thinking. Med. Educ. 28, 172–179.

Bowes, I., Jones, R.J., 2006. Working at the edge of chaos: understanding coaching as a complex interpersonal system. The Sport Psychologist 20, 235–245.

Cannon-Bowers, J.A., Sales, E., Pruitt, J.S., 1996. Establishing the boundaries of a paradigm for decision making research. Hum. Factors 38, 193–205.

Claxton, G., 1998. Knowing without knowing why. The Psychologist 11 (5), 217–220.

Côté, J., 1998. Coaching research and intervention: an introduction to the special issue. Avanti 4 (3), 1–15.

Côté, J., Salmela, J.H., Trudel, P., et al., 1995. The coaching model; A grounded assessment of expert gymnastic coaches knowledge. Journal of Sport and Exercise Psychology 17 (1), 1–17.

Currey, J., Botti, M., 2003. NDM: a model to overcome methodological challenges in the study of critical care nurses' decision making about patients' hemodynamic status. Am. J. Crit. Care 12 (3), 206–211.

Cushion, C., 2007. Modelling the complexity of the coaching process. International Journal of Sports Science & Coaching 2 (4), 395–401.

Devine, D.J., Kozlowski, S.W.J., 1995. Domain-specific knowledge and task characteristics in decision making. Organisational Behavior and Human Decision Processes 64 (3), 294–306.

Evans, J.S.B.T., 1989. Problem solving, reasoning and decision making. In: Baddeley, N.O., Bernsen, N.O. (Eds.), Cognitive psychology: research directions in cognitive science: European perspectives. Lawrence Erlbaum Associates, Hove, pp. 85–102.

Flin, R., Salas, E., Strub, M. et al. (Eds.), 1997. Decision making under stress: emerging themes and applications. Ashgate, Aldershot.

Gilbert, W., Trudel, P., 2004. Analysis of coaching science research published from 1970–2001. Res. Q. Exerc. Sport 75, 388–399.

Hall, T., Smith, M., 2006. Teacher planning, instruction and reflection: what we know about teacher cognitive processes. Quest 58, 424–442.

Jones, R.L., Turner, P., 2006. Teaching coaches to coach holistically: can Problem-Based Learning (PBL) help?

Physical Education and Sport Pedagogy 11 (2), 181–202.

Jones, R.L., Wallace, M., 2005. Another bad day at the training ground: coping with ambiguity in the coaching context. Sport, Education & Society 10, 119–134.

Jones, D.F., Housner, L.D., Kornspan, A.S., 1995. A comparative analysis of expert and novice basketball coaches' practice planning. Annual of Applied Research in Coaching and Athletics 10, 201–226.

Jones, D.F., Housner, L.D., Kornspan, A.S., 1997. Interactive decision making and behaviour of experienced and inexperienced basketball coaches during practice. Journal of Teaching in Physical Education 16, 454–468.

Kaempf, G.F., Klein, G., Thordsen, M.L., Wolf, S., 1996. Decision making in complex command-and-control environments. Hum. Factors 38, 206–219.

Kahneman, D., Tversky, A., 1982. The simulation heuristic. In: Kahneman, D., Slovic, A., Tversky, A. (Eds.), Judgement under uncertainty: heuristics and biases. Cambridge University Press, New York, pp. 201–208.

Klein, G.A., 1993. A recognition primed (RPD) model of rapid decision making. In: Klein, G.A., Orasanu, J., Calderwood, C.E., Sambok, C.E.

(Eds.), Decision making in action: models and methods. Ablex, Norwood, NJ, pp. 138–147.

Klein, G.A., 1998. Sources of power: how people make decisions. MIT, Cambridge, MA.

Klein, G.A., 2003. Intuition at work. Doubleday, New York.

Kushniruk, A.W., Patel, V.L., Fleiszer, D., 1995. Analysis of medical decision making: a cognitive perspective on medical informatics. In: Gardiner, R.M. (Ed.), Proceedings of the nineteenth annual symposium on computer applications in medical care. Hanley & Blefus, Philadelphia, pp. 193–197.

Lipshitz, R., Bar-Ilan, O., 1996. How problems are solved: reconsidering the phase theorem. Organisational Behavior and Human Decision Processes 65 (1), 48–60.

Lipshitz, R., Strauss, O., 1997. Coping with uncertainty: a naturalistic decision-making analysis. Organisational Behaviour and Human Decision Processes 6, 149–163.

Lipshitz, R., Klein, G., Orasanu, J., et al., 2001. Taking stock of Naturalistic Decision Making. Journal of Behavioural Decision Making 14, 331–352.

Lyle, J., 1999. Coaches' decision making. In: Cross, N., Lyle, J. (Eds.), The coaching process: principles and practice for sport. Butterworth Heinemann, Oxford, pp. 210–232.

Lyle, J., 2002. Sports coaching concepts: a framework for coaches' behaviour. Routledge, London.

Lyle, J., 2003. Stimulated recall: a report on its use in naturalistic research. British Educational Research Journal 29 (6), 861–878.

Meso, P., Troutt, M.D., Rudnicka, J., 2002. A review of NDM research with some implications for knowledge management. Journal of

Knowledge Management 6 (1), 63–73.

Montgomery, H., Lipshitz, R., Brehmer, B. (Eds.), 2004. How professionals make decisions. Lawrence Erlbaum Associates, Mahwah, NJ.

Nash, C., Collins, D., 2006. Tacit knowledge in expert coaching: science or art? Quest 58, 465–477.

Orasanu, J., 1997. Stress and naturalistic decision making: strengthening the weak links. In: Flin, R., Salas, E., Strub, M. et al. (Eds.), Decision making under stress: emerging themes and applications. Ashgate, Aldershot, pp. 149–160.

Payne, J.W., Bettman, J.R., Luce, M.F., 1996. When time is money: decision behaviour under opportunity–cost time pressure. Organisational Behavior and Human Decision Processes 66 (2), 131–152.

Randel, J.M., Pugh, H.L., Reed, S.K., 1996. Differences in expert and novice situation awareness in naturalistic decision making. International Journal of Human–Computer Studies 45, 579–597.

Readinger, W.O., Hutton, R.J.B., Klinger, D.W., 2005. Recognition-primed decision making in sport: improving individual, team and coaching decision making. In: Morris, P., Terry, P., Gordon, S. et al. (Eds.), Proceedings of the 11th World Congress of Sport Psychology (CD-ROM). International Society of Sport Psychology, Sydney, Australia.

Sadler-Smith, E., 2008. Inside intuition. Routledge, London.

Saury, J., Durand, M., 1998. Practical knowledge in expert coaches: on-site study of coaching in sailing. Res. Q. Exerc. Sport 69 (3), 254–266.

Schempp, P., McCullick, B., Mason, I.S., 1996. The development of expert coaching. In: Jones, R.L. (Ed.), The

sports coach as educator: reconceptualising sports coaching. Routledge, Abingdon, pp. 145–161.

Schmidt, H.G., Norman, G.R., et al., 1990. A cognitive perspective on medical expertise: theory and implications. Acad. Med. 65 (10), 61–621.

Schön, D.A., 1983. The reflective practitioner: how professionals think in action. Basic Books, New York.

Simon, H.A., 1990. Invariants of human behaviour. Annu. Rev. Psychol. 411–419.

Svenson, O., 1996. Decision making and the search for fundamental psychological regularities: what can be learned from a process perspective. Organisational Behavior and Human Decision Processes 65, 252–267.

Teigen, K.H., 1996. Decision making in two worlds. Organisational Behavior and Human Decision Processes 65 (3), 249–251.

Vergeer, I., Hogg, J.M., 1999. Coaches' decision policies about the participation of injured athletes in competition. The Sport Psychologist 13, 42–56.

Vergeer, I., Lyle, J., 2007. Mixing methods in assessing coaches' decision making. Res. Q. Exerc. Sport 78, 225–235.

Vergeer, I., Lyle, J., 2009. Coaching experience: examining its role in coaches' decision making. International Journal of Sport and Exercise Psychology 7 (4), 431–449.

Wierzbicki, A.P., 1997. On the role of intuition in decision making and some ways of multicriteria aid of intuition. Journal of Multi-criteria Decision Analysis 6, 65–76.

Zsambok, C.E., Klein, G. (Eds.), 1997. NDM. Lawrence Erlbaum Associates, Mahwah, NJ.

Coach behaviour

4

Chris Cushion

Introduction

Coaching is a social process, comprising a series of negotiated outcomes *between* structurally influenced agents within an ever-changing environment (Saury & Durand 1998, Poczwardowski et al 2002, Cushion et al 2003, Cushion & Jones 2006,). In this respect, the coaching process can be considered the result of the dynamic interaction between coaches, athletes and the socio-cultural context (Smith & Smoll 1993, Côté et al 1995a, 1995b, Langley 1997, Saury & Durand 1998, Cushion et al 2006,). In these constructed relationships neither coach, the player, nor the context has the capacity to unilaterally determine action; the key to understanding the coaching process lies in the relationships between the three variables (Cushion 2008). However, while coaching is best conceptualised and understood as a series of inter-related and interconnected relationships (Lyle 2002, Cushion et al 2006), at the heart of these relationships, and as a consequence the coaching process, the coach plays an essential and highly influential role. It seems a statement of the obvious, but it is a statement worth making nonetheless; the coach occupies a position of centrality and considerable influence in efforts to improve sporting performance (Cushion et al 2006, Smith & Smoll 2007).

Indeed, the coach has been identified as a powerful socialising agent in the physical domain (e.g. Amorose 2007, Horn 2002). The coach's behaviour impacts on athletes' behaviour, cognitions and affective responses, and coaches can influence whether athletes learn and achieve at a high level, enjoy their experience, demonstrate effort and persistence, and develop a sense of confidence and a self-determined motivational orientation (Smoll & Smith 2002, Mageau & Vallerand 2003, Amorose 2007). Moreover, coaching behaviour delivered or interpreted incorrectly or inappropriately can lead to negative outcomes (e.g. poor performance, low self-esteem, high levels of competitive anxiety, burnout) (Amorose 2007). Given this, it follows that through their words and actions (i.e. their behaviour), coaches will not just impact performance but also the social and emotional well-being and perspectives of their athletes (Miller 1992, DeMarco et al 1996a, 1996b, Jones et al 1997, Horn 2002).

With this in mind we can see that coaching practice has affective, cognitive, behavioural and social elements. On a strictly behavioural level coaching can also be considered in terms of antecedents (the stimuli prior to the event); the behaviour (what is done or said); and consequences or what follows from the behaviour. The traditional or common sense view of coaching has tended to focus solely on the observable behavioural elements, and has paid much less attention to the 'what' or 'why' of the behaviour. Indeed, the most common focus for coaching research since the 1970s has been concerned with the coach's behaviour. As a result this research has emerged as one of the largest single categories within the general body of coaching knowledge (Gilbert & Trudel 2004). This approach to coaches and their behaviour has resulted in coach behaviour being an area of significant research activity (Nash & Collins 2006). Research into this aspect of the coach's influential role has been rightly warranted. However, rather than embracing the complexity of the coaching role, both with the coach as a person and with how he or she engages with the wider pedagogical process, the majority of coaching research to date has been content simply to describe how coaches behave during practice, and to a lesser extent, competitive situations (Kahan 1999, Lyle 1999, Cushion & Jones 2001, McPhail & Kirk 2001). Even within the behavioural literature it is unlikely that we would find an exploration of the antecedents or consequences of coach behaviour. It is against this backdrop that the coach behaviour literature should be considered.

This approach can perhaps be attributed to coaching's traditional location within a dominant psychological discourse, which, in turn, has its epistemological roots in the positivistic natural sciences (Ward & Barret 2002). A key characteristic of behavioural analysis is the production of objective, reliable and valid data, free from the distortion of suggestion and perception, and as a result systematic descriptive-analytic systems have been widely used as research instruments to gather information on coaches while coaching (Kahan 1999). This approach can also be attributed to an initial desire by many early scholars for some dispassionate baseline data to find out 'what (good) coaches do' in what was, not so long ago, a very under-researched field. Despite its original popularity, in more recent times such methods and the resultant findings have somewhat fallen into disrepute as many authors have tended to highlight their weakness (e.g. Abraham & Collins 1998).

Clearly, coaching behaviours per se do not stand alone as predictors of effective coaching (Douge & Hastie 1993) nor do they 'embrace the entirety of the coaching process' (Lyle 1999a p 14). Since this was never their purpose, it would be wrong to criticise them for not doing so. However, given this, what is the value of a chapter considering coach behaviour and its related research? The initial rationale for this area of endeavour remains as valid today as it did in the 1970s; coaches are central to the coaching process and what they say and do continues to impact performers' achievement and well-being. Therefore, understanding which behaviours translate into positive experiences and functioning on the part of the athletes is critical for researchers and practitioners alike (Amorose 2007). Moreover, while coach behaviour may be portrayed as 'superficial' in one sense, we still know relatively little about coaching practice, good or bad,

across a variety of settings (Lyle 2002, Cushion et al 2006, Portac et al 2007), and thinking about what coaches do and why they do it, still offers much in developing our understanding about coaching.

A useful database of coach behaviour does exist, and what this body of work has done is to identify (within certain constraints) 'tried and tested coaching behaviours' (Douge & Hastie 1993 p 54). This has resulted in claims that 'instructors within sport have available to them an extensive and growing knowledge base from which to make decisions about their practice' (Hughes & Franks 1997 p 190). The term 'instructors' with its connotations of a more restricted performance improvement role is perhaps a revealing comment about the value of 'behavioural' evidence. Despite this knowledge base, however, coaching practice remains largely 'belief' as opposed to 'evidence based' (Rushall 2003). It is important therefore, that as our understanding of coaching becomes more sophisticated, and research priorities change, we should not disregard existing accumulated knowledge but, rather, consider ways to integrate new knowledge with what is already known (Cushion 2007). It is in the interests of coaching and its development that we integrate existing work and ideas into a more sophisticated knowledge base (Rink 1993, Cushion 2007). In essence, how can we use and integrate what we know about coach behaviour into contemporary debates about coaching practice and the nature of coaching? This chapter goes some way to addressing this question.

Finally, and perhaps most importantly, coaches are notoriously poor at describing their own behaviour. Indeed, research has demonstrated that coaches have limited awareness of how often they behave in various ways, and that performer's ratings correlate more strongly with observed behaviours than the coaches own self-ratings (Smoll & Smith 2006). Therefore, illustrating the actions performed by the coach in practice and competition situations (Borrie & Knowles 2003) can contribute to raising the awareness of coaches to what they are actually doing. The most sophisticated understandings of coaching practice and advances in coach education would seem fruitless if coaches lack seemingly basic levels of self-awareness.

In terms of this chapter, it is not the intention to provide a full comprehensive 'review' of all coaching behaviour research to date, a task which, if done to an insightful level of critical depth, would inevitably fall outside the constraints of a single chapter.

Rather, the objective here is first, to locate and critique key elements of coach behaviour, to attempt to identify principles for practice, and to identify where further research is required. Second, it is intended to examine critically the core concepts and assumptions associated with, and inferred through, such research. Such critical mapping provides us with a progressive way both to evaluate past and to process future research (Hart 1998). The significance of this work is also grounded in an attempt to improve the clarity and applicability of past and future findings for those who can then use them in the practical setting. Indeed, the utility of a body of knowledge such as coach behaviour lies in its usage in assisting everyday coaching practice. Hence, this chapter marks an attempt to develop further the relationship between academic presentation and dissemination and the concrete (reality) of coaching experience and need.

The chapter is divided into two parts. The first part examines current coach behaviour research; the objective is to identify key consistent behaviours identified in the research (what coaches do) and develop some explanations for this behaviour (why coaches behave this way) before going on to consider the gaps inherent in the knowledge produced to date. The second part of the chapter attempts to synthesise this discussion with more contemporary debates about coach behaviour and considers the dualism in coaching created by directive versus non-directive approaches. Finally, an attempt is made to draw these arguments together and develop some ideas about the nature of coaching behaviour with some consideration given to potential coach behaviour strategies.

The study of coach behaviour

Background

Initially, behaviour analysis and the use of descriptive analytical instruments were prominent in teaching where research focusing on the description and analysis of physical education instruction gathered momentum during the 1970s (Lawson 1990). This research was perceived as ushering sport pedagogy into 'an era of legitimacy, innovation, and unparalleled activity' (DeMarco et al 1996b, Kahan 1999 p 18) with the research resulting in a wealth of information on the type and quality of practitioners'

instruction (DeMarco et al 1996b). Investigations into coach behaviour grew from this foundation. These were perceived by some to have increased legitimacy as the behaviour of coaches was viewed as being more directly related to outcomes, such as win/loss (Claxton 1988). Considerable enthusiasm greeted this development, with many authors stressing its importance in establishing an empirical base for a future 'science' of coaching particularly related to coach behaviour (Lacy & Darst 1985, Lacy & Goldston 1990, Seagrave & Ciancio 1990, Trudel et al 1996).

A prominent feature of this work was and continues to be, the examination of observable coach intervention, in particular, coaches' instruction. Tharp and Gallimore (1976) were pioneers in this field, conducting a ground-breaking and extensive study of legendary UCLA basketball coach John Wooden (re-visited recently, see Gallimore & Tharpe 2004). This research was replicated and built upon by many others and further inspired the widespread development and use of systematic observation instruments for examining coaches' work in training and competition environments (Williams 1978, Langsdorf 1979, Smith et al 1979, Lucas 1980). Subsequently, a number of manual and computerised observation systems have been developed specifically to analyse coaching behaviour and have been used across a number of sports and at various levels of competition (e.g. Tharp & Gallimore 1976, Rushall 1977, Smith et al 1977, Langsdorf 1979, Smith et al 1979, Lucas 1980, Quarterman 1980, Metzler 1983, McKenzie & Carlson 1984, Crossman 1985, Lacy & Darst 1985, Franks et al 1988).

The constant production of articles since 1975, from different authors, using various observation instruments, and focusing on different aspects of coach behaviour, would appear to indicate that such a method is indeed appropriate for describing coaches' behaviour in training and competition (Trudel et al 1993, Kahan 1999, Gilbert & Trudel 2004). Undoubtedly, the studies conducted have yielded insights that have contributed greatly to the body of knowledge in sport pedagogy (DeMarco et al 1996a, 1996b, Jones 1997), providing a wide range of literature describing coach behaviour in an array of sports including for example: basketball, soccer, athletics, archery, tennis, American football, swimming, volleyball, and rowing (Dubois 1981, Lacy & Darst 1985, Claxton 1988, Lacy 1989, Lacy & Goldston 1990, Seagrave & Ciancio 1990, Van der

Mars et al 1991, Miller 1992, Salminen & Liukkonen 1995, Millard 1996, Potrac et al 1997, Vangucci et al 1997, Bloom et al 1999, Cushion & Jones 2001). Such studies represent the beginnings of a database of coaching behaviours, fulfilling in part the goal set by Lacy and Goldston (1990) that, to be meaningful, observation should be conducted in a variety of settings.

Part 1: Key behaviours (what coaches do and why)

This section considers coach behaviours that consistently appear in the findings of coach behaviour research. Of course the complex nature of coaching and the coaching process means that the different elements of coach behaviour are in fact interrelated and interdependent (Cushion et al 2006, Smith & Cushion 2006), and coaches will engage with and deploy a range of discrete behaviours. Moreover, in reality, behaviours overlap and do not occur in neat ordered ways, and whilst they are described as such here, these behaviours should not be thought of as separate or isolated.

The section is organised around three categories of behaviour: (1) instruction, (2) praise/scold, and (3) silence; and together these behaviours account for approximately 80% of what research has identified that coaches do. This analysis is by no means definitive, but attempts to locate these key behaviours within a number of analytical frameworks. What it does do, however, is to attempt to look beyond the superficiality of 'just behaviour' to offer insight into why these behaviours occur and go some way to demonstrate the complexity of the coaching task.

Instruction

There is evidence to link effective coaching and athlete learning to the quality of the coaches' instructional behaviour (Carreira et al 1992, DeMarco et al 1996a, 1996b, Gallimore & Tharp 2004, Hodges & Franks 2004). However, as the discussion here will illustrate, coaches validate the use of instructional techniques based on a variety of reasons, not solely upon their effectiveness for athlete learning. Moreover, there are principles that underlie the provision of effective instruction (Hodges & Franks 2004), but these principles alone would seem unable to account for the dominance of such

behaviour in coaching, both in terms of individual coaching sessions and across coaching sessions over time.

With this in mind, instruction remains the most frequently used 'active' coaching behaviour; a finding that consistently permeates research literature. Moreover, behaviours that relate to task accomplishment, e.g. training and instruction and positive feedback, are generally speaking the most preferred by athletes (Chelladurai & Riemer 1998, Reimer 2007). How can we account for this? Jones et al (2004) contend that coaches use behaviours that they perceive are congruent with the coaching role. Prior socialisation (as an athlete and a coach), along with established beliefs and traditions that validate and acknowledge certain behaviour as 'effective' serves to reinforce this image (Cushion & Jones 2006, Potrac et al 2007). Therefore, high levels of instruction reflect beliefs about effective and appropriate coaching behaviour that derive from previous playing (athlete as recipient) and coaching experiences, and reproduce and reinforce an 'instructional' and directive approach (Potrac et al 2007). As Goffman (1959) suggests, this behaviour is a performance shaped by the environment and audience, and constructed to provide others with impressions that are consonant with the desired goals of the actor (Potrac et al 2002).

This emphasis on instructional behaviour can also be seen in terms of fulfilling the requirements of the role, particularly when they are strongly associated with performance success. The pressure to succeed in sport and the accountability and kudos for such success (real or perceived) sees the coach attempting to control as many variables as possible through high levels of instructional behaviour (Bloom et al 1999, Coakley 2004, Potrac et al 2007). 'Responsibility for the outcome of performance is a notable determinant in understanding a coach's desire to be in control of his or her respective athletes and coaching situations' (Eitzen & Sage 1989, Potrac et al 2002 p 191).

To achieve success, coaches perhaps not only perceive the need to have the respect of their athletes, but also the capacity to impact significantly on their athletes' performances thus achieving the desired outcomes (Potrac et al 2002, 2007, Jones et al 2004). This means not being viewed as weak, indecisive or lacking in knowledge or expertise (i.e. asking athletes for solutions). As such they tend to rely on safer, tried and tested traditional methods that prove their knowledge and expertise, namely instruction (Coakley 1994, Potrac et al 2002, 2007, Jones et al 2004). 'The consequence of such action is that athletes are, in turn, increasingly socialised into expecting instructional behaviours from coaches, and thus resist other coaching methods' (Potrac et al 2007 p 40), as these behaviours are deemed consciously or subconsciously to be associated with performance accomplishment. As a result, coaching behaviours like instruction become a historical and traditional thread passed on through an 'apprenticeship of observation' (Schempp 1989, Cushion et al 2003) with experiences becoming a powerful, long-lasting, and continual influence over pedagogical perspectives, practices, beliefs and behaviours.

Silence

Silence has been identified as a significant behaviour within coaching practice and can account for up to 40% of a coach's total behaviours in both training and competition (Potrac 2001, Smith & Cushion 2006). This would seem logical as clearly coaches cannot constantly be engaged in 'active' coaching behaviours (Miller 1992). However, coaches whose observation has been interpreted as 'passive' have been described as 'off-task' (Claxton 1988). This suggestion has been superseded, with silence becoming increasingly understood as a deliberate coaching strategy, being used as a tool for promoting learning (Cushion & Jones 2001, Smith & Cushion 2006, Potrac et al 2007).

Indeed, research (Cushion & Jones 2001, Smith & Cushion 2006, Potrac et al 2007) describes a pattern of coaching behaviours in which periods of silence are punctuated with verbal cues, short reminders and specific commands or correction. When the coaches were not 'actively' providing feedback, they were in fact 'on-task', intently watching the action in silence. Therefore the research evidence would clearly indicate that the coaches' silence was indeed an intentional modus operandi.

Interestingly, the coaches in the Smith and Cushion (2006) study expressed concern that too much verbal intervention would deny the athletes not only opportunities to learn but also the opportunity to demonstrate what has already been learnt. Clearly, during moments of silence, coaches are involved in a number of cognitive processes. These include observing and analysing the athletes' performance, allowing opportunities for the athletes to learn for themselves, and checking learning and athletes' decision-making.

Positive reinforcement; praise and scold

Research suggests that coaches consider a positive working climate a vital part of delivering high-quality coaching practice (Jones et al 2004, Potrac et al 2007). Indeed, Smith and Smoll (2002) have identified a positive approach to coaching where 'effective' coaching behaviours include: high frequencies of reinforcement for effort and performance, encouragement following errors, mistake contingent and general instruction, while minimising punitive behaviours and non-responses. This approach is supported by Amorose and Horn (2000), who champion behaviour that contains high-frequency positive and informational feedback and low frequencies of punishment-oriented feedback.

With this in mind it appears that coaches frequently provide liberal support and encouragement to their performers. This is evidenced by behavioural research that reports praise as a substantial element in coaching practice, often being the second or third largest category of behaviour overall (e.g. Lacy & Darst 1985, Miller 1992, Bloom et al 1999, Cushion & Jones 2001, Portac et al 2007). In attempting to account for this, Potrac et al (2002) contend that coaches understand the significance of establishing a positive learning environment, recognising that athletes are more responsive to a positive coach and that positive behaviour can impact motivation and self-efficacy in athletes. More subtly than this, the coaches could use this behaviour to reinforce desired athlete behaviour. As Benfarri et al (1986) note, the method and style of transmission is critical in forming the recipients' perception of it. However, too much praise can be seen as losing its value and thus becoming meaningless to athletes. This suggests that the overuse of praise, especially general praise, can be interpreted as non-specific feedback that dilutes its effects (Schmidt 1991). This can usefully be understood in terms of reward power; the power that comes from a person's control over another's rewards (Slack 1997, Potrac et al 2002). Maintaining the legitimacy of reward power, in this case praise, will require that the recipient perceives the behaviour as having meaning. Thus, overusing praise or giving praise when not deserved, will reduce its value (Potrac et al 2002).

Alongside high levels of praise and contributing to a notion of a 'positive' coaching environment is a low level of scold behaviour, with some recorded praise to scold ratios recorded as high as 33:1 (Potrac et al 2002). The ability to punish another can be regarded as 'dysfunctional because it alienates people and builds up resentment' (Slack 1997 p 181). Hence coaches' restricted use of scold behaviour is perhaps evidence of recognition of the unproductive nature of such behaviour and the potential damage that can be caused to coach–athlete relationships (Jowett 2007).

What and why: expectancy effects

One factor that has been shown to influence coach behaviour is coaches' expectations or judgements of their players, which has been shown to 'influence the athletes' performance and behaviour' (Horn & Lox 1993 p 69). This is an important point because it illustrates the bi-directional or dialectic nature of coach behaviour (LaVoi 2007). It is often assumed that the athlete is a passive recipient, that the coach's behaviour is successfully received, and that neither coach nor athlete is affected by the interaction. However, Poczwardowski et al (2002), and Cushion (2008) and his colleagues (Cushion et al 2006) illustrate that coach behaviour is not benign and that there is a dialectic relationship with both coach and player influenced by their interaction.

Given the competitive and evaluative nature of sport, it is common for coaches to form expectations of athletes at the beginning of a season (Solomon 1998, Wilson et al 2006). These are initial judgements or assessments about the physical competence or sporting potential of each athlete and are based on certain information available to the coach. A coach's expectations develop from a variety of factors but generally fall into two categories; person cues and performance information (Horn & Lox 1993). Person cues include, for example, the player's age, social background, ethnicity, and physical attributes. These cues are not used exclusively but are combined with performance information about the player that could include: past performance, physical test scores, ability, and comments from other coaches (Horn & Lox 1993, Solomon et al 1996). Coaches also use initial impressions of athletes in practice situations informed by, for example, observation of the player's motivation, enthusiasm, pleasantness, response to criticism, and interaction with staff and team mates (Horn & Lox 1993). In addition, it is possible, if not likely, for two coaches to form different sets of expectations for an athlete based on which aspects of the available information they value most (Horn & Lox 1993). These expectations are expressed to the athlete through verbal and non-verbal behaviours (Solomon et al 1996).

The major sport research linking feedback and expectations has found that differential feedback is issued to high- and low-expectancy athletes but is not consistent. For example Cushion and Jones (2006) and Wilson et al (2006) identified significant differences in the nature of coach behaviour based on an athlete's position in the group with clear 'favourites' and 'rejects' suffering differential treatment within the coaching process. The conclusions from these and other works, have again shown that some coaches appear to be 'Pygmalion-like' with differences between the quality and frequency of athlete–coach interaction (Horn & Lox 1993). Expectancy theory, applied to the sport setting, assumes that coaches' feedback patterns will differ because athletes are perceived as high or low expectancy (Solomon et al 1996). However, this assumption is worth considering further. Put simply, expectation effects are responsible for some differences in coach behaviour, but not all.

Perception of ability may not be the only basis for differential treatment and behaviour patterns. In accordance with the principles of behaviour modification and reinforcement theory, coaches ordinarily use performance feedback to cultivate and shape desired athlete behaviours (Sinclair & Vealey 1989). Markland and Martinek (1988) noted that players of more successful coaches (defined by win/loss record) received more feedback than their less-successful peers. This finding was mirrored by Solomon et al (1996) who, while investigating expectancy effects, found that head coaches and assistants differed in the amount of feedback given. Here, head coaches gave feedback based on mistakes whereas assistant coaches delivered more general positive feedback. Moreover, Claxton (1988) found that expert coaches used more questioning behaviours and would give less instruction than their non-expert colleagues (Claxton 1988).

This research demonstrates other possible reasons for differential feedback, namely the coaches' 'success' or expertise. Indeed, differential feedback and differences in coach behaviour have been attributed to numerous factors related to the coach. These include for example job expectation, interaction opportunities, differentiation of roles, the philosophy of the programme, and the goals of the sessions (Solomon 1998).

Thinking about coach behaviour

The existing research evidence suggests that 'what coaches do' in terms of coaching behaviour is a judicious mix of the instructional and positive and that this is a considered approach with silence used as a deliberate behavioural strategy to enhance learning. Indeed, several authors advocate a positive approach to behaviour in general and link this positively with improved levels of performance, team cohesion, and player self-esteem (Dubois 1981, Wandzilak et al 1988, Amorose 2007, Smith & Smoll 2007). This notion is supported by Saury and Durand (1998), who further reported that expert coaches are empathetic, tactful, give autonomy and share knowledge and experience. There is an intuitive appeal to this positive approach but unfortunately effective coach behaviour is more complex than implied distinctions between positive or negative, directive and non-directive (Amorose 2007). Indeed, considering the application of these behaviours in practice provides a glimpse of coaching's complexity.

First, there is evidence that suggests that if it is used inappropriately negative affective outcomes can occur from praise and instruction, while if perceived incorrectly socially supportive behaviours can lower motivation (Amorose & Horn 2001, Mageau & Vallerand 2003, Amorose 2007). Thus, the skill or craft of the coach in applying appropriate behaviours is likely to be hugely influential.

Second, there are numerous 'negative cases' where the coaches' behaviour may be considered contrary to the principles espoused in the prevailing literature. For example, the coaches in research by d'Arrippe-Longueville et al (1998) investigating elite judo were highly autocratic, showed low levels of social support and used their behaviour as part of a 'toughening up' process for their players. The researchers found that the athletes did not like this autocratic coaching behaviour but acknowledged it to be the most effective. d'Arrippe-Longueville et al (1998) explain this by proposing that the culture of the sport strongly influences coach behaviour. Indeed echoing these sentiments, Parker (1996), Tomlinson (1993), Roderick (2006) and Cushion and Jones (2006) argue that there remains an underlying authoritarian character in some sporting sub-cultures and this has a pervasive and influential effect in the coaching process and on coach behaviour. Consequently, differences in coach behaviour may indeed be reflective of 'deep seated cultural differences, inherent differences in belief systems, value structure and underlying cultural patterns that are embedded' (Greendorfer 1982 p 198) within it.

Therefore, there would be merit in understanding how much coaching behaviour is 'traditional' and how the coach's current practice is related to a selectively remembered past, which acts to validate and acknowledge it as 'effective' (Cushion & Jones 2006). Moreover, we perhaps need to probe more deeply and examine processes of socialisation among other influencing factors, before trying to draw conclusions about coaches' good practice and the practice of the 'good'. In addition, despite their historical and sub-cultural connections within the context of athlete development and well-being, it might be pertinent to consider more critically the evidence supporting certain behaviours and whether these practices might be legitimately justified.

Identifying gaps and problematising existing knowledge

Clearly, the range and variety of opportunities to observe coach behaviour is considerable. Not only does this relate to observations within differing cultures but also to the number of different sports available and to the various levels or domains in each sport. Even within a particular sport and at specific levels of competition, coach behaviour could be examined in both contest and practice environments and at different times in the season. As these variables have been demonstrated to have an impact on coaches' actions, and despite the general volume of work undertaken (Kahan 1999, Potrac et al 2002), there appear to be several 'gaps' in existing coach behaviour knowledge.

For example, the majority of coaching research has been conducted in predominantly educational settings within North America. It would be naive to accept that this body of knowledge can be unproblematically applied to coaches in Europe as a consequence of an assumed transatlantic 'validity'. Coaching knowledge, however labelled, can never be so culture-proof (Nicholas 1983). Yet, despite this rather obvious limitation, there has been insufficient account taken of the culture and contextual differences in how the body of knowledge has been interpreted (Brewer & Jones 2002). Furthermore, professional as opposed to youth or university sport as a context for analysis remains very much under-researched. Clearly, the demands and pressures upon professional coaches in 'performance' sport

(Lyle 1999a, 2002) are different to those upon other coaches who operate within a more recreational ethos. Indeed, Lyle (2002) argues that performance coaches fulfil a distinctive role and are not part of a sporting continuum from participation to performance; hence, their functions and actions will reflect that uniqueness. Although the clarity of this distinction is open to debate (Jones 2006), certainly evidence exists that the performance coach is engaged differently within the coaching process in terms of time, detail and emotion than the 'participation'-orientated coach, who is not so nearly concerned with the result of the next competition. Gaps are clearly evident in the existing knowledge base, as coach behaviour within many coaching environments remains largely under-researched.

A principal shortcoming in this respect lies in the lack of research on coaches' in-competition behaviour. It is understandable that the actions of the coach have been observed more frequently in practice settings than in games or competitions. Simply there are fewer games than practices, and the coaches' behaviour in competition may be more variable, context-specific, and difficult to capture. The practice environment therefore, provides greater scope and opportunity to observe coach behaviour. This issue of availability has been reflected in the number of studies undertaken, with observations of how coaches manage the competitive 'game' environment being conspicuous by their absence (Kahan 1999, Smith & Cushion 2006). Those projects that have been carried out under both settings, have found that certain behavioural categories register differently under game as opposed to practice conditions, hence the findings from one can not be assumed for the other (Horn 1984, Chaumeton & Duda 1988, Wandzilak et al 1988, Trudel et al 1996). For example, coaches engage in less instruction and overall interaction with their athletes during competition (Salmela et al 1993). Speculative factors responsible for these differences include the greater time spent in practice which impacts on the nature of coach–athlete interaction, in addition to a general 'hardening' of the emotional climate during competition (Liukkonen et al 1996). Competition is also a time for predominantly reactive decision-making by coaches, as she or he must evaluate progress within the on-going event and act accordingly. It would appear that the nature of the competition experience and the pressures contained within it could well be an important factor that impacts on a coach's actions; a time that not only involves physical game engagement, but also that period spent in immediate preparation for it, time-outs, half-time talks, between attempts or points, full-time briefings, and managing other stoppages where opportunities exist for coach–athlete interaction. The examination of practice time alone then would appear to exclude an important and by its very nature spontaneous and 'creative' part of the coach's work (Gilbert et al 1999, Smith & Cushion 2006).

Despite the general volume of research carried out and an apparent 'pattern' of coach behaviour that emerges, when divided into context-specific studies, the scope for drawing meaningful conclusions from the work seems to be limited. However, this limitation does not seem to have inhibited the tendency towards proclaiming generalisations from the particular. Indeed, many conclusions about coach effectiveness have been drawn from only a few hours of observation of a very small number of coaches practising in a specific context (Horn 1984, Kahan 1999). These conclusions have often been assumed to be valid across all contexts and applicable to all coaches. Similarly, research that has compared behaviours across a season has been based on a limited number of observed hours of practice, which inevitably casts doubt on the validity of any generalisations drawn from it (Potrac et al 2002). The research evidence therefore needs to be treated with considerable caution.

Indeed, it could be argued that the resulting recommendations and subsequent strategies for coaches have been 'too absolutist for the complex coaching environment' (Abraham & Collins 1998 p 65). This echoes the point made earlier in relation to generalisations drawn from the particular, and perhaps highlights a fundamental problem with coaching knowledge so far and its accompanying 'models' approach. Indeed, it is becoming increasingly recognised that coaching scholars have not taken the time to acknowledge adequately and empirically explore the complex nature of coaching, before developing generalist explanations of, and recommendations for, 'good practice' (Jones 2006, Cushion 2008).

Part 2: How should coaches behave?

Given the discussion so far, what research-led behaviour guidelines can we give coaches in relation to their practice? This is a difficult question to address because, as highlighted, there are no definitive answers about how much of which behaviour a coach should use in any particular situation. Similarly, just because a 'successful' coach uses much of a specific behaviour or coaches in a particular 'style', does not mean that it will be either applicable or effective for another coach in a different context. Coaching prescriptions cannot be so simplistic.

The problem with the inability of the research to prescribe appropriate behaviour is partly rooted in the nature of behaviourist and reductionist study as it cannot by itself capture the complex and dynamic essence of coaching. Indeed, as already discussed most research only provides a very limited snapshot of coaches' behaviours, while much of the interaction which typifies the wider process including what transpires prior to, during, and after practice sessions or games, goes unrecorded (Jones et al 1997). A further problem in this respect lies in the assumption that the methodologies used have the ability to differentiate good coaches from bad (Abraham & Collins 1998), which has been found largely not to be the case.

These inconsistencies have led Abraham and Collins (1998) to suggest that coach behaviour relates to the specific situation rather than to global rules. Moreover, attempting to apply the findings of behavioural analysis in prescriptive ways ignores the particular context under which studies have been conducted (Douge & Hastie 1993, Kahan 1999); an important issue when considering the design and implementation of coach education. Importantly, however, certain behaviours do consistently permeate the findings of behavioural studies and provide a commonality of practice that cannot be ignored. Bearing this in mind, it is worthwhile considering some of the factors that can inform a considered approach to coach behaviour, and in doing so, to consider critically contemporary issues relating to this topic from a coach education perspective.

Coach behaviour: thinking philosophically

Although coaches may not necessarily articulate clear beliefs about it, their practice invariably rests upon basic often-unquestioned beliefs about learning (Light 2008). Indeed, all coaching is based upon some theory about how we learn. As has been discussed in this chapter so far, behaviourism strongly informs coaching (and its research) with a resulting instructional approach that emphasises the use of feedback and reward behaviour.

Epistemology refers to questions about the nature of knowledge and the relationship between the inquirer and the known (Sparkes 1992, Denzin & Lincoln 1994, 2000). Epistemological assumptions determine the issue of 'whether knowledge is something which can be acquired on the one hand, or something which has to be personally experienced on the other' (Burrell & Morgan 1979 p 2 cited in Sparkes 1992). Epistemologically, a behaviourist approach assumes that knowledge is objective and 'out there' and filtering or internalising objective knowledge requires a highly structured and technical pedagogical approach (Light 2008).

Recent developments in coaching research and coach education have tended to promote a more constructivist epistemology, where knowledge is assumed to be socially constructed in interaction, and has to be experienced rather than acquired (e.g. Cassidy et al 2004, Cushion 2006). This approach emphasises the coach's facilitative behaviour, not *instructing* per se but *constructing* experiences for athletes, an example being Teaching Games for Understanding (Bunker & Thorpe 1982).

It is not the intention here to square the philosophical circle, or indeed promote one approach as superior to another. Instead, as a starting point to a discussion around recommendations/ guidelines for coach behaviour, there is a need to emphasise that coaches should be aware of the assumptions about learning that underpin their behaviour and practice (Light 2008). This is crucial in raising coach self-awareness, a quality that the evidence suggests is lacking, but seems essential if coaches are to grasp the implications (good or bad) of their behaviour. More importantly perhaps, Butler (2005) identifies an 'epistemological gap' or 'cognitive dissonance' (Light 2008) where there is a difference between an embodied and unarticulated belief that informs behaviour and practice and an alternative set of assumptions, resulting in coaches struggling to adopt any alternative behaviour. This has manifested itself in coaches' 'impression managing' on coach education courses and paying lip service to alternative behaviour (Cushion et al 2003) by adopting the language of a particular approach but continuing to coach and behave in ways that are informed by a traditional objectivist approach to learning. Coaches can develop better conceptual understanding by reflecting on why they coach as they do and what assumptions underpin this. This, alongside critical reflection on their socialisation experiences and the culturally accepted coaching behaviours of their sport, puts coaches in a strong position to transcend 'traditional' coach behaviour and develop their own informed approach.

Much is written about the purposes and approaches to coaching and coach behaviour. The aim of the following section is to contribute to this discussion and set out some key tenets that impact and inform coach behaviour. Drawing on experiences as a coach and coach educator as well as relevant research sources referred to later I have attempted to set out issues through which a reflective dialogue that encourages critical thought about coach behaviour can be facilitated. This is by no means a 'how to' guide but attempts to give explicit recognition and examples as a means for coaches and coach educators to reflect on their practice, as well as supporting the development of informed self-awareness and consequent practice.

Coach behaviour *is* context specific

What are the outcomes?

Coach behaviour should be a way to connect athlete understanding with the concepts and skills relevant to the objectives of the session (Hall & Smith 2006). It is imperative therefore that the coach considers the objectives of the session, so that he or she can determine whether given behaviours are relevant to the task. Abraham and Collins (1998) posit this in terms of a simple question: 'is the coach's behaviour appropriate to the aim of the session?' (p 66). This seemingly important consideration in relation to good practice should be given due attention. Indeed, coaches need to give as much consideration to their behavioural strategy as they do to other parts of the session. For example, legendary UCLA basketball coach John Wooden's behaviour was in no sense ad hoc, but the product of extensive, detailed and daily planning based on continuous evaluation of team and individuals matched to the outcomes of the session (Gallimore & Tharp 2004). It is important to note also that coaches should not necessarily follow a plan or style either rigidly or 'blindly' without any consideration of what is happening in front of them. In aligning behaviour to objectives there remains a need to be flexible and adaptive. This key consideration can be overlooked by some coaches and is often devalued by coach education.

Research too can play a part through conducting studies that attempt to match behaviour and objectives, or at least acknowledge the coach's assumptions. This would appear necessary if an accurate picture of effective coaching is to emerge. Indeed, not unlike similar limitations in teaching research (Hiebert et al 2002) existing studies have not connected coaches' knowledge, planning, and philosophies to their behaviour, in terms of assessing athlete learning. Clearly, coach behaviour is the combination of thought with action. It is important therefore not to just look at observable behaviour or focus on cognition in isolation, but consider their relationship and interaction (Hall & Smith 2006).

Know your athletes, and yourself

To be truly 'athlete-centred' coach behaviour should be focused on the potential of the learner. Coach behaviour should create the possibilities for development through the kind of active participation that characterises collaboration; it should be socially negotiated and should entail transfer of control to the learner (Daniels 2001). Indeed, the purpose of coach behaviour is to enable athletes to 'consciously manipulate and voluntarily control crucial socio-cultural symbolic systems' (Moll & Whitmore 1993 p 20). This would suggest a facilitative rather than dominating role for the coach, which, in turn, needs to be responsive to the diversity of learners with an appropriately diverse range of approaches (Daniels 2001). Coaches should direct and guide individual athlete activity, but they should not force or dictate their own will onto them. Authentic coaching comes through collaboration. The most valuable behaviour corresponds with the athlete's developmental needs and individual particularities, and therefore these methods cannot be uniform. Indeed, Vygotsky argues 'the fundamental prerequisite of pedagogics inevitably demands an element of individualization, that is, conscious and rigorous determination of individualized goals' (Vygotsky 1997 p 324). This suggestion of responsiveness to diversity rather than imposition of sameness in coaching has still to permeate day-to-day practices in the field. Coaching is a complex activity that demands that the coach interpret athletes' constructions of opportunities for engagement and select responses that assist that engagement (Daniels 2001).

Curiously, however, approaches that appear to emphasise the individual often tend to take a 'one size fits all' approach to coach behaviour. That is, regardless of individual differences in the person, even significant ones, the same basic attitudinal and behavioural qualities in the coach are viewed as necessary and sufficient for all athletes (Cain 1989). Adopting one single approach means very little variation in interaction between coach and athlete. However, not all athletes are the same, nor are circumstances and contexts, and therefore a 'one size fits all' approach will not work for all athletes in all situations (Amorose 2007). Athletes have been shown to have different preferences and different responses to coach behaviour (Reiman 2007) and in complex social and interpersonal settings, individual differences are certain to play an important role (Smith & Smoll 2007). Advocating a singular approach to coach behaviour seems to contradict athlete-centredness and deny or minimise individual difference. While notions of different learning styles have been largely discredited for being reductionist (Davis & Sumara 1997, Light 2008), the idea that there are many approaches to coaching is a useful starting point.

Clearly then, coach behaviour will be more effective if it 'fits' the athletes and the context. Athletes do have the capacity to know or recognise that which promotes learning and growth (Cain 1989, Jones & Standage 2006). Athletes' perceptions of themselves and their worlds, must be viewed as a key criterion for determining whether the coach's attitude, manner of relating, or specific behaviours are facilitative or not. Truly athlete-centred coaches would be continuously receptive to learning how their athletes learn effectively. To create an optimal atmosphere for learning, coaches would be less concerned about a coaching style or behaviour and more concerned about whether whatever they do impairs or facilitates learning. Receptivity, flexibility and differentiated responses in coaches are likely to maximise learning (Cain 1989).

However, Potrac and Cassidy (2006) draw upon Floden's (1989) work from education, which suggests that there is a failure in coach education to provide coaches with the opportunity to explore how their behaviour looks to athletes, how athletes perceive what they are learning, and how athletes learn content that is in some way foreign to them. In essence we are largely ignoring a key aspect of the coaching role and function (Jones 2006). This reveals two key elements: first, that coaches are well advised to get to know their athletes (Chelladurai & Reimer 1998); second, that athletes respond to their own perceptions of the coach's behaviour therefore coaches need to understand how athletes interpret their behaviour (Reimer 2007). Hence, a key to behaving effectively involves awareness of one's own behaviour and its consequences, and as such, self-monitoring becomes a crucial skill (Smith & Smoll 2007). Indeed, Smith and Smoll (2007) argue that high levels of self-monitoring will impact coach behaviour because coaches become more responsive to situational cues, are able to recognise the differing needs of their athletes and situations and, are therefore are more flexible in their behaviours.

Role of the coach

After positioning the coach at the heart of the coaching process, it seems somewhat unnecessary to consider the role of the coach framed within a discussion of coach behaviour. However, as already discussed, coaches' behaviour will be informed, implicitly or explicitly, by their beliefs about learning (coaching). Practising and behaving according to one's beliefs will directly impact how the coach's role is perceived and enacted within the coaching process. Therefore, behaviour and role are inextricably linked with the coach's behaviour, depending on the role that they have adopted within the coaching process. More often than not, there is a 'default' role and the behaviours that coaches engage with are linked to the issues discussed previously; tradition of the sport, socialisation experiences, etc.

The traditional role for the coach has been highly directive, instructional or prescriptive (Kidman 2001, Cassidy et al 2004), with the coach deciding when and how athletes should perform specified skills or movements (Kidman 2001, Potrac & Cassidy 2006). This has led to the coach being regarded as the sole source of knowledge, transmitting this in a unidirectional way with athletes having a passive role in the learning process (Potrac & Cassidy 2006). Alternatively, the coach can be regarded as a facilitator who is entirely non-directive and where within certain constraints, athletes largely control their own development. In this case coaches would provide little or no instructional feedback (and therefore need no specialist or content knowledge), but be engaged in helping the athlete solve their problems and construct knowledge experientially through, for example, questioning, summarising, reflecting and listening (Downey 2003).

The ends of the continuum described here, directive/non-directive, coach-led/athlete-led, can be illustrated by coaches, coach educators and scholars alike who each advocate or even 'indoctrinate' (Nelson et al 2006) their 'right way' or indeed the 'only' way of coaching. The reality, of course, is that neither approach and related behaviours is problem- or issue-free, particularly when used solely and to the exclusion of any other. For example, the use of a directive approach *alone* has the potential to disempower athletes and impacts the development of decision-making, problem-solving and creative skills (Cassidy et al 2004, Potrac & Cassidy 2006). An entirely non-directive approach that allows unchecked development can result in the learner acquiring levels of knowledge and understanding that are immature, incorrect and may lead to the neglect of key skills (Butler 1997, Cushion 2006, Potrac & Cassidy 2006). Moreover, knowledge may be implicit in practice and an assumption that it is therefore entirely 'situated' renders knowledge objects invisible, and questions how any knowledge is personalised and how individuals' understanding can be transferred from one context to another (Bereiter 1997).

Potrac and Cassidy (2006) argue that to develop self-regulating and autonomous athletes (i.e. those who can perform when not under the direct control of the coach), the coaching role requires 'more than either the one-directional transmission of knowledge from coach to athlete or the total ownership by athletes of their own development' (p 40). As the argument in this chapter has suggested the role and behaviour the coach adopts is highly context-dependent, and therefore there is no 'one size fits all' approach. However, this does not seem to prevent zealous coach educators and indeed some coaches from forcefully advocating and rigidly adhering to a single role within the coaching process and with it, a singular way of behaving.

This rigid adherence to a certain set of behaviours may be experienced by athletes (and other coaches) as an imposition if this is the only way coaches are willing to behave and interact (Cain 1989, Nelson et al 2006). Despite well-intended notions of 'freedom' for the athlete, by maintaining one approach, and despite feedback (directly and indirectly) that this is not helpful, coaches are in fact constrained by a limited manner of behaving and

interaction. Consequently, any notions of 'empowerment' may well be lost as the athlete has less power and freedom because they perceive coaches as 'authorities' on how best they can change (Cain 1989). So from different theoretical perspectives there may be 'optimum' roles for the coach and related behaviour needed to promote learning, but these may not necessarily align for a given athlete, or athletes with specific goals or needs (Cain 1989, Amorose 2007). Indeed, there is no single behaviour, role or approach that is either a defining or essential component of athlete-centredness (Cain 1989, Popkewitz 1998). In fact, if coaches feel compelled to behave in a single and therefore restricted way, the *more* likely they are to impose limits on their athletes because their own behaviour is constrained (Cain 1989, Daniels 2001).

Coaches must be free to interact and behave in a variety of ways that may or may not include directive or non-directive behaviour. Attempting to adhere to a particular way of behaving, coaches may lose sight of the fact that they need to be free to act appropriately in order to create optimal conditions for learning. If behaviour and practice can be seen to be derived from an understanding of the athletes needs, then this is truly athlete-centred. Coaches need to consider if they are inadvertently imposing an ideology and value on the athlete rather than providing that which will best meet the athlete's individual needs in a manner compatible with their individual learning.

So the role of the coach and coach behaviour is not, and should not be, an 'either–or' scenario. Nor should it be a matter of behaving in a singular way. Coaches are presented with a directive/non-directive continuum, but there are of course many degrees of freedom between the two positions (Jones & Standage 2006). In reality, the coach has a role to play in identifying and addressing sporting problems and assisting athletes to deconstruct knowledge related to aspects of sporting performance (Potrac & Cassidy 2006). Moreover, the coach must provide the athlete with the personal and informational resources for learning (Cain 1989).

In this regard, a number of concepts are useful in guiding coaches. One example is Vygotsky's (1986) Zone of Proximal Development (ZPD). While subject to a range of interpretations (Cushion 2006), the ZPD is often linked with a 'scaffolding' analogy. The ZPD involves identifying between understood knowledge provided by instruction and active knowledge owned by individuals (Lave & Wenger 1991, Hedegaard 1996). The coach (or more capable other) plays a critical guiding role for participation in activities designed to increase understanding of a particular concept (Emihovich et al 1995 p 378). Coach behaviour in this sense is conceptualised as 'assisted performance' with the assistance being given where required (Tharp & Galimore 1988). The amalgam of the assistance provided, utilises a process of diagnosis of the learner's understanding and skill level and estimation on the support needed (Stone 1998). Crucially, the support is not a uniform prescription and importantly it may vary in mode (e.g. instruction, demonstration, question, prompt, dialogue) as well as amount. Throughout, the support is contingent on the response of the athlete; progressive success toward given outcomes reduces the support, while issues or mistakes raise the level of support (Wood 1998, Daniels 2001). Essentially, the level of support is contingent on the learner's progress within the interaction. The coach looks to ensure progress while reducing the level of support, thus gradually withdrawing control over the task and transferring to the learner. Scaffolding coach behaviour in this way is a form of assistance enabling athletes to solve problems, carry out a task, or achieve a goal, which would be beyond unassisted efforts (Wood 1998). The coach's behaviour focuses on controlling those elements beyond the athlete's capacity, thus allowing the athlete to complete those that were within their capabilities. In this sense, scaffolding coach behaviour involves simplifying the learner's role rather than the task (Daniels 2001).

Usefully, the notion of ZPD and scaffolding are helpful tools when thinking about behavioural strategies as they allow coaches to move beyond the dilemma of 'directive' versus 'non-directive' and focus on the needs of the athlete. Coach behaviour becomes centred upon the current knowledge level and potential of the athlete, appropriateness of the behaviour to that current level, the structure of the behaviour with a sequence of thought and action, and gradual withdrawal and transfer of control (Langer & Applebee 1986) from the coach to the athlete.

Central to this approach is the role of the coach, who is perceived to be a 'more capable other', a notion that has received some support in coaching (Cassidy & Potrac 2006). Indeed, as a more capable other, Vygotsky was convinced of the need for instructional behaviour, suggesting that instruction in a system of knowledge enables the learner to be guided toward things that are not immediately apparent; that far exceed the limits of their current knowledge and their potential immediate experience (Vygotsky 1987).

This 'active' view of the coach is also highlighted by Jones and Standage (2006) who usefully discuss the distinction between autonomy and independence suggesting that autonomy does not reflect independence but volitional control, and as such suggests and embraces continued necessary support (Ryan 1993) by the coach. Drawing on another useful concept, Deci and Ryan's Self-Determination Theory (1991), Jones and Standage (2006) argue that autonomy-supportive environments support choice and choice initiation, and understanding and are not authoritarian, pressurised and dictating. Total independence in these circumstances is tantamount to neglect as the coach should provide professional support for the athlete's progression (Jones & Standage 2006). Importantly, autonomy-supportive environments are enhanced in circumstances of unequal power relations (i.e. coach and athlete) (Sheldon et al 2003, Jones & Standage 2006). Autonomy support is facilitated by structure (feedback, clear expectations, understandable behaviour-outcome contingencies) where coach authority exists via promoting athlete choice but within specific rules and limits (Mageau & Vallerand 2003).

Concluding thoughts

Clearly, coaches are central to the coaching process and play a crucial role therein. DeVito (1986) identified three principles of communication that when applied to coach behaviour demonstrate this and reinforce the importance of developing an in-depth understanding of coach behaviour. First, it is inescapable. Even doing or saying nothing, not responding or ignoring is a form of behaviour subject to interpretation. Second, coach behaviour is irreversible. Once said or done it cannot be taken back, and coaches can only deal with the consequences. Finally, as this chapter has gone some way to demonstrate, coach behaviour is complex, involving the interplay of the individual's perceptions of self, other and the relationship (LaVoi 2007). The functional significance of any interaction/behaviour does not lie solely with 'what' the coach says or does, but depends on how the athlete perceives, interprets and evaluates a coach's behaviour (Horn 2002). Athletes are remarkably perceptive at detecting differences in treatment or reactions from coaches; differences that coaches themselves would either be unaware of or at times deny (Solomon 1998, Cushion & Jones 2006, Wilson et al 2006). Indeed, as Tudge and Rogoff (1989) remind us, social interaction does not carry 'blanket benefits' and the circumstances in which coach behaviour facilitates development and learning need to be carefully planned and considered. Therefore, coaches need 'relational expertise', a capacity to observe patterns of connection and disconnection including an awareness of self, other and relationship (Jordan 1995, LaVoi 2007).

Despite the seemingly 'muddy water', research confirms that coaching behaviour is 'very situation specific and dependent on the interaction of a myriad of influencing variables' (Jones 1997 p 30), only some of which are beginning to be studied. Many reasons for this specificity have been cited and the behavioural literature has assisted in identifying mediating factors. Some of these include the gender of coach and athlete (Lacy & Goldston 1990, Millard 1996), if the sport is team or individual in nature (Claxton 1988), the age of the athlete (Lacy & Darst 1985, Wandzilak et al 1988, Seagrave & Ciancio 1990, Smith & Smoll 1993) the type of sport (Claxton 1988, Wandzilak et al 1988), if the athlete is characterised by high or low expectations (Solomon et al 1996, Solomon 1998), the skill level of the athlete (Lacy & Darst 1985, Markland & Martinek 1988), the aims of the coaching session (Krane et al 1991), the coach's level in the coaching structure (Solomon et al 1996, Solomon 1998), the stage in the season (Lacy & Darst 1985, Potrac et al 1997), the coach's philosophy (Cushion 2001), and if the context is that of practice or game (Wandzilak et al 1988, Trudel et al 1996). Therefore, it remains logical to conclude that there is 'no stereotypic coaching personality or set of behaviours which leads to success in coaching' (Markland & Martinek 1988 p 299).

As has been argued, the coach's behaviour will often reflect more deep-seated values, and coaching practice, an essentially social practice, does not occur in a vacuum and therefore cannot be value-free (Schinke et al 1995, Schempp 1998, Lyle 1999b, McAllister et al 2000). Values are always represented in and through coach behaviour, although coaches may or may not be conscious of them. All coaches will have developed a personal set of views on coaching, on issues regarding their sport, and about interpersonal relationships (Lyle 1999b, Cushion 2006). These views will have evolved over time and will be derived from experience and other kinds of education (Gilbert & Trudel 2001, Cushion et al 2003, Cushion 2006). Therefore coaches need to reflect critically on why they behave as they do in order that they are able to make coaching judgements that are meaningful within their particular situation and challenge, rather than reinforce, certain beliefs or practices.

Because coach behaviour should vary across athletes and situations, providing specific recommendations on how to behave becomes difficult. However, it is important to see beyond the directive/non-directive debate and position the needs of the athlete as paramount. Arguably, effective coaches are able to focus on the needs of individual athletes; and behaviour should be shaped around individual athletes' progress and responses, and also the context at any given moment. The intent should always be to connect coach behaviour to athlete learning. Therefore, the quality of the support and behaviour provided by the coach is the key. There is not a 'one size fits all' approach and the optimal behaviour will depend on the characteristics of the situation and the athlete. Regardless of the 'style' of coach behaviour, directive or non-directive, if this is perceived by the athlete as imposing the coach's way of thinking, feeling or acting and is not aligned with the athlete's needs, then it will be seen as controlling and will not be positively received. In this sense, the coach needs to be *an* authority rather than *in* authority (Bergman-Drewe 2000, Jones & Standage 2006) while being active rather than passive in the coaching process.

References

Abraham, A., Collins, D., 1998. Examining and extending research in coach development. Quest 50, 59–79.

Amorose, A.J., 2007. Coaching effectiveness exploring the relationship between coaching behaviour and self-determined motivation. In: Hagger, MS., Chatzisarantis, N.L.D. (Eds.), Intrinsic motivation and self-determination in exercise and sport. Human Kinetics, Champaign, IL, pp. 209–227.

Amorose, A.J., Horn, T.S., 2000. Intrinsic motivation: relationships with collegiate athletes' gender, scholarship status, and perceptions of their coaches' behaviour. Journal of Sport and Exercise Psychology 22, 63–84.

Amorose, A.J., Horn, T.S., 2001. Pre- to post season changes in the intrinsic motivation of first year college athletes: relationships with coaching behaviour and scholarship status. Journal of Applied Sport Psychology 13, 355–373.

Benfarri, R., Wilkinson, H., Orth, C., 1986. The effective use of power. Bus. Horiz. 29, 12–16.

Bereiter, C., 1997. Situated cognition and how to overcome it. In: Whitson, J.A., Kirshner, D. (Eds.), Situated cognition: social, semiotic and psychological perspective. Lawrence Erlbaum, Mahway, NJ.

Bergman-Drewe, S., 2000. An examination of the relationship between coaching and teaching. Quest 52, 79–88.

Bloom, G.A., Crumpton, R., Anderson, J.E., 1999. A systematic observation study of the teaching behaviors of an expert basketball coach. The Sport Psychologist 1, 157–170.

Borrie, A., Knowles, Z., 2003. Coaching science and soccer. In: Reilly, T., Williams, M. (Eds.), Science and Soccer. E & FN Spon, London, pp. 187–197.

Brewer, C.J., Jones, R.L., 2002. A five-stage process for establishing contextually valid systematic observation instruments: the case of rugby union. The Sport Psychologist 16 (2), 139–161.

Bunker, D., Thorpe, R., 1982. A model for the teaching of games in secondary schools. Bulletin of Physical Education 18 (1), 5–8.

Burrell, G., Morgan, G., 1979. Sociological paradigms and organizational analysis. Teacher Educator 29 (1), 43–52.

Butler, J., 1997. How would Socrates teach games? A constructivist approach. Journal of Physical Education Recreation and Dance 68 (9), 42–47.

Cain, D.J., 1989. The paradox of nondirectiveness in the person centred approach. In: Cain, D. (Ed.), Classics in the person-centred approach. PCCS Books, Ross on Wye, pp. 365–370.

Carreira Da Costa, F., Pieron, M., 1992. Teaching effectiveness: comparison

of more and less effective teachers in an experimental teaching unit. In: Williams, L., Almond, L., Sparkes, A. (Eds.), Sport and physical activity: moving towards excellence. E & FN Spon, London, pp. 169–176.

Cassidy, T., Jones, R., Potrac, P., 2004. Understanding sports coaching: the social, cultural and pedagogical foundations of coaching practice. Routledge, Abingdon.

Chaumeton, N.R., Duda, J.D., 1988. Is it how you play the game or whether you win or lose? The effect of competitive level situation on coaching behaviours. Journal of Sport Behaviour 11, 157–174.

Chelladurai, P., Reimer, H.A., 1998. Measurement of leadership in sport. In: Duda, J. (Ed.), Advances in sport and exercise psychology measurement. Fitness Information Technology, Morgantown, WV.

Claxton, D., 1988. A systematic observation of more or less successful high school tennis coaches. Journal of Teaching in Physical Education 7, 302–310.

Coakley, J., 2004. Sports in society: issues and controversies, eighth ed. McGraw-Hill, New York.

Côté, J., Salmela, J., Russell, S., 1995a. The knowledge of high performance gymnastic coaches: Competition and training considerations. The Sport Psychologist 9, 76–95.

Côté, J., Salmela, J., Trudel, P., et al., 1995b. The coaching model: a grounded assessment of expert gymnastic coaches knowledge. Journal of Sport and Exercise Psychology 17 (1), 1–17.

Crossman, J.E., 1985. The objective and systematic categorisation of athlete and coach behaviour using two observational codes. Journal of Sport Behaviour 8, 195–207.

Cushion, C.J., 2001. The coaching process in professional youth football: an ethnography of practice. Unpublished Ph.D. thesis, Brunel University, UK.

Cushion, C.J., 2006. Mentoring harnessing the power of experience. In: Jones, R.L. (Ed.), The sports coach as educator re-conceptualising sports coaching. Routledge, London, pp. 128–144.

Cushion, C.J., 2007. Modelling the complexity of the coaching process: a response to commentaries.

International Journal of Sport Science and Coaching 2 (4), 427–433.

Cushion, C.J., 2008. Understanding the coaching process in elite youth soccer. In: Paper presented at the World Congress of Science and Soccer May 15th–May 16th, Liverpool John Moores University, Liverpool UK.

Cushion, C.J., Jones, R.L., 2001. A systematic observation of professional top-level youth soccer coaches. Journal of Sport Behaviour 24, 354–376.

Cushion, C.J., Jones, R.L., 2006. Power, discourse and symbolic violence in professional youth soccer: The case of Albion FC. Sociology of Sport Journal 23 (2), 142–161.

Cushion, C.J., Armour, K.M., Jones, R.L., 2003. Coach education and continuing professional development: experience and learning to coach. Quest 55 (3), 215–230.

Cushion, C.J., Armour, K.M., Jones, R.L., 2006. Locating the coaching process in practice: models 'for' and 'of' coaching. Physical Education and Sport Pedagogy 11 (1), 1–17.

Daniels, H., 2001. Vygotsky and pedagogy. Routledge, London.

d'Arrippe-Longueville, F., Fournier, J.F., Dubois, A., 1998. The perceived effectiveness of interactions between expert French judo coaches and elite female athletes. The Sport Psychologist 12, 317–332.

Davis, A., Sumara, J., 1997. Cognition, complexity and teacher education. Harvard Educational Review 67 (1), 105–125.

Deci, E.L., Ryan, R.M., 1991. A motivational approach to self: integration in personality. In: Dienstbier, R.A. (Ed.), Nebraska symposium on motivation: perspectives on motivation, vol. 38. University of Nebraska, Lincoln, NE.

DeMarco, G., Mancini, V., Wuest, D., 1996a. Reflections on change: A qualitative and quantitative analysis of a baseball coach's behaviour. Journal of Sport Behaviour 20 (2), 135–163.

DeMarco, G., Mancini, V., Wuest, D., et al., 1996b. Becoming reacquainted with a once familiar tool: systematic observation methodology revisited. International Journal of Physical Education 32 (1), 17–26.

Denzin, N.K., Lincoln, Y.S., 1994. Handbook of qualitative research. Sage, Thousand Oaks, CA.

Denzin, N.K., Lincoln, Y.S., 2000. The discipline and practice of qualitative research. In: Denzin, N.K., Lincoln, Y.S. (Eds.), Handbook of qualitative research. second ed. Sage, London, pp. 1–29.

DeVito, J.A., 1986. The interpersonal communication book. Harper & Row, New York.

Douge, B., Hastie, P., 1993. Coach effectiveness. Sport Science Review 2 (2), 14–29.

Downey, M., 2003. Effective coaching: lessons from the coach's coach. Thomson, London.

Dubois, P.E., 1981. The youth sport coach as an agent of socialisation: an exploratory study. Journal of Sport Behaviour 4, 95–107.

Eitzen, D.S., Sage, G.H., 1989. Sociology of North American sport, fourth ed. WM C Brown, Dubuque, IA.

Emihovich, C., Souza, L., Lima, E., 1995. The many facets of Vygotsky. Anthropology and Education Quarterly 25, 375–385.

Floden, R., 1989. What teachers need to know about learning. In: Proceedings from an NCRTE Seminar for Policy Makers, 24–26 February, USA.

Franks, I., Johnson, R., Sinclair, G., 1988. The development of computerized coaching analysis system for recording behaviour in sporting environments. Journal of Teaching in Physical Education 8, 23–32.

Gallimore, R., Tharp, R., 2004. What a coach can teach a teacher, 1975–2004: reflections and reanalysis of John Wooden's teaching practices. The Sport Psychologist 18, 119–137.

Gilbert, W., Trudel, P., 2001. Learning to coach through experience: reflection in model youth sport coaches. Journal of Teaching in Physical Education 21, 16–34.

Gilbert, W., Trudel, P., 2004. Analysis of coaching science research published from 1970–2001. Res. Q. Exerc. Sport 75, 388–399.

Gilbert, W., Trudel, P., Haughian, L.P., 1999. Interactive decision making factors considered by coaches of youth hockey players during games.

Journal of Teaching in Physical Education 18, 290–311.

Goffman, E., 1959. The presentation of self in everyday life. Doubleday, Garden City, NY.

Greendorfer, S.L., 1982. Shaping the female athlete: the impact of the family. In: Boutilier, M.A., San Giovanni, L. (Eds.), The sporting woman. Human Kinetics, Champaign IL, pp. 135–156.

Hall, T.J., Smith, M.A., 2006. Teacher planning and reflection: What we know about teacher cognitive processes. Quest 58, 424–442.

Hart, C., 1998. Doing a literature review: releasing the social science research imagination. Sage, London.

Hedegaard, M., 1996. The zone of proximal development as basis for instruction. In: Daniels, H. (Ed.), An introduction to Vygotsky. Routledge, London, pp. 171–195.

Hiebert, J., Gallimore, R., Stigler, J., 2002. A knowledge base for the teaching profession: what would it look like and how can we get one? Educational Researcher 31 (5), 3–15.

Horn, T.S., 1984. Expectancy effects in the interscholastic setting: methodological considerations. Journal of Sport Psychology 6, 60–76.

Horn, T.S., 2002. Coaching effectiveness in the sport domain. In: Horn, T.S. (Ed.), Advances in sport psychology. Human Kinetics, Champaign, IL, pp. 309–354.

Horn, T.S., Lox, C., 1993. The self fulfilling prophecy theory: when coaches' expectations become reality. In: Williams, J.M. (Ed.), Applied sport psychology: personal growth to peak performance. Mayfield, Palo Alto, CA, pp. 66–81.

Hughes, M., Franks, I.M., 1997. Notational analysis of sport. E & F N Spon, London.

Jones, R.L., 1997. Effective' instructional coaching behaviour: a review of literature. International Journal of Physical Education 24 (1), 27–32.

Jones, R.L., 2004. An educational endeavour: Coaching redefined. In: Paper presented as part of a symposium, 'Exploring educational relationships' at the British Education Research Association (BERA) Conference, 15th–17th

September, UMIST, Manchester, UK.

Jones, R.L., 2006. How can educational concepts inform sports coaching? In: Jones, R.L. (Ed.), The sports coach as educator: re-conceptualising sports coaching. Routledge, London, pp. 3–13.

Jones, R.L., Standage, M., 2006. First among equals: shared leadership in the coaching context. In: Jones, R.L. (Ed.), The sports coach as educator re-conceptualising sports coaching. Routledge, London, pp. 65–76.

Jones, D.F., Housner, L.D., Kornspan, A.S., 1997. Interactive decision making and behaviour of experienced and inexperienced basketball coaches during practice. Journal of Teaching in Physical Education 16, 454–468.

Jones, R.L., Armour, K.M., Potrac, P., 2004. Sports coaching cultures: from practice to theory. Routledge, London.

Jordan, J.V., 1995. Transforming disconnection, working paper no 75. Stone Center, Wellesly, MA.

Jowett, S., 2007. Interdependence analysis and the 3+1 C's in the coach–athlete relationship. In: Jowett, D., Lavallee, D. (Eds.), Social psychology in sport. Human Kinetics, Champaign, IL, pp. 15–29.

Kahan, D., 1999. Coaching behaviour: a review of the systematic observation research literature. Applied Research in Coaching and Athletics Annual 14, 17–58.

Kidman, L., 2001. Developing decision makers: An empowerment approach to coaching. Innovative Print Communications, Christchurch, New Zealand.

Krane, V., Eklund, R., McDermott, M., 1991. Collaborative action research and behavioral coaching intervention: a case study. Applied Research in Coaching and Athletics Annual 119–147.

Lacy, A.C., 1989. Behaviour analysis of youth sport soccer coaches. In: Paper presented at the American Alliance for Health, Physical Education, Recreation and Dance, National Convention, Boston, MA.

Lacy, A.C., Darst, P.W., 1985. Systematic observation of behaviors of winning high school head football coaches. Journal of Teaching in Physical Education 4, 256–270.

Lacy, A.C., Goldston, P.D., 1990. Behaviour analysis of male and female coaches in high school girls' basketball. Journal of Sport Behavior 13 (1), 29–39.

Langer, J.A., Applebee, A.N., 1986. Reading and writing instruction: toward a theory of teaching and learning. In: Rothkopf, E.Z. (Ed.), Review of research in education, vol. 13. AERA, Washington, pp. 171–194.

Langley, D., 1997. Exploring student skill learning: a case for investigating subjective experience. Quest 49, 142–160.

Langsdorf, E.V., 1979. Systematic observation of football coaching in a major university environment. Unpublished masters thesis, Arizona State University, USA.

Lave, J., Wenger, E., 1991. Situated learning: legitimate peripheral participation. Cambridge University Press, Cambridge.

LaVoi, N.M., 2007. Interpersonal communication and conflict in the coach–athlete relationship. In: Jowett, D., Lavallee, D. (Eds.), Social psychology in sport. Human Kinetics, Champaign, IL, pp. 75–90.

Lawson, H.A., 1990. Sport pedagogy research: From information gathering to useful knowledge. Journal of Teaching in Physical Education 10, 1–21.

Light, R., 2008. Complex learning theory – its epistemology and its assumptions about learning: implications for physical education. Journal of Teaching in Physical Education 27, 21–37.

Liukkonen, J., Laasko, L., Telama, R., 1996. Educational perspectives of youth sport coaches: analysis of observed coaching behaviors. International Journal of Sport Psychology 27, 439–453.

Lucas, W.G., 1980. Coaching communication patterns: a pilot study utilising methods for determining patterns of communication among Canadian College championship coaches. In: Shilling, W., Baur, W. (Eds.), Audiovisuelle medien in sport. Birkhauser Verlag, Basel, pp. 301–311.

Lyle, J., 1999a. The coaching process: an overview. In: Cross, N., Lyle, J. (Eds.), The coaching process: principles and practice for sport. Butterworth-Heinemann, Oxford, pp. 3–24.

Lyle, J., 1999b. Coaching philosophy and coaching behaviour. In: Cross, J., Lyle, J. (Eds.), The coaching process: principles and practice for sport. Butterworth-Heinemann, Oxford, pp. 25–46.

Lyle, J., 2002. Sports coaching concepts: a framework for coaches' behaviour. Routledge, London.

McAllister, S.G., Blinde, E.M., Weiss, W.M., 2000. Teaching values and implementing philosophies: dilemmas of the youth sport coach. Physical Educator 57 (1), 35–45.

MacPhail, A., Kirk, D., 2001. The coach as committed volunteer. In: Poster presentation at 6th Annual Congress of the European College of Sport Science, Cologne, July 2001.

Mageau, G.A., Vallerand, R., 2003. The coach–athlete relationship: a motivational model. Journal of Sport Sciences 21, 883–904.

Markland, R., Martinek, T.J., 1988. Descriptive analysis of coach augmented feedback given to high school varsity female volleyball players. Journal of Teaching in Physical Education 7, 289–301.

McKenzie, T.L., Carlson, B.R., 1984. Computer technology for exercise and sport pedagogy: recording, storing, and analysing interval data. Journal of Teaching in Physical Education 3, 17–27.

Metzler, M., 1983. An interval recording system for measuring academic learning time in physical education. In: Darst, P.W., Mancini, V.H., Zakrajsek, D.B. (Eds.), Systematic observation instrumentation for physical education. Leisure Press, West Point, NY, pp. 181–195.

Millard, L., 1996. Differences in coaching behaviors of male and female high school soccer coaches. Journal of Sport Behavior 19 (1), 19–31.

Miller, A.W., 1992. Systematic observation behavior similarities of various youth sport soccer coaches. Physical Educator 49 (3), 136–143.

Moll, L.C., Whitmore, K.F., 1993. Vygotsky in classroom practice: moving from individual transmission to social transaction. In: Forman, E., Minick, C.A., Stone, C.A. (Eds.), Contexts for learning: socio-cultural dynamics in children's development. Oxford University Press, New York, pp. 19–42.

Nash, C., Collins, D., 2006. Tacit knowledge in expert coaching: science or art? Quest 58 (4), 465–477.

Nelson, L.J., Cushion, C.J., Potrac, P., 2006. Formal, nonformal and informal coach learning. International Journal of Sport Science and Coaching 1 (3), 247–259.

Nicholas, E.J., 1983. Issues in education: a comparative analysis. Harper & Row, London.

Parker, A., 1996. Chasing the big-time: football apprenticeship in the 1990s. Unpublished Doctoral Thesis, Warwick University, UK.

Poczwardowski, A., Barott, J.E., Henschen, K.P., 2002. The athlete and coach: their relationship and its meaning. Results of an interpretive study. International Journal of Sport Psychology 33, 116–140.

Popkewitz, T.S., 1998. Dewey, Vygotsky, and the social administration of the individual: constructivist pedagogy as systems of ideas in historical spaces. American Educational Research Journal 35 (4), 533–570.

Potrac, P., 2001. A comparative analysis of the working behaviours of top-level English and Norwegian soccer coaches. Unpublished doctoral dissertation, Brunel University, UK.

Potrac, P., Cassidy, T., 2006. The coach as 'more capable other'. In: Jones, R.L. (Ed.), The sports coach as educator re-conceptualising sports coaching. Routledge, London, pp. 39–50.

Potrac, P., Jones, R.L., Armour, K., 1997. A comparison of the early and mid season coaching behaviours of top level English soccer coaches. In: Paper presented at the AIESEP '97 (International Association of Physical Education in Higher Education) World Conference, 4–6 December, Singapore.

Potrac, P., Jones, R.L., Armour, K., 2002. It's all about getting respect': the coaching behaviours of an expert English soccer coach. Sport Education and Society 7 (2), 183–202.

Potrac, P., Jones, R.L., Cushion, C.J., 2007. Understanding power and the coach's role in professional English soccer: a preliminary investigation of coach behaviour. Soccer and Society 8 (1), 33–49.

Quarterman, J., 1980. An observational system for observing the verbal and nonverbal behaviors emitted by physical educators and coaches. The Physical Educator 37, 15–20.

Rink, J.E., 1993. Teacher education: a focus on action. Quest 45, 308–320.

Roderick, M., 2006. The work of professional football: a labour of love? Routledge, London.

Ryan, R.M., 1993. Agency and organization: intrinsic motivation autonomy and the self in psychological development. In: Jacobs, J. (Ed.), The self: interdisciplinary approaches. Springer-Verlag, New York, pp. 208–238.

Reimer, H.A., 2007. Multi-dimensional model of coach leadership. In: Jowett, D., Lavallee, D. (Eds.), Social psychology in sport. Human Kinetics, Champaign, IL, pp. 57–73.

Rushall, B.S., 1977. Two observational schedules for sporting and physical education environments. Can. J. Appl. Sport Sci. 2, 15–21.

Rushall, B.S., 2003. Coaching development and the second law of thermodynamics (or belief-based versus evidence-based coaching development). Online Available: http://rohan.sdsu.edu/dept/coachsci/csa/thermo/thermo.htm.

Rushall, B.S., Smith, K.C., 1979. The modification of the quality and quantity of behavior categories in a swimming coach. Journal of Sport Psychology 1, 138–150.

Salmela, J.H., Draper, S.P., La Plante, D., 1993. Development of expert coaches of team sports. In: Serpa, J., Alves, J., Ferreira, V. et al., Proceedings of the VIII World Congress of Sport Psychology. FMH, Lisbon, pp. 296–300.

Salminen, S., Liukkonen, J., 1995. Coach athlete relationship and evaluation of training sessions. Paper presented at IXth European Congress on Sport Psychology, Brussels.

Saury, J., Durand, M., 1998. Practical knowledge in expert coaches:

on site study of coaching in sailing. Res. Q. Exerc. Sport 69 (3), 254–266.

Schempp, P., 1989. Apprenticeship of observation and the development of physical education teachers. In: Templin, T., Schempp, P. (Eds.), Socialisation into physical esducation: learning to Teach Benchmark Press, Indianapolis, pp. 13–37.

Schempp, P., 1998. The dynamics of diversity in sport pedagogy scholarship. Sociology of Sport On Line 1 (1). http://physed.otago.ac.nz/sosol/v1i1/v1i1a8.htm.

Schinke, R.J., Bloom, G.A., Salmela, J.H., 1995. The evolution of elite Canadian basketball coaches. Avante 1, 48–62.

Schmidt, R.A., 1991. Motor control and performance: from principles to practice. Human Kinetics, Champaign, IL.

Seagrave, J., Ciancio, C.A., 1990. An observational study of a successful Pop Warner football coach. Journal of Teaching in Physical Education 9, 294–306.

Sheldon, K.M., Williams, G.C., Joiner, T., 2003. Self-determination theory in the clinic: motivating physical and mental health. Yale University Press, New Haven, CT.

Sinclair, D.A., Vealey, R.S., 1989. Effects of coaches' expectations and feedback on the self-perceptions of athletes. Journal of Sport Behaviour 12, 77–91.

Slack, T., 1997. Understanding sport organisations: the application of organisation theory. Human Kinetics, Champaign, IL.

Smith, M., Cushion, C.J., 2004. An investigation of the in-game behaviours of professional, top-level youth soccer coaches. Unpublished paper.

Smith, R.E., Smoll, F.L., 1993. Educating youth sport coaches: an applied sport psychology perspective. In: Williams, J.M. (Ed.), Applied sport psychology: personal growth to peak performance. second ed. Mayfield, Mountain View CA, pp. 36–57.

Smith, R.E., Smoll, F.L., 2002. Way to go coach! A scientifically proven approach to coaching effectiveness, second ed. Warde, Portolla Valley, CA.

Smith, R.E., Smoll, F.L., 2007. Social-cognitive approach to coaching behaviours. In: Jowett, S., Lavallee, D. (Eds.), Social psychology in sport. Human Kinetics, Champaign IL, pp. 75–90.

Smith, R.E., Smoll, F.L., Hunt, E.B., 1977. A system for the behavioral assessment of athletic coaches. Res. Q. Exerc. Sport 48, 401–407.

Smith, R.E., Smoll, F.L., Curtis, B., 1979. Coach effectiveness training: a cognitive-behavioral approach to enhancing relationship skills in youth sport coaches. Journal of Sport Psychology 1, 59–75.

Smith, R.E., Zane, N.W., Smoll, F.L., et al., 1983. Behavioral assessment in youth sports: coaching behaviors and children's attitudes. Med. Sci. Sports Exerc. 15 (3), 208–214.

Smoll, F.L., Smith, R.E., 1980. Psychologically oriented coach training programs: design, implementation, and assessment. In: Nadeau, C.H., Halliwell, W.R., Newell, K.M. et al., (Eds.) Psychology of motor behaviour and sport. Human Kinetics, Champaign, IL, pp. 112–129.

Smoll, F.L., Smith, R.E., 1984. Leadership research in youth sports. In: Silva III, J., Smith, R.E. (Eds.), Psychological foundations of sport. Human Kinetics, Champaign, IL, pp. 371–386.

Smoll, F.L., Smith, R.E., 2002. Coaching behaviour research and intervention in youth sport. In: Smoll, FL., Smith, R.E. (Eds.), Children and youth in sport. Kendall/Hunt, Dubuque, IA, pp. 211–231.

Smoll, F.L., Smith, F.E., 2006. Development and implementation of a coach training program: cognitive behavioural principles and techniques. In: Williams, J.M. (Ed.), Applied sport psychology: personal growth to peak performance. fifth ed. McGraw-Hill, New York, pp. 458–480.

Solomon, G.B., 1998. Coach expectations and differential feedback: perceptual flexibility revisited. Journal of Sport Behaviour 21 (3), 298–310.

Solomon, G.B., Striegel, D.A., Eliot, J.F., et al., 1996. The self fulfilling prophecy in college basketball: implications for effective coaching. Journal of Applied Sport Psychology 8, 44–59.

Sparkes, A.C., 1992. The paradigms debate. In: Sparkes, A.C. (Ed.), Research in physical education and sport: exploring alternative visions. Falmer Press, London, pp. 9–60.

Stone, C.A., 1998. The metaphor of scaffolding: its utility for the field of learning disabilities. J. Learn. Disabil. 31 (4), 344–364.

Tharp, R.G., Gallimore, R., 1976. What a coach can teach a teacher. Psychology Today 9 (8), 75–78.

Trudel, P., Côté, J., Donohue, J., 1993. Direct observations of coaches' behaviors during training and competition: a literature review. In: Serpa, S., Alves, J., Ferreira, V. et al., (Eds) Proceedings of the VIII World Congress of Sport Psychology. FMH, Lisbon, pp. 316–319.

Trudel, P., Côté, J., Bernard, D., 1996. Systematic observation of youth ice hockey coaches during games. Journal of Sport Behaviour 19 (1), 50–65.

Tomlinson, A., 1983. Tuck up tight lads: structures of control within football culture. In: Tomlinson, A. (Ed.), Explorations in football culture. Leisure Studies Association, Eastbourne, pp. 149–174.

Tudge, J.R.H., Rogoff, B., 1989. Peer influences on cognitive development: Piagetian and Vygotskyian perspectives. In: Bornstein, M.H., Bruner, J.S. (Eds.), Interaction in human development. Lawrence Erlbaum, Hillsdale NJ, pp. 213–248.

van der Mars, H., Darst, P.W., Sariscany, M.J., 1991. Practice behaviors of elite archers and their coaches. Journal of Sport Behaviour 14 (2), 103–112.

Vangucci, M., Potrac, P., Jones, R.L., 1997. A systematic observation of elite women's soccer coaches. Journal of Interdisciplinary Research in Physical Education 1 (2), 1–17.

Vygotsky, L.S., 1986. Thought and language (A. Kouzilin, Ed. and Trans.). MIT Press, Cambridge, MA.

Vygotsky, L.S., 1987. The collected works of L S Vygotsky, vol 1: problems of general psychology. In: Rieber, R.W., Caron, A.S. (Eds.), (N. Minick, Trans.). Plenum Press, New York.

Vygotsky, L.S., 1997. The collected works of L S Vygotsky, vol 4: the history of the development of higher mental functions. In: Rieber, R.W. (Ed.), (M.J. Hall, Trans.). Plenum Press, New York.

Wandzilak, T., Ansorge, C.J., Potter, G., 1988. Comparison between selected practice and game behaviors of youth sport coaches. Journal of Sport Behavior 11 (2), 78–88.

Ward, P., Barrett, T., 2002. A review of behavior analysis research in physical education. Journal of Teaching in Physical Education 21, 242–266.

Williams, J.K., 1978. A behavioral analysis of a successful high school basketball coach. Unpublished masters thesis, Arizona State University, USA.

Wilson, M., Cushion, C.J., Stephens, D., 2006. "Put me in coach...I'm better than you think!" Coaches perceptions of their expectations in youth sport. International Journal of Sport Science & Coaching 1 (2), 149–162.

Wood, D.J., 1998. How children think and learn: the social contexts of cognitive development. Blackwell, Oxford.

Athlete development and coaching

5

Jean Côté, Mark Bruner, Karl Erickson,
Leisha Strachan and Jessica Fraser-Thomas

Introduction

There is growing concern about the healthy development of today's children, adolescents, and young adults. Researchers and policy makers alike have expressed distress and alarm around issues such as the growing epidemic of childhood obesity (Tremblay et al 2002), increases in adolescents' problem behaviours (Igra & Irwin Jr 1996), and young adults' failure to develop initiative and become productive members of society (Larson 2000). While acknowledging these challenges, researchers in developmental psychology have proposed that young people's strengths need to be fostered appropriately for optimal development to occur (Peterson 2004). Given that young people spend almost half their waking hours in leisure (Larson & Verma 1999), organised leisure activities have been suggested as an effective vehicle to promote positive development (Larson 2000). In particular, sport has consistently been found to be the most popular and time-consuming organised leisure activity in which young people participate (e.g. Eccles & Barber 1999, Hansen & Larson 2007).

However, not all children, adolescents, and young adults have positive experiences in sport programs. While an extensive body of literature associates sport involvement with positive experiences and outcomes, a considerable body of literature also associates sport involvement with negative experiences and outcomes. Specifically, sport has been linked to increased self-esteem, confidence, citizenship, academic achievement, and decreased delinquency (e.g. Mahoney 2000, Broh 2002) as well as increased aggression, alcohol consumption, stress, dropout, burnout, and low morality reasoning and self-esteem (e.g. Shields & Bredemeier 1995, Gould et al 1996, Eccles & Barber 1999). Further, negative experiences in sport such as lack of playing time, negative coach experiences, and pressure to win have consistently been associated with dropout in youth sport settings (Weiss & Williams 2004).

Researchers in both sport and developmental psychology emphasise the coaches' critical role in promoting athletes' healthy development through sport. For example, the essential role of coaches, as well as parents, sport programmers, and policy makers is highlighted by Fraser-Thomas et al (2005). These authors argue that delivering positive developmental experiences and outcomes is dependent on conducting programs in appropriate settings that consider developmental stage, and aim to develop personal attributes. Similarly, researchers in developmental psychology (e.g. Lerner et al 2000, Benson et al 2006) consistently highlight supportive relationships, relationships with adults, appropriate role models, and connections with community members as elements of youth activity contexts that facilitate positive development. Moreover, Peterson (2004) points out that while youth development programs such as sports have the potential to 'build a better kid' (p 9), it is the personal characteristics of group leaders that are critical for the success of all youth development programs.

However, clear guidelines for coaches aiming to optimise athletes' development through sport have been lacking (Petitpas et al 2005). Youth sport coaches have been left largely on their own to develop their coaching styles (Gilbert & Trudel 2004), while more expert coaches have received little formal training related to athlete development (Erickson et al 2007). Coaches clearly have the powerful and unique potential to influence athletes' development (Poczwardowski et al 2006), but significantly more understanding of appropriate athlete-centred coaching is necessary to ensure that coaches are positively influencing athletes' development.

The purpose of this chapter therefore, is to discuss and highlight coaches' roles in the development of athletes of different ages and competitive levels in sport. The positive youth development literature suggests that the base of healthy development in sport lies in favourable relationships between participants and coaches, with coaches supporting and promoting healthy growth and excellence. In this context, coaching excellence should be defined by the highly variable roles that coaches assume and should reflect the quality of the constant personal exchanges and interactions between athletes and their coaches in training and competition settings. Consequently, research that focuses on what coaches do and think is valuable and important; however, this descriptive work is often not carried out against the backdrop of athlete outcomes. There are already several reviews of research on the impact of the coaching process (Côté et al 1995, Abraham & Collins 1998, Lyle 2002, Potrac et al 2002, Cushion et al 2003) and the aim of this chapter is *not* to repeat the work covered in these. Instead we focus on research that links athletes' outcomes and coaches' practices, using athlete age and competitive level as a framework. Specifically this chapter: (a) summarises coaching frameworks related to athlete development, (b) proposes a modified coaching model centred around athletes' development, (c) proposes a typology of coaches based on athletes' age, competitive levels, and developmental needs, (d) discusses research on athletes' developmental needs within each coaching typology, and (e) outlines practical implications for coaches within each typology, in order to foster athletes' development.

Coaching frameworks related to athletes' development

Empirical research has led to the conceptualisation of various frameworks that focus on the outcomes of coach and athlete interactions in sport (e.g. Chelladurai 1984, Smoll & Smith 1989, Côté et al 1995). The Multidimensional Model of Leadership (Chelladurai 1984) has generated a large number of studies on coaching effectiveness and athletes' outcomes. The central component of the Multidimensional Model of Leadership features three states of coaches' behaviours: (a) actual behaviours, (b) athletes' preferred behaviours, and (c) required behaviours. Three 'antecedent' variables labelled as the characteristics of the coach, athletes, and situation influence these coaching behaviours. The model suggests that performance and satisfaction are positively related to the degree of congruence among the three states of coach behaviours. To test the model, Chelladurai and Saleh (1980) developed the Leadership Scale for Sport (LSS). The LSS has been used extensively to assess the influence of selected variables such as gender, age, or personality on perceived and/or preferred coach behaviours, and the congruence between perceived and preferred leadership in relation to athletes' performance and/or satisfaction (Chelladurai & Reimer 1998). It is important to note that the LSS is a psychometric instrument that assesses a limited scope of coaching behaviours. Furthermore, the relationships specified in the multidimensional model have primarily focused on adult competitive sports. For detailed reviews of the studies conducted using the Multidimensional Model of Leadership and the LSS see Chelladurai (2007) and Chelladurai and Riemer (1998).

Smoll and Smith (1989) proposed the mediational model of leadership to investigate coaching behaviours and athletes' outcomes, based on findings gathered with the Coaching Behaviour Assessment System (CBAS) (Smith et al 1977). A distinguishing feature of the CBAS is its focus on youth sport coaches. Further, in addition to the coach, athlete, and situational factors, the model specifies that coach behaviours are influenced by players' perceptions and recall, coaches' perceptions of players' attitudes, and players' evaluative reactions. Smoll and Smith suggest a series of coach, athlete, and situational variables such as coaches' goals/motives, athletes' levels of self-esteem, and the level of competition are likely to affect coaches' and players' behaviours. Although, specific coaching behaviours have been linked to positive and negative outcomes in young athletes, the specific context of the studies conducted with the mediational model of leadership is limited to the youth sport environment. For a thorough review of the literature using the CBAS see Smith and Smoll (2007).

The Coaching Model (CM) (Côté et al 1995) provides another useful model to conceptualise the variables that should be considered in designing an optimal learning environment for athlete development. The CM identifies the conceptual and operational knowledge of coaching and was developed around the following six components: (a) competition, (b) training, (c) organisation, (d) coach's personal characteristics, (e) athletes' characteristics, and (f) contextual factors. The CM can be divided into two levels of variables: those that *represent* actual coaching behaviours and that have a direct influence on athletes' development (i.e. competition, training, and organisation) and those that *affect* coaching behaviours (i.e. coach's personal characteristics, athletes' characteristics, and contextual factors). The CM has been used as a conceptual framework for several studies conducted with coaches and athletes (e.g. Côté & Salmela 1996, Gilbert & Trudel 2000, Côté & Sedgwick 2003). Furthermore, the Coaching Behaviour Scale for Sport (CBS-S) (Côté et al 1999) was developed from items based around the behavioural components of the CM. The CBS-S is an evaluative instrument of coaches' work, beneficial both for research and intervention with coaches at the competitive level (Mallett & Côté 2006).

The theoretical frameworks proposed by Chelladurai (1984), Smoll and Smith (1989), and Côté and colleagues (1995) share common variables. The three models propose that the athletes' characteristics, the coach's characteristics, and the context are determinants of coach–athlete interactions. The way coach–athlete interactions are conceptualised in each model is, however, different, and characterises diverse methodological approaches. Each model described above can, however, be incorporated into a more comprehensive framework that highlights the centrality of athletes' personal characteristics and the centrality of athletes' desired outcomes that result from the interaction of coaches and athletes in sport settings.

The Coaching Model revisited

More recently, Côté and colleagues (Côté 2006, Côté & Gilbert 2007) systematically defined the main components and variables of the CM by providing a thorough description of the six main components of the model (competition, training, organisation, coach's personal characteristics, athletes' characteristics, and contextual factors). Using a cognitive approach, these components and their specific relationships were organised to explain how coaches work towards their objective of 'developing athletes'. Generally, the coaches evaluated their personal characteristics (i.e., what they could and could not do), the athletes' and/or team's characteristics, and additional contextual influences, in order to have an estimation of athletes' potential. This estimation, or 'mental model', was then used as a basis to define which coaching knowledge and behaviours were important for use in competition, training, and organisation. The notion of mental models was used to link coaches' knowledge to their actual behaviours, and interactions with athletes.

One component of the CM that has yet to be described is the actual objective of coaches, defined generally as 'developing athletes' (Côté et al 1995). The positive youth development literature provides different frameworks that could be used for conceptualising the development of athletes from a coaching perspective. In particular, the 5Cs – Competence, Confidence, Connection, Character, and Caring/Compassion (Lerner et al 2000) – can be hypothesised as desirable outcomes that should emerge from the interactions of coaches and athletes in a sporting environment. A general definition of the 5Cs according to Jelici and colleagues (Jelici et al 2007) is provided in Table 5.1. In this chapter, discussion of the 5Cs will centre on a collapsed framework of 4Cs (Competence, Confidence, Connection, Character/Caring) and hereon it will be referred to as the 4Cs. This step was taken in response to the integration of caring and compassion within the character development literature in sport (Hellison 1995, Shields & Bredemeier 1995) and the general relatedness of these three constructs (i.e., character, caring, and compassion). A brief overview of each of the 4Cs may be informative at this point to offer theoretical and empirical support for the inclusion of each one as a developmental outcome and as a focus for coaches.

Competence

Self-determination theory (Deci & Ryan 1985) asserts that humans have a basic psychological need for competence, which can be defined as individuals' perceptions of their abilities in specific domains (e.g. academic, athletic, physical, social) (Weiss & Ebbeck 1996). Social contexts that support the satisfaction of competence are proposed to facilitate growth and intrinsically motivated behaviour, while those that hinder competence are associated with poorer motivation, performance, and well-being (Deci & Ryan

Table 5.1 'Working definitions' of the 5Cs of positive youth development

C	Definition
Competence	A positive view of one's actions in domain-specific areas including social, cognitive, academic, and vocational. Social competence pertains to interpersonal skills (e.g., conflict resolution). Cognitive competence pertains to cognitive abilities (e.g., decision making). Academic competence includes school grades, attendance, and test scores. Vocational competence involves work habits and career choice explorations
Confidence	An internal sense of overall positive self-worth and self-efficacy; one's global self-regard, as opposed to domain-specific beliefs
Connection	Positive bonds with people and institutions that are reflected in bidirectional exchanges between the individual and peers, family, school, and community, in which both parties contribute to the relationship
Character	Respect for societal and cultural rules, possession of standards for correct behaviours, a sense of right and wrong (morality), and integrity
Caring or compassion	A sense of empathy and sympathy for others

2000). Within the youth sport and developmental psychology literature, higher perceptions of competence are associated with a number of salient outcomes including: (a) greater intrinsic motivation, (b) higher levels of achievement, (c) more positive achievement-related cognitions (e.g. self-esteem) and behaviours (e.g., effort, persistence), (d) higher levels of positive affect (e.g. happiness), and (e) lower levels of negative affect (e.g. anxiety) (see Weiss & Ebbeck 1996, Weiss & Ferrer-Caja 2002 for reviews).

Confidence

Confidence can be defined as the degree of certainty individuals possess about their ability to be successful (Feltz & Chase 1998). This construct can be viewed in relation to a particular context (i.e. task self-efficacy) (Maddux 1995) or it can be viewed more generally to encompass a number of domains (Horn 2004). According to Jelici et al's (2007) broader conceptualisation, confidence represents an individual's global self-worth. In the developmental psychology literature, low levels of self-worth among children and adolescents have been associated with depression, suicide ideations, eating disorders, antisocial behaviours, delinquency, and teen pregnancy (see reviews by Mecca et al 1989, Harter 1999). Within the sport domain, confidence has been identified as being fragile and critical to the cognitions, affect, and behaviours of athletes (see Vealey & Chase 2008 for a review).

Connection

Humans hold a 'pervasive drive' to form and maintain lasting, positive interpersonal relationships which originates from an innate, fundamental need for belonging (Baumeister & Leary 1995). Self-determination theory identifies this psychological need as relatedness, the need to feel connected and cared for, and the need to be close to others and one's community (Deci & Ryan 1985). Within the sport psychology literature, there is a growing body of research that supports the importance of connections that young people have with significant others (e.g. peers, coaches) in contributing to well-being (see Jowett & Poczwardowski 2007, Smith 2007 for reviews).

Character/caring

Sport has long been celebrated as an activity that builds character. However, sport has also been the subject of much criticism, often being viewed as a pursuit that undermines character (Weiss & Smith 2002b). The distinct, opposing views of character development in sport have led to a considerable amount of research (see Weiss et al 2007 for a review). In the sport literature, character development is often discussed in terms of moral development and sportspersonship. The final C of caring/compassion is commonly viewed as a goal of moral development. Past work highlighting the potential impact of sport in fostering moral development, has led to the implementation of a number of initiatives and interventions such as Personal-Social Responsibility (Hellison 1995).

By integrating the 4Cs into the CM, the model is strengthened by providing concrete outcomes that coaches should aim to develop in their athletes. This integration re-affirms the three key variables that must be considered in any kind of coaching environment: the coach's personal characteristics, the athletes' personal characteristics, and other contextual factors. In particular, individuals who are initiated into coaching come from different backgrounds, experiences, and knowledge (i.e. the coach's personal characteristics). Second, coaches work with athletes who vary in terms of age, developmental level, and goals (i.e. the athletes' personal characteristics). Finally, coaches work in various types of contexts with varying resources, equipment, and facilities (i.e. contextual factors). As in the original model, one can see that any changes in one of these three key variables may affect the learning environment and the interactions that a particular coach may have with his or her athletes, thus affecting athletes' development in training, competition, and organisation settings. Although the coach's personal characteristics and the contextual factors are important in affecting coaching, any coaching system should start by examining the varying developmental needs of athletes of different ages and competitive levels. Figure 5.1 is an adaptation of the original CM emphasising the athletes' personal characteristics as the foundation of coaching effectiveness and highlighting the specific developmental outcomes (i.e. the 4Cs) that should be facilitated through an athlete's sport involvement. In the section that follows, a typology of coaches, which is built on athletes' developmental needs at various ages and competitive levels, is proposed.

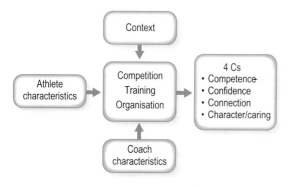

Figure 5.1 • An adaptation of the original CM

A coaching typology built on the Developmental Model of Sport Participation

A recent review of the sport psychology literature (Alfermann & Stambulova 2007) identified a number of models of athlete development in sport. One of the models, the Developmental Model of Sport Participation (DMSP), highlights the importance of developmentally appropriate training patterns and social influences (Côté 1999, Côté et al 2003, Côté et al 2007a, Côté & Fraser-Thomas 2007). The DMSP proposes three possible sport participation trajectories: (a) recreational participation through sampling; (b) elite performance through sampling; and (c) elite performance through early specialisation. The different stages within each trajectory are based on changes in the type and amount of involvement in sport activities and also highlight the changing roles of social influences (i.e., parents, coaches, peers) at each stage of development. In particular the DMSP differentiates the amounts of two types of sport activities – deliberate play and deliberate practice. Côté (1999) defined 'deliberate play' as sporting activities that are intrinsically motivating, provide immediate gratification, and are specifically designed to maximise enjoyment. Deliberate play activities such as street hockey or backyard soccer are regulated by rules modified according to the needs of the participants and typically monitored by the participants themselves. In contrast, Ericsson et al (1993) defined deliberate practice activities as structured activities typical of organised sport, with the goal of improving performance and often strictly monitored by the coach.

The DMSP proposes that recreational participation and elite performance through sampling have the same activity and training foundation from ages 6 to 12 (i.e. sampling years). After the sampling years, sport participants can either choose to stay involved in sport at a recreational level (i.e. recreational years, ages 13+) or embark on a path that focuses primarily on performance (i.e. specialising years, ages 13–15; investment years, ages 16+). While these two distinct trajectories have different outcomes in terms of performance, the aim of each path should be to yield similar personal developmental outcomes in young athletes (i.e. 4Cs) through appropriate, research-based coaching strategies.

Côté et al (2007b) proposed a typology of four different categories of coaches based on developmentally appropriate sport contexts as outlined by the DMSP: (a) participation coaches for children (sampling years); (b) participation coaches for adolescents (recreational years); (c) performance coaches for young adolescents (specialising years); and (d) performance coaches for older adolescents and adults (investment years). Each of the four categories of coaches according to this typology is elaborated upon in the sections that follow. In particular, the athletes' developmental needs in the areas of competence, confidence, connection, and character/caring are discussed, and implications for coaches are explored.

Four categories of coaching: athletes' developmental needs and implications for coaches

Participation coaches for children

Sampling years

The sampling years of the DMSP (ages 6–12), encompassing middle to late childhood, provide the foundation for both the recreational participation and elite performance through sampling trajectories. Characterised by participation in or 'sampling' of a number of different sports as opposed to specialising in one sport year-round, the sampling years usually involve high amounts of deliberate play and lower amounts of deliberate practice.

Competence

For children to develop physical competence during the sampling years, it is important that they engage in a variety of fundamental physical and cognitive skills associated with later sporting ability (Martindale et al 2005). These fundamental skills are not sport-specific and are not usually developed through deliberate practice in any single sport, as deliberate practice is typically characterised by a relatively limited range of required movements and decisions (Côté 2007). In judging their own physical competence, Harter (1999) noted that children tend to start with an overall sense of physical competence based on concrete and observable skills and abilities, generally taking an all-or-none evaluative approach (i.e. either 'good' or 'bad'). In later childhood,

young athletes progress to a more differentiated perception of competence.

Thus, in order to develop feelings of physical competence, children in the sampling years need to be developing fundamental skills, and having concrete mastery experiences with tangible outcomes (Chase 1998). The direct promotion of deliberate play may be an effective way for coaches to address these developmental needs in sport. High amounts of deliberate play can provide children with the diversity and freedom to try new and alternative approaches necessary for fundamental skill development (Wiersma 2000, Côté 2007), while the child-centred nature of deliberate play (i.e., modified rules, focus on enjoyment) allows children many opportunities to experience success.

Recent work in the field of talent development has suggested that competence at very young ages is most often not predictive of future ability (Martindale et al 2005). In Bloom's (1985) landmark study of talent development, very few elite-level performers reported a similar elite level of performance in relation to their peers at age 11 or 12. Kaplan (1996) echoed this sentiment, noting that performance in childhood is an unreliable predictor of future performance. As such, an inclusive focus as opposed to a focus on selection of only the most physically competent top performers appears the most appropriate developmental approach during the sampling years (Martindale et al 2007).

It is important to note that substantial changes in children's sources of information used to judge physical or athletic competence occur during the sampling years (Horn & Weiss 1991, Weiss et al 1997). In particular, children first become capable of peer comparison during this stage. Further, while children initially take adult feedback as in independent source of information, adult feedback is gradually integrated with feedback from other sources during this time (i.e. peer comparison), such that it is no longer automatically taken at face value (Horn 2004). Use of performance outcomes as a source of competence information also develops from middle to late childhood. It is only in later childhood when young people develop the ability to integrate a number of different sources of personal competence information that they are able to separate their own competence from team performance (Horn 2004). Therefore, as children develop, they need individualised competence information from adults that is positive, but that is also realistic in relation to what they can observe through peer comparison.

Past research by Smith, Smoll and colleagues (see Smith & Smoll 2007 for a review) has examined coaches for their provision of individualised competence information. Their work found strong support for the positive influence of coach supportiveness and instructiveness and for the negative effects of punitive coach behaviour. These findings were further validated through intervention studies implementing a coach training program (Coach Effectiveness Training: CET) (Smith et al 1979, Smith & Smoll 2002). Coaches trained to be more supportive and to provide more technical instruction with limited use of punishment were consistently found to produce more positive outcomes related to perceived competence and confidence in their athletes (i.e. lower competitive anxiety, higher self-esteem) than untrained coaches (Smith & Smoll 2007).

Confidence

Children's confidence, equated with a global sense of self-esteem or self-worth, and associated with feelings of competence, begins as a behavioural pattern during the sampling years (Harter 1990). Specifically, children thought to exhibit high self-confidence express a behaviour pattern characterised by curiosity, initiative, and independence, as well as a capacity for flexibility in response to environmental change. Thus, children in the sampling years need to be encouraged to demonstrate curiosity, initiative, and independence. The intrinsic motivation associated with deliberate play is characterised by and encourages this behavioural pattern (Ryan & Deci 2000). As such, deliberate play is a potentially fruitful means by which to develop children's confidence.

Judgements of self-worth may also be significantly influenced by goal orientations in sport (Duda 1993), given the increasing awareness of peer comparison that children develop during the sampling years. Children employing an ego-orientation, with a focus on evaluating competence in relation to the performance of others, may be at an increased risk for damage to self-confidence, especially in the presence of more skilled peers. In contrast, the confidence of children with a task-orientation, whereby competence is evaluated according to self-referenced improvement and effort, may be more resilient to fluctuations in relative performance. This resilient confidence may, in turn, encourage persistence in skill learning efforts and increased perceptions of competence (Harwood et al 2008).

Given the positive influence of a task goal-orientation on confidence and competence in childhood, the promotion of such an orientation in children's sport contexts is of utmost importance. In particular, the development of a task orientation in individuals has been linked to a perceived mastery motivational climate as created by the coach (Harwood et al 2008). A mastery climate is one in which improvement, effort, and learning are valued and rewarded (Ames 1992). A performance climate, on the other hand, is one in which evaluation is relative to others and defeating others is of primary importance. Treasure (2001) suggests that a mastery-oriented motivational climate can be created in children's sport, in accordance with Epstein's (1989) TARGET model: *Tasks* that are diverse and appropriately challenging, *Authority* that is flexible and allows for children's input, *Recognition* that is private and personal, *Groupings* that are varied and heterogeneous in ability, *Evaluation* that is self-referenced and considers fun, effort, and participation, and *Timing* that provides an appropriate pace of instruction and adequate time for tasks.

Connection

Positive peer relationships and friendships have been identified as a key reason why many children participate in sport (Scanlan et al 1993, Weiss 1993). These early peer relationships and friendships also play a critical role in the development of vital social skills, such as intersubjectivity or shared understanding (Goncu 1993). During the sampling years, children tend to define friendship quality according to characteristics related to loyalty, mutual liking, and helping or taking care of each other (Newcomb & Bagwell 1995). However, Zarbatany and colleagues (1992) noted that children's friendship expectations differ by context. Within the sport context, Weiss, Smith, and Theeboom (1996) found that loyalty and prosocial behaviour were rated as most important by children under 12.

Thus, to promote the development of positive peer connections, children in the sampling years need the time and opportunity to develop friendships. In developing these friendships, children need encouragement to demonstrate loyalty and prosocial helping behaviours. The child-driven nature of deliberate play (Côté 1999) can provide opportunities for both positive peer interaction and the demonstration of prosocial behaviours by encouraging cooperation and recognition of the needs and abilities of others.

In addition to connections with peers, connections with adults are also important during the sampling years. Parents are typically the individuals of most influence in children's lives (Siegler et al 2003). With regard to sport participation, parents in the sampling years '...have a greater and more lasting effect on children's sport involvement than in other periods of development' (Wylleman et al 2007 p 239). As such, the positive participation and supportive involvement of parents in their children' sport experiences should be encouraged. Further, this may help to ensure consistency of developmental messages across contexts, what Benson and colleagues (2006) refer to as developmental redundancy.

Finally, while parents tend to be most influential in children's lives overall, coaches are the primary adults in the sport setting and their connections with young athletes should not be overlooked. Positive relationships with coaches are predictive of children's enjoyment of their sport participation (Scanlan et al 1993), while negative feedback and lack of interaction have been linked to non-enjoyment (McCarthy & Jones 2007). As such, active coaches who promote positive relationships with their young athletes are essential to developing healthy coach connections (Smith & Smoll 2007).

Character/caring

It has been argued that sport participation can lead to both positive and negative character development (Shields & Bredemeier 1995), a consideration of utmost importance for children in the sampling years who are still developing their moral reasoning skills and abilities. Siegler and colleagues (2003) suggest that the primary environmental influence on the development of prosocial behaviour in children is socialisation through interactions with significant adults. This socialization takes three general forms: (a) modelling and communication of values; (b) opportunities for prosocial activities; and (c) discipline style (i.e. reasoning and drawing attention to consequences of behaviour for others). In the sport context, Shields and Bredemeier (1995) posit that compassion, a key component of moral character, is manifested through the psychological competencies of role taking, perspective taking, and empathy. Similar to the socialisation of prosocial behaviour, Shields and Bredemeier argue that leaders in sport settings (i.e. coaches) can promote the development of these competencies through

their interaction style and the appropriate structuring of activities. Thus, in order to develop character and caring, children in the sampling years need positive role models, interactions with adults that promote moral reasoning, and opportunities to demonstrate character and caring.

Deliberate play may again provide a fertile context to demonstrate character and caring. The intrinsically motivating structure and emphasis on fun typical of deliberate play (Côté 1999) may promote a more adaptive and ethical view of competition, whereby focus is placed on the process of competing to the best of one's abilities rather than on the outcome of competition (Hochstetler 2003). Sport is inherently competitive; however, competition during childhood should not lead to negative character development (e.g. Eccles & Barber 1999) unless the outcome is over-emphasized and instrumental antisocial behaviours are subsequently more likely to be justified.

The development of character and caring in children may also be facilitated by goal orientation and climate. By defining success as competing to the best of one's own abilities, opponents may be more likely to be seen as fellow competitors, necessary for the game or competition to occur (Harwood et al 2008). In contrast, an increase in ego-orientation may promote the view of opposition as enemy, standing in the way of the desired outcome. With this ego-oriented perspective, one may therefore feel more justified in demonstrating unsportspersonship-like behaviour, or injurious acts towards the opposition in order to win (Harwood et al 2008).

Implications

Below are five strategies emerging from the literature that highlight how coaches can facilitate the 4Cs in athletes during the sampling years, through appropriate competition, training, and organisational strategies. First, coaches can best encourage children's development by structuring competition and training to include high amounts of deliberate play. Second, coaches should promote a mastery-oriented motivational climate through the use of Epstein's (1989) TARGET activity guidelines (discussed earlier). Third, in implementing these strategies, coaches should seek to interact with their athletes in a supportive and instructive manner, while limiting punitive interactions. Fourth, with regard to organisation, coaches should include parents in positive and supportive roles. Finally, coaches should adopt an inclusive developmental focus, as opposed to an exclusive team selection policy based on current performances, to provide all children with opportunities to develop the 4Cs.

Participation coaches for adolescents

Recreational years

Adolescent participants electing not to pursue an elite developmental trajectory but remaining involved in sport seek a context that promotes fun, challenge and enjoyment (Côté et al 2007a). To this end, participation coaches for adolescents must be cognisant of the specific developmental and contextual needs of their athletes. This may be particularly relevant for participation coaches, as their young athletes are in a critical period of growth and development, and engaging in a number of activities to build their personal identity (Wagner 1996). As such, the 4Cs framework (Jelicic et al 2007) can once again serve to help coaches identify adolescent's developmental needs.

Competence

An adolescent's perceived abilities or competence have been found to be associated with a number of positive outcomes in several domains including sport (see Weiss & Ebbeck 1996, Weiss & Ferrer-Caja 2002 for reviews). As a child moves into adolescence, he or she begins to integrate competence information from various sources, with a greater emphasis on information from peers and coaches (Horn & Weiss 1991, Weiss et al 1997). Young adolescents' perceptions of competence develop as a function of two separate but interrelated factors: cognitive maturation and social-cultural environment. The contextual setting of sport can be critical to an adolescent's cognitive maturation. This is exemplified particularly by adolescents' differentiation of self-competence into several sub-domains. Specifically, teenagers begin to compartmentalise themselves as being 'different' people in the different domains. This ability to develop higher-order abstractions about self permits adolescents to evaluate themselves as having differing levels of ability in different contexts. For example, athletes may feel competent in one sport (e.g. basketball) yet not in another (e.g. soccer) or view themselves as being

competent in one skill (e.g. jump shot) but not in another (e.g. lay-up). However, this developmental process is not seamless, and frequently involves adolescents reconciling 'cognitive confusion' of one self (Harter 1999). It is during these trying times that young athletes look to their social-cultural environment, specifically the feedback of significant others such as coaches and peers, to resolve conflicting information about the self.

Confidence

Another related developmental construct of self is confidence. Jelicic and colleagues (2007) operationalise confidence as a global construct such as self-worth. As previously outlined, low levels of self-worth among adolescents have been linked to a number of negative outcomes such as depression, delinquency, and antisocial behaviours (see reviews by Mecca et al 1989, Harter 1999). Based upon studies in school settings, physical appearance and social acceptance are primary personal antecedents of global self-confidence at this age (Harter 1999). As such, it is critically important that adolescents' sport environments foster a culture of social acceptance of all teammates, and intolerance of negative comments directed toward a young athlete's physical appearance.

Connection

During adolescence, positive ties with peers become increasingly important as young people develop personal identity and a sense of self (Harter 1999, McLellan & Pugh 1999). In a sport setting, peers are particularly important given their direct involvement in most young athlete's day-to-day experiences. Quite surprisingly, research investigating the developmental significance of peer connections and relationships in sport is relatively underdeveloped (Weiss & Stuntz 2006, Smith 2007). As such, considerable theoretically driven research is needed to understand the role of peer relationships (i.e. peer acceptance, friendship) on a young athlete's development (Weiss & Stuntz 2006).

Alongside the salient role of peers, adolescents' connections with their families and schools are important. Adolescents' perceptions of family closeness or cohesion have been found to be positively associated with a number of health-promoting behaviours (e.g. decreased alcohol usage) (Bray et al 2001), and negatively associated with adolescent problem behaviours (e.g. delinquency, aggression)

(Barber & Buehler 1996). Further adolescents' school cohesion, operationalised as the level of mutual support, belonging, and connectedness of the school, has been found to offer a protective, moderating effect for adolescents experiencing low family and peer support (Botcheva et al 2002). However, similar to the lack of research on peers in sports, additional research is necessary to further explore the role of family and school connections on the development of the young athlete.

Over the last decade, the athlete–coach relationship has received a considerable amount of attention in the literature. Several conceptual models have been proposed (e.g., LaVoi 2004, Jowett 2005) highlighting the importance of the connections between the coach and athlete (see Jowett & Poczwardowski 2007 for a review). LaVoi's (2004) conceptual framework of coach–athlete relationships proposes how feelings of belonging and close, inter-dependent relationships with coaches and teammates lead to athletes' healthy psychological development. Jowett's (2005) integrated model of coach–athlete relations also includes the psychological construct of closeness. Jowett (2007) describes closeness as the affective component of the coach–athlete relationship that is reflected in mutual feelings of trust and respect. While there is a need for significantly more research on connections in adolescent sport context, it is clear that the supportive, dynamic, and diverse connections of athletes with their peers, coaches, families, and wider communities are an essential component of adolescents' healthy development in their sport environment.

Character/caring

Research on adolescents has shown that experiences in sport can promote prosocial behaviour and reduce antisocial behaviours (e.g. aggression, lack of responsibility) (Weiss et al 2007). Two primary theoretical perspectives dominate the field: (a) social learning theory (Bandura 1986) and (b) structural development approaches (Weiss et al 2007). In brief, social learning theory suggests that moral development is learned through individuals' interactions with socialising agents such as adults and peers. Specifically, appropriate behaviours that conform to societal norms and regulations occur as a result of modelling and reinforcement from significant others (e.g. adults, peers). Social learning theory identifies self-regulation skills as being critical in displaying moral behaviour. These self-regulating skills include

monitoring, judgement, evaluation, strong beliefs in one's capabilities to achieve personal control, and self-regulatory efficacy to adhere to moral standards (Weiss et al 2007).

Structural developmental theories focus on how individuals reason or judge values and behaviour (Weiss et al 2007). Shields and Bredemeier (1995) proposed a conceptual model that outlines factors that may explain variations in moral thoughts and behaviours in physical activity and sport settings. Within the model, Shields and Bredemeier identify several important contextual factors that coaches can modify to play a vital role in shaping young athletes' moral thoughts and behaviours. Two salient contextual factors include moral atmosphere and motivational climate. A considerable amount of research has investigated the influence that moral atmosphere, conceptualised as team norms, can have on adolescent athletes' beliefs about appropriate and inappropriate behaviour (e.g., Smith 1974, Stephens et al 1997, Stephens 2000). As previously discussed, motivational climate typically identifies what is recognised, rewarded and emphasised within the context of the team environment (Ames 1992). A mastery-oriented climate generally emphasises effort, improvement, and personal mastery, while a performance-oriented climate focuses more on peer comparison and final outcome. Several studies with youth soccer teams (e.g. Ommundsen et al 2003, Miller et al 2005) have found support for participants' perceptions of a more mastery-oriented motivational climate being associated with higher levels of moral-reasoning and a more performance-oriented climate being associated with lower level of moral reasoning (e.g. greater perceived legitimacy of aggression and injurious acts).

Along with the identified contextual factors, Shields and Bredemeier's (1995) model suggests a number of individual factors such as moral reasoning, achievement goal-orientation, moral identity, and self-regulation skills as essential for understanding moral development in sport. The early work of Bredemeier and Shields (1984, 1986) on moral reasoning in sport led to the introduction of several key concepts such as game reasoning or bracketing one's morals in a sport setting (e.g. legitimising aggression in pursuit of winning). Individuals' achievement goal orientations (i.e. task versus ego) (Duda 1993) have also been linked to moral attitudes, intentions, and behaviours. Research examining the linkages between goal orientations and sportsperson-like attitudes have consistently found that young athletes (high school, college), who are higher on task-orientation report higher sportsperson-like attitudes. In contrast, athletes higher on ego-orientation report greater approval of unsportsperson-like play (e.g. Lemyre et al 2001, Kavussanu & Ntousmanis 2003). A promising implication for coaches from this area of research has been the recommendation to implement social goals (e.g. bring honour to the group, be a productive member of society, be a good person) along with task and ego goals (e.g. Urdan & Maehr 1995, Jarvien & Nicholls 1996, Wentzel 1998). It has been suggested that this integrated goal perspective may be particularly important for recreational adolescent athletes, and an area in need of further research (Weiss et al 2007). Furthermore, empirical evidence has begun to demonstrate how an adolescent's moral identity (i.e. a person's use of moral beliefs to define the self) (Damon 1984, 2004) and self-regulatory skills may influence a young athlete's moral thoughts and actions (e.g. Aquino & Reed 2003, Bandura et al 2003).

Collectively the research on contextual and individual factors has increased the awareness of character development in sport. Stemming from this research, a number of theoretically driven interventions have been developed to promote moral development in sport. Among these interventions, the Personal-Social Responsibility Model (Hellison 1995) may be particularly useful for coaches of adolescent recreational athletes. The model outlines five levels of personal-social responsibility: (a) respecting the rights and feelings of others; (b) being self-motivated; (c) being self-directed; (d) caring about others and working together for the group's welfare; and (e) applying these and other responsibilities to domains outside the gym. While the model was originally developed to target underserved youth, the five levels of responsibility specified in the model warrant consideration in all adolescent sport environments, with the goal of developing character and caring in sport and other life contexts.

Implications

Participation coaches for adolescents should be viewed as being instrumental gatekeepers in the development of young athletes' 4Cs. First, within competition and training settings, coaches should create a social context that supports athletes' competence and confidence development. In particular, coaches should foster an environment of social acceptance of all teammates and provide appropriate feedback to support young athletes. Second, coaches should place an emphasis on personal growth rather than athletic excellence in competition and training, through the creation of a mastery rather than performance-oriented motivational climate. Third, to strengthen coach–athlete relations, coaches should foster close, interdependent relationships by demonstrating trust and respect for their young athletes. Fourth, in line with the social learning theory, coaches should model appropriate moral behaviour for youth and demonstrate self-regulatory skills during challenging situations in competition.

Fifth, from an organisational perspective, coaches should provide opportunities for teammates to develop strong connections within and outside of sport. Sixth, coaches should promote an environment rich in character development and social responsibility. For example, coaches can facilitate the goal-setting process among athletes, through continued encouragement and monitoring of social goals along with task (process) and ego (performance) goals. The social goals may be set in practice after engaging in coach–athlete discussions of potential moral dilemmas that may arise in competition; such discussions should foster moral development and enhance youth's self-regulatory efficacy. Finally, coaches should consider adopting a moral development framework such as Hellison's (1995) Personal-Social Responsibility Model to promote athletes' development of personal responsibility within the sporting context and beyond the sport context, as contributing members of society.

Performance coaches for young adolescents

Specialising years

Young adolescents who have decided to focus on attaining high levels of performance have different motives for participation to their recreational peers. While non-elite youth athletes participate in sport for fun, to develop skills, and to make friends (Gould et al 1985, Coetzee & Viljoen 2002), young elite athletes participate in sport to increase competence, fitness, and for challenge (Klint & Weiss 1986). Further, although enjoyment is still an important aspect of participation for elite adolescent athletes, the acquisition of sport-specific skills becomes increasingly important (Côté et al 2007a). As such, it is suggested that specialising adolescent athletes have specific developmental needs that differ from those of recreational adolescent athletes. As an increased number of young athletes are specialising in sport (Gould & Carson 2004), further comprehension of what constitutes a healthy training and competition environment for this group of athletes is of critical importance. In the sections that follow, research related to adolescent performance athletes' developmental needs according to the 4Cs framework is reviewed.

Competence

Within elite youth sport programs, competence is a key developmental focus. During the specialising years, young performance athletes spend a considerable amount of time in deliberate practice activities, as their training shifts to include approximately equal amounts of deliberate practice and deliberate play (e.g. Côté et al 2007a, Côté & Fraser-Thomas 2007). Deliberate practice is comprised of activities that are repetitive, well-defined, at a level of difficulty that is appropriate for the individual, and provide opportunities for feedback, proper error detection, and correction (Ericsson et al 1993, Ericsson 2003). More specifically, deliberate practice activities require concerted effort with the goal of improving performance, and are not always inherently enjoyable. Ericsson et al (1993) suggest that in order to become an expert (i.e. develop very high levels of competence), an individual must spend ten years or 10 000 hours in deliberate practice activities. There has been much research support for the deliberate practice framework in the sport domain (e.g. Helsen et al 1998, Hodge & Deakin 1998). As such, the more time an individual spends in deliberate practice activities throughout his or her development in sport, the higher his or her skill level is likely to be, and thus inevitably, the more likely athletes are to experience athletic competence (Harter 1999).

Psychological skills also play an important role in facilitating competence development during the specialising years. Even at a young age, athletes can experience the benefits of psychological skills training (i.e. goal setting, imagery, arousal regulation; Munroe-Chandler & Hall 2007). In fact, the earlier athletes can learn to put psychological skills into practice, the more effective they will be at using these skills to enhance performance and competence.

As previously discussed, adolescence is a critical period of transition, which must also be considered in adolescent performance athletes' development.

While more deliberate practice will ultimately lead to an increased skill level, there have also been negative outcomes linked to increased training for young athletes. For example, in some cases the hours spent in sport-specific training have been found to be not enjoyable for young athletes (Law et al 2007). Further, injuries appear more prevalent in young performance athletes than their less-competitive peers (Micheli et al 2000, Law et al 2007). Finally, burnout has been associated with intense youth sport participation (e.g. Coakley 1992, Gould et al 1996). Three dimensions have been found to impact young athletes: reduced accomplishment, physical/emotional exhaustion, and sport devaluation (Raedeke 1997). This research highlights the importance of appropriate sport environments to alleviate potential negative outcomes (Raedeke & Smith 2004).

Confidence

Adolescents' confidence is associated with self-perceptions related to athletic competence, physical appearance, and overall self-worth (Harter 1999). As such, performance athletes must develop and experience confidence, not only in specific sport skills, but also in other domains such as social skills. While there is a reduction of time spent in other sport and non-sport activities (Baker et al 2003) and a marked decrease in deliberate play activities during the specialising years, the important role of deliberate play activities in performance athletes' sport of specialisation, and in other sport activities should not be undermined. Deliberate play is important in the growth of sport-specific skills (Côté 1999) and offers additional benefits related to talent development including increased creativity, enjoyment, and emotional regulation (Strachan et al 2008). Deliberate play activities, through their loosely structured nature, also offer an ideal platform for performance adolescent athletes to develop confidence in their social skills such as communication and leadership (Fraser-Thomas et al 2005).

Connection

Past research suggests that connections may be fostered through the appropriate modeling and mentoring of coaches (Sedgwick et al 1997). In particular, high-quality coach–athlete relationships may lead to less antisocial behaviour and more prosocial behaviour due to the important roles coaches play in modelling and supporting athletes (Rutten et al 2007). While a limited body of research has explored the role of sport peers in contributing to adolescent athletes' development, perceptions of peer acceptance and the development of close friendships are critically important to youth of this age. Specifically, friendship quality in sport is a key factor in the development of close connections for youth (Weiss & Smith 2002a). Further, positive peer relationships in youth sport are closely connected to the youth's motivation for continued sport engagement (Patrick et al 1999, Allen 2003). As such, more time spent in elite sport may allow for the growth of close friendships and relationships which may in turn lead to athletes' persistence in their chosen sport.

Character/caring

Adolescents' participation in high-performance sports may also facilitate character development. Character attributes such as sportspersonship, positive values, resilience, optimism, and a good work ethic have been noted to be fostered through sport participation (Gould et al 2002, Fraser-Thomas et al 2005). In retrospective interviews with Olympic champions, Gould and colleagues (2002) found that these elite athletes were typified by these characteristics and highlighted the important role that coaches played in the emergence of these traits. Further, caring may be viewed as a byproduct of character development. Caring in youth sport may be observed through athlete interactions such as displays of empathy in both training and competitive situations (Côté 2002, Fraser-Thomas et al 2005). As empathy may be more easily facilitated in deliberate play situations (Strachan et al 2008), the presence of play in competitive youth sport programs has the potential to enable the development of caring; however, more research is needed to examine how caring is fostered in high-performance youth sport.

Implications

Performance coaches for young adolescents have unique considerations to ponder in the delivery of high-performance programs. First, with regard to training, coaches should increase quantities of deliberate practice activities in order to develop competence. In particular, coaches need to be knowledgeable and have the ability to give technical corrections and feedback (Smoll & Smith 2002). Further, coaches must work to develop not only athletes' physical skills but also cognitive skills (e.g. decision-making, memory) (Gallagher et al 2002). However,

coaches must not forget that deliberate practice activities should be balanced with deliberate play activities, even for athletes of this age and level (Côté et al 2007b). Specifically, an infusion of opportunities for deliberate play enables athletes continued motivation for sport through enjoyment. Finally, while adolescent performance coaches should encourage specialisation in order to build skills, they should also allow athletes to 'sample' effectively within their sport by encouraging them to attempt other roles and positions, and thus allowing them more diversity and growth in their sport experience and skill development.

Second, through training and competition, coaches should facilitate athletes' competence development in other areas (i.e. psychological and social). This can be achieved by training athletes' psychological skills (e.g. imagery, goal setting) as well as through the introduction of diverse peer groups (i.e. various age and cultural groups). Further, coaches can provide opportunities for recognition through sport travel and participation in appropriate competitions (Côté et al 2007b). Third, adolescent-performance coaches must develop character and connections in training and competition settings, by demonstrating leadership, modelling appropriate behaviours, interacting closely with athletes, and fostering safe peer–peer interactions. For example, coaches should encourage athletes to display sportspersonship and show empathy to their teammates and other competitors.

Finally, from an organisational perspective there are a number of initiatives that adolescent-performance coaches can undertake to develop the 4Cs in their athletes. For example, to facilitate connections, character, and caring in high-performance youth sport, coaches should deliver social events and create team or club unifiers (e.g. team colors, tracksuits), establish athlete mentor programs within clubs, link elite sport programs to other contexts (e.g. school, community) and facilitate positive growth opportunities (e.g. volunteerism, civic responsibility). These types of connections may empower athletes to contribute to the development of not only their athletic clubs, but also the communities in which they live.

Performance coaches for late adolescents and adults

Investment years

During the investment years, athletes (approximately ages 16+) usually commit to only one sport activity and engage primarily in deliberate practice. Athletes in the investment years are often motivated by extrinsic factors such as winning, being chosen for an international team, or establishing a sport career. Ideally, this type of motivation should be self-determined and integrated in the athlete's whole life (Deci & Ryan 2000). The DMSP suggests that elite athletes that have the resources, ability, and desire for competitive performance at the national or international level increase their deliberate practice hours and decrease their deliberate play hours even further during the investment years (Côté et al 2007a). Elite-level athletes in the investment years need quality structured training in large quantities, however this type of training should be conducted in an environment that is conducive to the development of the 4Cs.

Competence

Competence in elite sport necessitates the integration of several skills including motor, perceptual, cognitive, and psychological. Larson (2000) points to the acquisition of initiative as the essential ingredient in the development of competence or efficacy in any domain. The initiative perspective highlights three features of competent behaviours: (a) intrinsic motivation; (b) the ability to mobilise one's attention on a deliberate course of action; and (c) the ability to devote cumulative effort for a long period of time (Larson 2000). This framework is similar to Ericsson et al's (1993) notion of expertise through deliberate practice, which explicitly links the amount and type of training performed to the level of competence attained in a specific domain. According to Ericsson et al (1993) deliberate practice activities that require effort and attention do not lead to immediate social or financial rewards and are performed for the purpose of performance enhancement rather than enjoyment. The ability to accumulate the quantity and quality of training required for competent performance in sport during the investment years is directly linked to accessibility of essential resources such as training facilities and coaches (Ericsson 2003).

The development of a competent elite-level athlete is, however, much more than developing motor, perceptual, cognitive, and psychological skills. Walton (1992) revealed that great coaches of elite athletes do not simply master the teaching of their sport, but are also champions of wisdom and understanding. The coaches examined by Walton not only produced excellent athletes, but also educated and contributed to the human competence of these athletes. For instance, all of the coaches were committed to the athletes' integrity, values, and personal growth, and were profound thinkers who saw themselves as educators of social values, not just trainers of physical skills. This commitment to holistic athlete development has recently been encouraged by coaching researchers (e.g. Bergmann Drewe 2000, Jones 2006).

Confidence

Confidence refers to an internal sense of positive self-worth and self-efficacy (Jelicic et al 2007) and is essential for athletes in the investment years striving towards elite performance (Sedgewick et al 1997). Studies of coaching behaviours in swimming (Black & Weiss 1992), figure skating (Hall & Rodgers 1989), field hockey (Grove & Hanrahan 1988), and wrestling (Gould et al 1987) have shown that confidence building is one of the most important characteristics that coaches want to hone in their athletes. Accordingly, authors agree that the relationship between coaches and athletes is an important determinant of the way in which athletes' confidence is affected by their participation in competitive sport (e.g. Côté & Salmela 1996, Hays et al 2007). Although athletes during the investment years may appear to be autonomous and independent, they still appreciate the attention they receive from their coaches about their sport and other aspects of their life. The coach–athlete relationship and effective communication with coaches influence athletes' confidence and should be at the forefront of coaching strategies in the investment years (Sedgwick et al 1997).

Connection

Deci and Ryan (2000) suggested that the development of highly motivated, self-determined, and invested individuals in any domain requires an environment that provides opportunities to make autonomous decisions, develop competence, and feel connected to others. Because athletes are so highly invested during this period, coaches have a crucial role in providing optimal learning and social conditions in which athletes feel supported (Kalinowski 1985, Côté et al 1995, Salmela 1996, Côté 2002). In general, coaches of athletes in the investment years have been shown to provide both physical and social resources to help athletes overcome the effort and motivational constraints associated with deliberate practice (Salmela 1996). Jowett (2007) proposed that the quality of coach–athlete relationships in providing these resources is determined by the degree of closeness, commitment to the relationship, complementarity, and co-orientation between both parties. An effective sporting environment during the investment years will also support athletes' basic need to belong to a social group whose members are mutually supportive. To maintain a healthy perspective on sport and life, elite-level athletes in the investment years should be encouraged to constantly nourish their relationships with their coach, peers inside and outside of sport, community, and parents.

Character/caring

In the realm of elite sports, coaches have a crucial role in enabling athletes to develop their character, become a constructive and caring member of a team, and ultimately, a productive member of society. For many competitive athletes, sport stimulates a change in social values and moral reasoning patterns (Bredemeier & Shields 1996). Coaches of athletes in the investment years should not 'use language or techniques that might encourage participants to separate their sport experiences from "real life"' (Bredemeier & Shields p 396). Rather, like any other sport settings, elite sports should be seen as a medium by which social values are learned and transferred to real life situations.

Implications

To meet athletes' training needs in the investment years, coaches must construct a regime that is grounded in deliberate practice. Specifically, training should be structured purposefully to improve current performance levels and to circumvent arrested skill development (Ericsson 2003). During training, coaches should focus on structured drills and activities with well-defined learning goals, provide regular feedback for skill improvement, and create ample opportunities for repetitions. Within the deliberate practice framework, training activities should be carefully monitored by coaches, and coaches' interventions should be aimed at correcting errors and improving athletes' performances. Thus, coaches must be keenly in tune with each athlete's skill-set and, based on systematic task analyses, should be able to prescribe sport-specific drills accordingly. Since deliberate practice is physically and mentally taxing, performance coaches for late

adolescents and adults should help athletes negotiate these effort constraints by scheduling proper work-to-rest ratios and by encouraging athletes to find time for recovery (Young & Salmela 2002). Further, coaches should include supplementary training activities (e.g. weight, plyometric, aerobic training) that are aimed at improving sport-specific performance (Côté et al 2007b).

In competition, coaches of athletes in the investment years should promote situations that are likely to have a direct effect on their athletes' progress towards elite performance in their main sport and their personal development. Although competition is not the most important activity to improve performance in all sports, competitive situations are critical for the development of perceptual and decision-making skills, skill execution, and physical fitness in many sports (Baker et al 2003). Furthermore, through competitive situations that lead to winning or losing, athletes have the opportunities to develop their 4Cs by gaining social reinforcement and confidence, increasing their perceived competence, developing their character and relationships, and caring for others.

From an organisational perspective, coaches should surround each athlete with the physical and social resources they will need to overcome the effort and motivational constraints associated with deliberate practice. Coaches should recognise that their relationship with an athlete will likely change during the investment years, often becoming more collaborative, less top-down in nature, and relying on more continuous interchange of ideas between the coach and the athlete (Kalinowski 1985, Côté & Sedgwick 2003). Coaches should encourage athletes to commit fully to their one sport on a year-round basis, and the rigorous training that is demanded. However, coaches should also try to encourage athletes to stay involved in a small amount of deliberate play activities so that they are reminded of the intrinsic enjoyment that results from sport participation. Coaches could also encourage their athletes to participate in another sport in the off-season for relaxation or cross-training purposes. Finally, coaches should acknowledge and respect that their athletes are sacrificing other life opportunities for their one sport, and thus should make efforts to promote the benefits of such an investment rather than the costs associated with it.

The effectiveness of coaches during the investment years lies in their specific knowledge of the sport and the way they transmit that knowledge in training and in competition. By demonstrating enthusiasm in training and fostering a training environment that nurtures athletes' learning and motivation, coaches create a positive training environment, as illustrated in this quote by an international level rower:

> I think a coach that is willing to be in training at 5:30 in the morning and always be there is a big motivator for an athlete. It makes a big difference compared to a coach that sort of comes out maybe three or four times a week and doesn't really like coaching...I think if you see a coach that is willing to do everything that you are doing, it just makes that much more drive. I mean, you have to be down at practice because there is someone waiting for you... It's nice to have a coach that's as fully motivated as you.

(Sedgwick et al 1997)

Conclusion

This chapter highlights the coach's role in the development of athletes of different ages and competitive levels. The content of this chapter focuses on research that aligns athletes' outcomes, defined as the 4Cs, and associated recommended coaching practice. Four typologies of coaches initially suggested by Côté et al (2007b) were elaborated on: (a) participation coaches for children; (b) participation coaches for adolescents; (c) performance coaches for young adolescents; and (d) performance coaches for older adolescents and adults. These four generic types of coaches require distinct knowledge and skill sets to meet specific athletes' developmental needs. This suggests fundamental differences in the competencies that should be acquired for coaches working in different contexts (i.e., participation or performance, with young and older athletes). Therefore, coach education and training should be tailored to meet the specific experiential needs of individual coaches, given the context in which they coach.

It is also important to note that, in line with the sampling years of the DMSP (Côté & Fraser-Thomas 2007), we suggest that all children involved in sports between the ages of 6 and 12 should have coaches that focus on participation instead of performance, minimise competition and deliberate practice, and

emphasise involvement in various sports and deliberate play. This type of 'participation coach for children' builds a foundation of motivation and motor skills in children that can be translated into a sport participation or performance trajectory in the adolescent and adult years for most sports (Côté et al 2007b). In sports where peak performance occurs before maturation (e.g. women's gymnastics, figure skating) children may need to have performance coaches: however, there are costs such as dropout, burnout, and injuries associated with a performance environment in childhood (Baker & Côté 2006, Law et al 2007). Generally, problems will arise when a coach's knowledge and skills are associated with a context (e.g. a competitive performance model) that is incongruous with the contextual needs of the athletes (e.g., athletes in the recreational category). In most cases, coaching behaviours based on such incongruence will likely result in athletes' dissatisfaction, dropout, burnout, anxiety, or boredom, and a less than ideal sporting environment (Fraser-Thomas et al 2008a, 2008b).

Excellent coaches are aware of the necessity for congruence between their own knowledge and skills and a specific athlete's developmental needs including competitive level and age. A coach's behaviours in training, competition, and organisational settings should be in line with a specific athlete's competence, confidence, connection, and character needs (i.e., the 4Cs). Based on the literature on athletes' development in sport, we suggest that the 4Cs are universal needs that coaches of athletes of any competitive level or ages should strive to develop. However, a coach's ability to develop competence, confidence, connection, and character in athletes of different ages and competitive levels requires different types of knowledge, skills, and training. Each of the four typologies of coaches suggests different behaviours from coaches in training, competition, and organisation roles. In sum, this chapter underscores the importance of defining the athletes' development and coaching contexts, and the congruence between the two, in any discussion of coaching excellence.

References

Abraham, A., Collins, D., 1998. Examining and extending research in coach development. Quest 50, 59–79.

Alfermann, D., Stambulova, N., 2007. Career transitions and career termination. In: Tenenbaum, G.,

Eklund, R.C. (Eds.), Handbook of sport psychology. John Wiley & Sons, Hoboken, pp. 712–733.

Allen, J.B., 2003. Social motivation in youth sport. Journal of Sport and Exercise Psychology 25, 551–567.

Ames, C.A., 1992. Achievement goals, motivational climate, and motivational processes. In: Roberts, G.C. (Ed.), Motivation in sport and exercise. Human Kinetics, Champaign, pp. 161–176.

Baker, J., Côté, J., 2006. Shifting training requirements during athlete development: the relationship among deliberate practice, deliberate play and other sport involvement in the acquisition of sport expertise. In: Hackfort, G., Tenenbaum, G. (Eds.), Essential processes for attaining peak performance. Meyer & Meyer, Oxford, pp. 92–109.

Baker, J., Côté, J., Abernethy, B., 2003. Learning from the experts: practice activities of expert decision makers in sport. Res. Q. Exerc. Sport 74, 342–347.

Bandura, A., 1986. Social foundation of thought and action: a social cognitive theory. Prentice-Hall, Englewood Cliffs.

Bandura, A., Caprar, G.V., Barbanelli, C., et al., 2003. Role of affective self-regulatory efficacy in diverse spheres of psychosocial functioning. Child Dev. 74, 769–782.

Barber, B.K., Buehler, C., 1996. Family cohesion and enmeshment: different constructs, different effects. Journal of Marriage and the Family 58, 433–441.

Baumeister, R.F., Leary, M.R., 1995. The need to belong: desire for interpersonal attachments as a fundamental human motivation. Psychol. Bull. 117, 497–529.

Benson, P.L., Scales, P.C., Hamilton, S.F., et al., 2006. Positive youth development: theory, research, and applications. In: Damon, W., (series ed.), Lerner, R.M. (vol. ed.), Handbook of child psychology: Vol. 1. Theoretical models of human development. sixth ed. Wiley & Sons, New York, pp. 894–941.

Bergmann Drewe, S., 2000. An examination of the relationship between coaching and teaching. Quest 52, 79–88.

Black, S.J., Weiss, M.R., 1992. The relationship among perceived coaching behaviors, perceptions of ability and motivation in competitive age-group swimmers. Journal of Sport and Exercise Psychology 14, 309–325.

Bloom, B.S., 1985. Developing talent in young people. Ballantine, New York.

Botcheva, L.B., Feldman, S.S., Leiderman, P.H., 2002. Can stability in school processes offset the negative effects of sociopolitical

upheaval on adolescents' adaptation. Youth & Society 34, 55–88.

Bray, J.H., Gerald, A.J., Getz, J.G., et al., 2001. Developmental, family, and ethnic influences on adolescent usage: a growth curve approach. J. Fam. Psychol. 15, 301–314.

Bredemeier, B.J., Shields, D.L., 1984. The utility of moral stage analysis in the investigation of athletic aggression. Sociology of Sport Journal 1, 138–149.

Bredemeier, B.J., Shields, D.L., 1986. Moral growth among athletes and nonathletes: a comparative analysis. J. Genet. Psychol. 147, 7–18.

Bredemeier, B.J., Shields, D.L., 1996. Moral development and children's sport. In: Smoll, F.L., Smith, R.E. (Eds.), Children and youth sport: a biopsychosocial perspective. Brown & Benchmark, Chicago, pp. 381–404.

Broh, B.A., 2002. Linking extracurricular programming to academic achievement: who benefits and why? Sociology of Education 75, 69–91.

Chase, M.A., 1998. Sources of self-efficacy in physical education and sport. Journal of Teaching in Physical Education 18, 76–89.

Chelladurai, P., 1984. Leadership in sport. In: Silva, J.M., Weinberg, R.S. (Eds.), Psychological foundations of sport. Human Kinetics, Champaign, pp. 329–339.

Chelladurai, P., 2007. Leadership in sport. In: Eklund, R., Tenenbaum, G. (Eds.), Handbook of sport psychology. John Wiley, Hoboken, pp. 113–135.

Chelladurai, P., Reimer, H.A., 1998. Measurement of leadership in sport. In: Duda, J.L. (Ed.), Advances in sport and exercise psychology measurement. FIT, Morgantown, pp. 227–256.

Chelladurai, P., Saleh, S.D., 1980. Dimensions of leader behavior in sports: development of a leadership scale. Journal of Sport Psychology 2, 34–45.

Coakley, J.J., 1992. Burnout among adolescent athletes: a personal failure or social problem? Sociology of Sport Journal 9 (3), 271–285.

Coetzee, M., Viljoen, L., 2002. Reasons for youth participation in underwater hockey in South Africa. South African Journal for Research in

Sport, Physical Education and Recreation 24 (2), 13–22.

Côté, J., 1999. The influence of the family in the development of talent in sport. The Sport Psychologist 13, 395–417.

Côté, J., 2002. Coach and peer influence on children's development through sport. In: Silva, J.M., Stevens, D. (Eds.), Psychological foundations of sport. Allyn and Bacon, Boston, pp. 520–540.

Côté, J., 2006. The development of coaching knowledge. International Journal of Sports Science and Coaching 1 (3), 217–222.

Côté, J., 2007. Opportunities and pathways for beginners to elite to ensure optimum and lifelong involvement in sport. In: Hooper, S., Macdonald, D., Phillips, M. (Eds.), Junior sport matters: briefing papers for Australian junior sport. Australian Sports Commission, Belconnen.

Côté, J., Fraser-Thomas, J., 2007. Youth involvement in sport. In: Crocker, P. (Ed.), Sport psychology: a Canadian perspective. Pearson, Toronto, pp. 270–298.

Côté, J., Gilbert, W., 2007. Coaching and officiating for junior sport participants. In: Hooper, S., Macdonald, D., Phillips, M. (Eds.), Junior sport matters: briefing papers for Australian junior sport. Australian Sports Commission, Belconnen, pp. 49–60.

Côté, J., Salmela, J.H., 1996. The organizational tasks of high-performance gymnastics coaches. The Sport Psychologist 10 (3), 247–260.

Côté, J., Sedgwick, W., 2003. Effective behaviors of expert rowing coaches: a qualitative investigation of Canadian athletes and coaches. International Sports Journal 7, 62–78.

Côté, J., Salmela, J., Trudel, P., et al., 1995. The coaching model: a grounded assessment of expert gymnastic coaches' knowledge. Journal of Sport and Exercise Psychology 17 (1), 1–17.

Côté, J., Yardley, J., Hay, J., et al., 1999. An exploratory examination of the Coaching Behavior Scale for Sport. Avante 5, 82–92.

Côté, J., Baker, J., Abernethy, B., 2003. From play to practice: a developmental framework for the acquisition of expertise in team sports. In: Starkes, J., Ericsson, K.A. (Eds.), Expert performance in sports: advances in research on sport expertise. Human Kinetics, Champaign, pp. 89–110.

Côté, J., Baker, J., Abernethy, B., 2007a. Practice and play in the development of sport expertise. In: Eklund, R., Tenenbaum, G. (Eds.), Handbook of sport psychology. third ed. Wiley, Hoboken, pp. 184–202.

Côté, J., Young, B., North, J., et al., 2007b. Towards a definition of excellence in sport coaching. International Journal of Coaching Science 1 (1), 3–17.

Cushion, C.J., Armour, K.M., Jones, R.L., 2003. Coach education and continuing professional development: experience and learning to coach. Quest 55, 215–230.

Damon, W., 1984. Self-understanding and moral development from childhood to adolescence. In: Kurtines, W.M., Gerwirtz, J.L. (Eds.), Morality, moral behavior, and moral development. Wiley, New York.

Damon, W., 2004. What is positive youth development? Ann. Am. Acad. Pol. Soc. Sci. 591, 13–24.

Deci, E.L., Ryan, D.M., 1985. Instrinsic motivation and self-determination in human behavior. Plenum, New York.

Deci, E.L., Ryan, R.M., 2000. The "what" and "why" of goal pursuits: human needs and the self-determination of behaviour. Psychological Inquiry 11, 227–268.

Duda, J.L., 1993. Goals: a social-cognitive approach to the study of achievement motivation in sport. In: Singer, R.N., Murphy, M., Tennent, L.K. (Eds.), Handbook of research on sport psychology. Macmillan, New York, pp. 421–436.

Eccles, J.S., Barber, B.L., 1999. Student council, volunteering, basketball, or marching band: what kind of extracurricular involvement matters? Journal of Adolescent Research 14, 10–43.

Epstein, J., 1989. Family structures and student motivation: a developmental perspective. In: Ames, C., Ames, R. (Eds.), Research on motivation in education. Academic Press, New York, pp. 259–295.

Ericsson, K.A., 2003. Development of elite performance and deliberate practice: an update from the perspective of the expert performance approach. In: Starkes, J.L., Ericsson, K.A. (Eds.), Expert performance in sports: advances in research on sport expertise. Human Kinetics, Champaign, pp. 50–83.

Ericsson, K.A., Krampe, R.T., Tesch-Römer, C., 1993. The role of deliberate practice in the acquisition of expert performance. Psychol. Rev. 100 (3), 363–406.

Erickson, K., Côté, J., Fraser-Thomas, J., 2007. Sport experiences, milestones, and educational experiences associated with high performance coaches' development. The Sport Psychologist 21, 302–316.

Feltz, D.L., Chase, M.A., 1998. The measurement of self-efficacy and confidence in sport. In: Duda, J.L. (Ed.), Advances in sport and exercise psychology measurement. Fitness Information Technology, Morgantown, pp. 65–80.

Fraser-Thomas, J., Côté, J., Deakin, J., 2005. Youth sport programs: an avenue to foster positive youth development. Physical Education and Sport Pedagogy 10 (1), 19–40.

Fraser-Thomas, J., Côté, J., Deakin, J., 2008a. Examining adolescent sport dropout and prolonged engagement from a developmental perspective. Journal of Applied Sport Psychology 20, 318–333.

Fraser-Thomas, J., Côté, J., Deakin, J., 2008b. Understanding dropout and prolonged engagement in adolescent competitive sport. Psychology of Sport and Exercise 9, 645–662.

Gallagher, J.D., French, K.E., Thomas, K.T., et al., 2002. Expertise in youth sport: relations between knowledge and skill. In: Smoll, F.L., Smith, R.E. (Eds.), Children and youth in sport: a biopsychosocial perspective. Kendall/Hunt Publishing Company, Dubuque, pp. 475–500.

Gilbert, W., Trudel, P., 2000. Validation of the Coaching Model (CM) in a team sport context. International Sports Journal 4 (2), 120–128.

Gilbert, W.D., Trudel, P., 2004. Analysis of coaching science research published from 1970 to 2001. Res. Q. Exerc. Sport 75, 388–399.

Goncu, A., 1993. Development of intersubjectivity in the dyadic play of preschoolers. Early Childhood Research Quarterly 8, 99–116.

Gould, D., Carson, S., 2004. Fun and games? Myths surrounding the role of youth sports in developing Olympic champions. Youth Studies Australia 23 (1), 19–26.

Gould, D., Feltz, D., Weiss, M., 1985. Motives for participating in competitive youth swimming. International Journal of Sport Psychology 16, 126–140.

Gould, D., Hodge, K., Peterson, K., et al., 1987. Psychological foundations of coaching: similarities and differences among intercollegiate wrestling coaches. The Sport Psychologist 1, 293–308.

Gould, D., Udry, E., Tuffey, S., et al., 1996. Burnout in competitive tennis players: I. A quantitative psychological assessment. The Sport Psychologist 10, 322–340.

Gould, D., Dieffenbach, K., Moffett, A., 2002. Psychological characteristics and their development in Olympic champions. Journal of Applied Sport Psychology 14, 172–204.

Grove, J.R., Hanrahan, S.J., 1988. Perceptions of mental training needs by elite field hockey players and their coaches. The Sport Psychologist 2, 222–230.

Hall, C.R., Rodgers, W.M., 1989. Enhancing coaching effectiveness in figure skating through a mental skills training program. The Sport Psychologist 3, 142–154.

Hansen, D.M., Larson, R.W., 2007. Amplifiers of developmental and negative experiences in organized activities: dosage, motivation, lead roles, and adult–youth ratios. Journal of Applied Developmental Psychology 28, 360–374.

Harter, S., 1990. Causes, correlates, and the functional role of global self-worth: a lifespan perspective. In: Sternberg, J., Kolligian Jr., J. (Eds.), Competence considered. Yale University Press, New Haven, pp. 67–98.

Harter, S., 1999. The construction of the self: a developmental perspective. Guildford Press, New York.

Harwood, C., Spray, C., Keegan, R., 2008. Achievement goal theories in sport. In: Horn, T.S. (Ed.), Advances in sport psychology. third ed. Human Kinetics, Champaign, pp. 157–186.

Hays, K., Maynard, I., Thomas, O., et al., 2007. Sources and types of confidence identified by world class sport performers. Journal of Applied Sport Psychology 19, 434–456.

Hellison, D.R., 1995. Teaching personal and social responsibility through physical activity. Human Kinetics, Champaign.

Helsen, W.F., Starkes, J.L., Hodges, N.J., 1998. Team sports and the theory of deliberate practice. Journal of Sport and Exercise Psychology 20 (1), 12–34.

Hochstetler, D.R., 2003. Process and the sport experience. Quest 55, 231–243.

Hodge, T., Deakin, J., 1998. Deliberate practice and expertise in the martial arts: the role of context in motor recall. Journal of Sport and Exercise Psychology 20, 260–279.

Horn, T.S., 2004. Developmental perspectives on self-perceptions in children and adolescents. In: Weiss, M.R. (Ed.), Developmental sport and exercise psychology: a lifespan perspective. Fitness Information Technology, Morgantown, pp. 101–144.

Horn, T.S., Weiss, M.R., 1991. A developmental analysis of children's self-ability judgements in the physical domain. Pediatric Exercise Science 3, 310–326.

Igra, V., Irwin Jr., C.E., 1996. Theories of adolescent risk-taking behavior. In: DiClemente, J.R., Hansen, W.B., Ponton, L.E. (Eds.), Handbook of adolescent health-risk behavior. Plenum Press, New York, pp. 35–51.

Jarvien, D.W., Nicholls, J.D., 1996. Adolescents' social goals, beliefs about the causes of social success, and satisfaction in peer relations. Dev. Psychol. 32, 435–441.

Jelicic, H., Bobek, D.L., Phelps, E., et al., 2007. Using positive youth development to predict contribution and risk behaviors in early adolescence: findings from the first two waves of the 4-H study of positive youth development. International Journal of Behavioural Development 31, 263–273.

Jones, R.L., 2006. How can educational concepts inform sports coaching? In: Jones, R.L. (Ed.), The sports coach as educator. Routledge, Abingdon, pp. 3–13.

Jowett, S., 2005. On enhancing and repairing the coach–athlete relationship. In: Jowett, S., Jones, M.

(Eds.), The psychology of coaching. British Psychological Society, Leicester, pp. 14–26.

Jowett, S., 2007. Interdependence analysis and the 3 + 1 C's in the coach-athlete relationship. In: Jowett, D., Lavallee, D. (Eds.), Social psychology in sport. Human Kinetics, Champaign, pp. 15–28.

Jowett, S., Poczwardowski, A., 2007. Understanding the coach–athlete relationship. In: Jowett, S., Lavallee, D. (Eds.), Social psychology in sport. Human Kinetics, Champaign, pp. 3–13.

Kalinowski, A.G., 1985. The development of Olympic swimmers. In: Bloom, B.S. (Ed.), Developing talent in young people. Ballantine, New York, pp. 139–192.

Kaplan, T., 1996. Myths in the training of young athletes. Sports Medicine in Primary Care 2, 87–89.

Kavussanu, M., Ntousmanis, N., 2003. Participation in sport and moral functioning: does ego orientation mediate their relationship? Journal of Sport & Exercise Psychology 25, 501–518.

Klint, K.A., Weiss, M.R., 1986. Dropping in and dropping out: participation motives of current and former youth gymnasts. Can. J. Appl. Sport Sci. 11, 106–114.

Larson, R.W., 2000. Toward a psychology of positive youth development. Am. Psychol. 55, 170–183.

Larson, R.W., Verma, S., 1999. How children and adolescents spent time across the world: work, play, and developmental opportunities. Psychol. Bull. 125, 701–736.

LaVoi, N.M., 2004. Dimensions of closeness and conflict in the coach–athlete relationship. In: Paper presented at the meeting of the Association for the Advancement of Applied Sport Psychology, Minneapolis.

Law, M.P., Côté, J., Ericsson, K.A., 2007. Characteristics of expert development in rhythmic gymnastics: a retrospective study. International Journal of Sport and Exercise Psychology 5, 82–103.

Lemyre, P.N., Roberts, G.C., Ommundsen, U., 2001. Achievement goal orientations, perceived ability, and sportspersonship in youth soccer.

Journal of Applied Sport Psychology 14, 120–136.

Lerner, R.M., Fisher, C.B., Weinberg, R.A., 2000. Toward a science for and of the people: promoting civil society through the application of developmental science. Child Dev. 71, 11–20.

Lyle, J., 2002. Sports coaching concepts: a framework for coaches' behaviour. Routledge, London.

McCarthy, P.J., Jones, M.V., 2007. A qualitative study of sport enjoyment in the sampling years. The Sport Psychologist 21, 400–416.

McLellan, J.A., Pugh, M.J., 1999. The role of peer groups in adolescent society identity: exploring the importance of stability and change. Jossey-Bass, Stanford.

Maddux, J., 1995. Looking for common group: a comment on Bandura and Kirsch. In: Maddux, J. (Ed.), Self-efficacy, adaptation, and adjustment: theory, research and application. Plenum, New York, pp. 377–385.

Mahoney, J.L., 2000. School extracurricular activity participation as a moderator in the development of antisocial patterns. Child Dev. 71, 502–516.

Mallett, C., Côté, J., 2006. Beyond winning and losing: guidelines for evaluating high performance coaches. The Sport Psychologist 20, 213–218.

Martindale, R.J.J., Collins, D., Daubney, J., 2005. Talent development: a guide for practice and research within sport. Quest 57, 353–375.

Martindale, R.J.J., Collins, D., Abraham, A., 2007. Effective talent development: the elite coach perspective in UK sport. Journal of Applied Sport Psychology 19, 187–206.

Mecca, A.M., Smelser, N.J., Vascancellos, J. (Eds.), 1989. The social importance of self-esteem. University of California Press, Berkeley.

Micheli, L.J., Glassman, R., Klein, M., 2000. The prevention of sports injuries in children. Clin. Sports Med. 19 (4), 821–834.

Miller, B.W., Roberts, G.C., Ommundsen, Y., 2005. Effect of perceived motivational climate on moral functioning, team moral atmosphere perceptions, and the legitimacy of intentionally injurious acts among competitive youth football players. Psychology of Sport and Exercise 6, 461–477.

Munroe-Chandler, K., Hall, C., 2007. Sport psychology interventions. In: Crocker, P. (Ed.), Sport psychology: a Canadian perspective. Pearson, Toronto, pp. 184–213.

Newcomb, A.F., Bagwell, C.L., 1995. Children's friendship relations: a meta-analytic review. Psychol. Bull. 117, 306–347.

Ommundsen, Y., Roberts, G.C., Lemyre, P.N., et al., 2003. Perceived motivational climate in male youth soccer: relations to social-moral functioning, sportspersonship and team norm perceptions. Psychology of Sport and Exercise 4, 397–413.

Patrick, H., Ryan, A.M., Alfeld-Liro, C., et al., 1999. Adolescents' commitment to developing talent: the role of peers in continuing motivation for sports and the arts. Journal of Youth and Adolescence 28, 741–763.

Peterson, C., 2004. Positive social science. Ann. Am. Acad. Pol. Soc. Sci. 591, 186–201.

Petitpas, A.J., Cornelius, A.E., Van Raalte, J.L., et al., 2005. A framework for planning youth sport programs that foster psychosocial development. The Sport Psychologist 19, 63–80.

Poczwardowski, A., Barott, J.E., Jowett, S., 2006. Diversifying approaches to research on athlete–coach relationships. Psychology of Sport and Exercise 7, 125–142.

Raedeke, T.D., 1997. Is athlete burnout more than just stress? A sport commitment perspective. Journal of Sport & Exercise Psychology 19, 396–417.

Raedeke, T.D., Smith, A.L., 2004. Coping resources and athlete burnout: an examination of stress mediated and moderation hypotheses. Journal of Sport & Exercise Psychology 26, 525–541.

Rutten, E.A., Stams, G.J.J.M., Biesta, J.B., et al., 2007. The contribution of organized youth sport to antisocial and prosocial behavior in adolescent athletes. Journal of Youth and Adolescence 36, 255–264.

Ryan, R.M., Deci, E.L., 2000. Self-determination theory and the facilitation of intrinsic motivation,

social development, and well-being. Am. Psychol. 55, 68–78.

Salmela, J.H., 1996. Great job coach: getting the edge from proven winners. Potentium, Ottawa.

Scanlan, T.K., Carpenter, P.J., Lobel, M., et al., 1993. Sources of enjoyment for youth sport athletes. Pediatric Exercise Science 5, 275–285.

Sedgwick, W., Côté, J., Dowd, J., 1997. Confidence building strategies used by high-level rowing coaches. AVANTE 3 (3), 81–93.

Shields, D.L., Bredemeier, B.J., 1995. Character development and physical activity. Human Kinetics, Champaign.

Siegler, R., DeLoache, J., Eisenberg, N., 2003. How children develop. Worth, New York.

Smith, M.D., 1974. Significant others' influence on the assaultive behavior of young hockey players. International Review of Sport Sociology 3–4, 45–56.

Smith, A., 2007. Youth peer relationships in sport. In: Jowett, S., Lavallee, D. (Eds.), Social psychology in sport. Human Kinetics, Champaign, pp. 41–53.

Smith, R.E., Smoll, F.L., 2002. Way to go, coach! A scientifically-proven approach to coaching effectiveness, second ed. Warde, Portola Valley.

Smith, R.E., Smoll, F.L., 2007. Social-cognitive approach to coaching behaviors. In: Jowett, S., Lavallee, D. (Eds.), Social Psychology in Sport. Human Kinetics, Champaign, pp. 75–90.

Smith, R.E., Smoll, F.L., Hunt, B., 1977. A system for the behavioral assessment of athletic coaches. Res. Q. 48, 401–407.

Smith, R.E., Smoll, F.L., Curtis, B., 1979. Coach effectiveness training: a cognitive-behavioral approach to enhancing relationship skills in youth sport coaches. Journal of Sport Psychology 1, 59–75.

Smoll, F.L., Smith, R.E., 1989. Leadership behaviors in sport: a theoretical model and research paradigm. Journal of Applied Social Psychology 19, 1522–1551.

Smoll, F.L., Smith, R.E., 2002. Coaching behavior research and intervention in youth sports. In: Smoll, F.L., Smith, R.E. (Eds.), Children and youth in sport: a biopsychosocial perspective. Kendall/Hunt Publishing Company, Dubuque, pp. 211–233.

Stephens, D.E., 2000. Predictors of aggressive tendencies in girls' basketball: an examination of beginning and advanced participants in a summer skills camp. Res. Q. Exerc. Sport 72, 257–266.

Stephens, D.E., Bredemeier, B.J.L., Shields, D.L.L., 1997. Construction of a measure designed to assess players' descriptions and prescriptions for moral behavior in youth sport soccer. International Journal of Sport Psychology 28, 370–390.

Strachan, L., MacDonald, D., Fraser-Thomas, J., Côté, J., 2008. Youth sport: talent, socialisation, and development. In: Fisher, R., Bailey, R. (Eds.), Perspectives: Volume 9. Talent identification and development – The search for sporting excellence. H&P Druck, Germany, pp. 201–216.

Treasure, D.C., 2001. Enhancing young people's motivation in youth sport: an achievement goal approach. In: Roberts, G.C. (Ed.), Advances in motivation in sport and exercise. Human Kinetics, Champaign, pp. 79–100.

Tremblay, M.S., Katzmaryzk, P.T., Willms, J.D., 2002. Temporal trends in overweight and obesity in Canada 1981–1996. Int. J. Obes. 26, 538–543.

Urdan, T.C., Maehr, M.L., 1995. Beyond a two-goal theory of motivation and achievement: a case for social goals. Review of Educational Research 65, 213–243.

Vealey, R.S., Chase, M.A., 2008. Self-confidence in sport. In: Horn, T. (Ed.), Advances in sport psychology. Human Kinetics, Champaign, pp. 65–97.

Wagner, W.G., 1996. Facilitating optimal development in adolescence. The Counseling Psychologist 24, 357–359.

Walton, G.M., 1992. Beyond winning: the timeless wisdom of great philosopher coaches. Human Kinetics, Champaign, IL.

Weiss, M.R., 1993. Children's participation in physical activity: are we having fun yet? Pediatric Exercise Sciences 5, 205–209.

Weiss, M.R., Ebbeck, V., 1996. Self-esteem and perceptions of competence in youth sport: theory, research and enhancement strategies. In: Bar-Or, O. (Ed.), The encyclopedia of sports medicine, vol. VI: the child and adolescent athlete. Blackwell Science, Oxford, pp. 364–382.

Weiss, M.R., Ferrer-Caja, E., 2002. Motivational orientations and sport behaviour. In: Horn, T. (Ed.), Advances in sport psychology. second ed. Human Kinetics, Champaign, pp. 101–184.

Weiss, M.R., Smith, A.L., 2002a. Friendship quality in youth sport: relationship to age, gender, and motivation variables. Journal of Sport and Exercise Psychology 24, 420–437.

Weiss, M.R., Smith, A.L., 2002b. Moral development in sport & physical activity: theory, research, and intervention. In: Horn, T. (Ed.), Advances in sport psychology. second ed. Human Kinetics, Champaign, pp. 243–280.

Weiss, M.R., Stuntz, C.P., 2006. A little friendly competition: peer relationships and psychosocial development in youth sport and physical activity contexts. In:

Weiss, M. (Ed.), Developmental sport and exercise psychology: a lifespan perspective text. Fitness Information Technology, Morgantown, pp. 165–196.

Weiss, M.R., Williams, L., 2004. The *why* of youth sport involvement: a developmental perspective on motivational processes. In: Weiss, M.R. (Ed.), Developmental sport and exercise psychology: a lifespan perspective. Fitness Information Technology, Morgantown, pp. 223–268.

Weiss, M.R., Smith, A.L., Theeboom, M., 1996. "That's what friends are for": children's and teenagers perceptions of peer relationships in the sport domain. Journal of Sport & Exercise Psychology 18, 347–379.

Weiss, M.R., Ebbeck, V., Horn, T.S., 1997. Children's self-perceptions and sources of competence information: a cluster analysis. Journal of Sport & Exercise Psychology 19, 52–70.

Weiss, M.R., Smith, A.L., Stuntz, C.P., 2007. Moral development in sport & physical activity. In: Horn, T. (Ed.), Advances in sport psychology. third

ed. Human Kinetics, Champaign, pp. 187–210.

Wentzel, K., 1998. Social relationships and motivation in middle school: the role of parents, teachers, and peers. J. Educ. Psychol. 90, 202–209.

Wiersma, L.D., 2000. Risks and benefits of youth sport specialization: perspectives and recommendations. Pediatric Exercise Science 12, 13–22.

Wylleman, P., De Knop, P., Verdet, M., et al., 2007. Parenting and career transitions of elite athletes. In: Jowett, D., Lavallee, D. (Eds.), Social psychology in sport. Human Kinetics, Champaign, pp. 233–247.

Young, B.W., Salmela, J.H., 2002. Perceptions of training and deliberate practice of middle distance runners. International Journal of Sport Psychology 33 (2), 167–181.

Zarbatany, L., Ghesquire, K., Mohr, K., 1992. A context perspective on early adolescents' friendship expectations. Journal of Early Adolescence 12, 111–126.

Planning for team sports

6

John Lyle

Introduction

There can be little doubt that planning should be a central feature of the coaching process and of coaches' practice. This is true both of the single session within the short-term introductory programme and of the multi-year major games preparation cycle. In fact, planning has come to have a taken-for-granted place in coach education, analyses of practice, and prescriptions for good practice. When coaches have been asked to identify the most significant elements in the coaching process, a number of studies have confirmed the central role of planning (Gould 1990, Lyle 1992).

It is important to ask why a focus on planning is important. The context is the emerging and ongoing debate about the nature of the coaching process and the extent to which coaching behaviours and decisions are based firmly on planned interventions or more problematically subject to such a dynamic and 'messy' environment that there is a high level of contingency and immediate originality (Jones & Wallace 2005, Cushion et al 2006). This debate focuses not only on questions about how planning might take place, but also on what 'can be planned for'. Recently, Cushion (2007a) has argued that coaching expertise has 'limited roots' in planning or reason, and I have countered that there is a strong foundation of planned intervention (Lyle 2007), albeit subject to what I would argue is the everyday applied expertise of the coach in managing the vagaries of intervention. I have pointed out that there may be a difference between individual sports, particularly those that are not 'circuit' (an extended series of tournaments of events) or league sports, in

which the planning intention may be more systematically applied, and team sports, in which the complexity of the process presents further challenges. Cushion's rejoinder (2000b) was that there is a need for more evidence that has been derived 'from' practice in order to improve our understanding as a precursor to prescription. This implicitly draws a distinction between building a model 'of' practice, one that is based on evidence of coaches' practice, and a model 'for' practice that is more derivative and prescriptive. This chapter is a result of the quest to base an understanding of planning behaviour in team sports on evidence from coaches' 'real time' experiences. One of the key characteristics of this enquiry is that it was based on planning processes that had been identified in advance, applied over the course of the season, and subject to reflection.

At this stage it is necessary to clarify a number of assumptions. First, the focus within the chapter is on 'planning the intervention', that is, the training and competition programme directed by the coach towards identified targets and goals. Second, this is not a question of 'systematic coaching' versus 'structured improvisation' (Cushion et al 2003) as some of the literature has mistakenly labelled the debate. There may be some sports in which the planning intentions and intervention practice are unproblematically similar, and there are relatively few factors that interfere with a tightly planned and principled athlete workload. However, depending on the context, we might assume that coaching delivery requires an active process in which coaches make an almost continuous series of decisions about the most appropriate conduct and progression of the intervention in the context of a set of individual, group and organisational goals. This management of content and momentum is not the sole prerogative of the coach, but for the sake of simplicity, we can use this shorthand and assume that some of the decision making involves the players/athletes and other coaching personnel. Common sense tells us that often the conduct of the intervention will match the detailed intentions of the planning process, and at other times the coach will depart from the plan, or perhaps operate within more flexible guidelines. The vagaries of human effort, emotions, and motives, the response to training stimuli, the diverse interpretations of the technical model, and the complex interactions of team sport performance each and all combine to create a dynamic coaching environment. This may have contributed to a lack of coaching research focused on planning.

There is an absolute dearth of literature examining the planning process in coaching in any rigorous or conceptual way. To sports scientists applying, for example, physiological research and consequent principles to training schedules this may seem overstated. However, to understand this we have to look at how planning 'knowledge' has been developed and to appreciate the language or discourse that has developed around it. Planning to improve performance was subject to the application of 'training theory' (Schmolinsky et al 1983, Dick 1997). It is not a coincidence that each of these authors was focused on athletics. The training principles were primarily derived from principles of physical conditioning and underpinned by exercise physiology. They applied most readily to sports in which the outcomes were determined by energy outputs (and technique). Intricate and sophisticated cyclical combinations of volume, intensity and duration of training were prescribed, and a great deal of attention was paid to peaking for maximum performance. Sports-specific literature identified different coaches' approaches to the most appropriate balance and manipulation of performance factors (for example, in swimming, Councilman 1968). Perhaps the most significant influence was the work of Tudor Bompa (Bompa 1999). He provided a catalogue of 'menus' under the general rubric of 'periodisation'. Bompa's work also referred to team sport planning. General principles were provided that suggested a balance of technical, tactical and physical components in pre- and competition cycles. Although this 'bio-scientific driver' for coaching practice was based on sound principles, it might be argued that it was often

divorced from application, and contributed to a formulaic approach to some aspects of intervention. In some sports it may also have created a 'separateness' between physical conditioning and coaching.

The term periodisation has come to be synonymous with planning, although it will be clear later in the chapter that there is a tendency for this to be conceptualised in its diagrammatic form, rather than as a planning process. Within periodisation the preparation and competition programmes and training contents are shaped (normally) by the competition schedule, and the plan operates on the premise that the optimum performance will be facilitated by a cyclical, progressive, incremental, and selective attention to interdependent components of performance. The extent to which this framework needs to be amended as objectives change or the environment changes, and the extent to which daily or weekly planning is derived directly from this plan are problematic issues for team sports. There are unresolved issues about the optimum length of the planning period and whether (some) team sports are susceptible to detailed content planning. This refers to the fact that sports with a high level of performer interaction (the 'invasion sports') and significant degrees of freedom in execution may find it difficult to identify and regulate 'loading factors' (volume and intensity of practice).

There are also obvious questions for the researcher about how planning can be 'represented', how coaching's multiple objectives can be reconciled, whether or not 'plans' can be compared, and how the coaching context can be given a weighting. As a result, we have a planning 'literature' that is sports-specific, driven by physical conditioning, more obviously applied to individual sports, and based on prescription rather than research. There is remarkably little about planning in the refereed journals – perhaps a reflection of a lack of conceptual or theoretical depth. It tends to be dealt with in books and in coach education materials. This is in part a function of the methodological challenges in demonstrating comparative effectiveness and in experimenting with such a complex mix of planning variables, particularly over extended periods of time. There may also be an element of coaches not wishing to share more widely the detail of their plans. One of the most obvious factors is that the planning process and the success of the outcomes are likely to be influenced by the intensity of and commitment to the preparation process by players. Without prejudging our conclusions, it seems inevitable that the different coaching 'domains' (Lyle 2002, Trudel & Gilbert 2006) will demand different approaches to planning. Whether or not the planning prerequisites (evidence rich, clear goals, technical model, sufficient duration) are in place may become clearer as the planning models emerge.

The aim of this chapter

This chapter process specifically for team examines the planning process for team sports coaches. In particular it identifies the lessons to be learned from the planning practice of experienced rugby union coaches. I suggest that there is relatively little merit in treating planning as a generic or abstract process, other than to identify planning principles in a context-less fashion. To progress the field, we need the detail-rich experiences of coaches who exercised a measure of accountability for the plans they were executing. It needs to be made clear that the chapter is not about the technical matters that form the foundation of the planning content. The emphasis is on the process that coaches engage with in their planning and the range of planning models that emerge from the coaches' practice. The substance of the chapter is derived from an analysis of the planning intentions, implementation and subsequent reflections on a season's planning by coaches who were taking part in the Rugby Football Union's Level 4 coach education programme (this is the highest of four levels of coach education and is designed for experienced coaches). The author delivered a workshop for coaches on this course; part of the process was that coaches had to prepare plans for the coming season. These were submitted and feedback was given on some of the issues that might arise. The coaches implemented their plans, and prepared a summary document that reflected on the season's planning and the lessons they had learned. The author received these reports and provided feedback (permission was received from the Coaching Development Manager at the Rugby Football Union to use these coach education submissions for analysis. I'm very grateful to the RFU and to the coaches concerned).

The purpose of the chapter is to contribute to the literature available on this element of coaches' practice by describing models of coaches' planning in a team sport, and discussing the issues that arise in their implementation. The first part of the chapter presents an overview of planning principles. This is intended to create a vocabulary and a context for the rugby union coaches' practices. This part of the chapter is derived from the author's experience as a coach and a coach educator, and the 'working' of this material over many years. This is followed by the analysis and interpretation of the rugby union coaches' planning reflections.

The planning process in coaching

Planning for coaching implies a degree of pre-determination of preparation and an accounting for the consequences of actions over a given period of time. The underlying premise is that benefits can be achieved from the accumulation, integration, sequencing and aggregation of the various elements of preparation for performance; in addition, that this management of the intervention process is necessary for these benefits to be achieved effectively and efficiently. One way of conceptualising the coaching process is to recognise the intention to reduce chance and the unpredictability of performance, and that this requires the harmonisation of the contributory elements of the process. If we accept that there is an intentional aspect to achieving this (and undirected practice is unlikely to lead to optimum progress), planning becomes a prerequisite for coaching, although the practice of planning will be shown to vary enormously in its application.

Planning like coaching more broadly cannot be presumed to be unproblematic. The coaching process operates in an unstable environment, performance is made up of a challenging range of components, there are often multiple goals, and these are contested by others. Jones (2006) sums this up by suggesting that coaches and athletes often work with unattainable goals in a context in which they are not fully in control of all the factors involved. Interactive team sports are a particular subset of the coaching process and bring their own challenges for the planner.

A schematic of the planning process is provided in order to establish the vocabulary and illustrate something of the issues involved in planning (Figure 6.1). As the evidence from rugby will further demonstrate there are a number of options in how planning is conceived of and used, and these are determined by a series of largely contextual matters. Planning can range from the episodic (session by session approach) to integrated cyclical planning using a training principles-informed periodisation. The session or phase of sessions may also be characterised by the level of

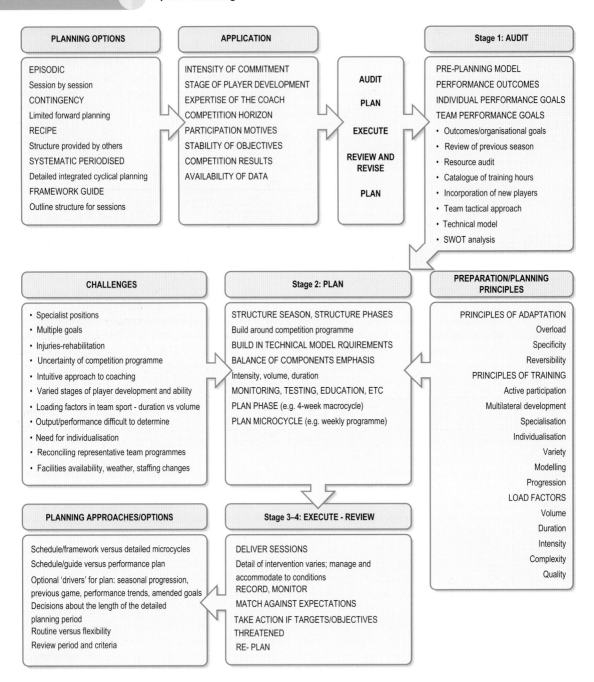

Figure 6.1 • A schematic of the planning process

contingency involved (ranging from the completely 'seat of the pants', to a guiding structure, and to detailed training workloads). An additional layer of analysis is provided by a continuum from 'recipe planning' to continual redevelopment and innovation. Recipe planning implies the use of existing or 'borrowed' session plans from published sources, sport-specific technical materials, fellow coaches, or the coach's own repertoire. Coaches may elect to employ a combination of these variations as a matter of habit, education, situated learning, rational choice, pragmatism or ideology.

Nevertheless, it is possible to identify a range of contributory factors, most of which emanate from the scope and scale of the coaching process. An intensity of engagement (with a requirement for planning over the longer term, and preparation for specific games/competitions) can be gauged from a combination of the stage of player development, participation motives, and intensity of commitment. Data follow from continual monitoring and evaluation of performance, and the presence or absence of detailed performance data will ultimately limit the range of planning and planning implementation practices.

Planning procedures

The most basic and often-cited process in coaching is described as 'plan–do–review'. This is a useful reminder that planning is important and that it is an iterative and cyclical process. A more elaborate description would be 'audit, plan, execute, review and revise, execute'. This cyclical process implies that there is a strategic blueprint that is subject to revision, and that the implementation of the coaching process is being monitored and fed back into the planning process at regular intervals. In this case, the plan itself may be a guiding template or a more detailed predetermination of activity.

The audit stage involves identifying the extent of the intervention programme (this is termed the pre-planning model in which the number of hours are identified), the existing feedback on performance, individuals' progress from the previous season, and the goals for the coming season. These goals or objectives provide a direction for the planning but have to be understood in the context of longer-term ambitions, changes of personnel, re-interpretation of the performance model, and the anticipated performance demands implied by the goals (how will we need to play to achieve our outcome goals and what does that mean for individual players). The audit stage is important, partly to understand subsequent changes to the conditions, and partly because detail (e.g. total coaching hours, individual goals) is often assumed, rather than specified. This stage also assumes an extensive (relative to context) knowledge and awareness of technical matters, of the likely opposition, and of the players. The audit should embrace the coaching and support staff, organisational resources, known competition markers, facilities, equipment, and other building blocks. Coaching effectiveness and expectation about outcomes need to be understood in relation to the planning audit. The interesting issue is the extent to which these 'conditions' can be influenced or altered by the coach. Coaches' accountability and employment may be based on outcomes that are influenced by conditions about which the coach has limited control. The coach may control training content, game preparation and intensity of preparation, in addition to awareness of the environment. However, there will be less control over personnel, organisational goals, resources, and competitor progress.

The next part of the planning process is the design of the coaching intervention. This is often represented in diagrammatic form and this 'plan' has come to be symbolic of the planning function. It should be noted, however, that there are many important steps before this stage, and, assuming that planning is an active process, a continuous process of implementation, review, and re-planning. Our purpose at this point is merely to outline the planning process and not to construct a primer on design and content. The illustrative examples from the rugby coaches will identify some of their planning practice.

The season's plan is usually built around the competition programme, although there may be some adjustments as a result of additional or delayed fixtures. This provides a simple differentiation into pre-season (or preparatory), competition season, and post-season (or 'off'). However, there are many potential variations. The pre-season will typically be characterised by an emphasis on physical preparation with technical work remaining high in terms of volume and tactical preparation moving from general to specific and gradually assuming greater importance. This phase is also characterised by 'pre-season games'. These are an opportunity for rehearsal, experimentation and a gradual development of readiness for competition. Coaches will often differ in their approach to this menu of games. The competition season may be quite extensive and there is merit in dividing it into sub-phases. This may be assisted by mid-season breaks, by cup competitions, by representative matches, or by a particular series of (perceived) difficult and less-difficult games. These sub-phases are important because they can provide a framework for physical preparation which itself needs to be periodised.

The subdivision of each of the phases creates a series of macrocycles, for example, the first half of a season, say 12–16 weeks, which is then divided into mesocycles of, perhaps, 4 weeks. These mesocycles are then divided into smaller planning units – usually one week microcycles. At various stages the plan will be populated by testing/monitoring dates, medical screening, review periods and so on. However, the implication from planning in this integrated and sophisticated way is that the physical, technical and tactical (and to some extent psychological) components will differ in their character and content in each phase. However, they are inter-dependent, both from one cycle to another, and on the other components. The training interventions will manipulate volume, duration, intensity and complexity, according to training prescriptions. The various energy systems are similarly balanced, and the coach's technical model is rehearsed and developed. There is an assumption that longer- and shorter-term needs are being accommodated within the plan.

For some team coaches this attempt to create an integrated plan, with its high level of detail on workloads may seem like an unattainable or undesirable process. Nevertheless, it provides a set of expectations against which we can contrast the coaches' practice. It should not be assumed, however, that the planning process as described here is unproblematic. The following list of confounding factors will not only apply to all coaches but also in concert create a dynamic environment, which makes it difficult both to prescribe training content and to evaluate its effectiveness:

- The need to deal with specialist position within teams and the consequent demands on performance components.
- The complex interaction of individual, team and organisational goals over the longer- and short-term.
- The inevitability that many goals will become unattainable as the season progresses.
- Player availability in terms of injury, rehabilitation, illness, re-location, transfers, retirement (and by implication the absorption of new players).
- Changes to the competition programme may be weather postponements, extended success in cup competitions, or simply fixture congestion. It may be possible to plan for some of these possibilities.
- Team sports will inevitably have a mixture of player abilities and stages of development. This will impact significantly on physical preparation and the technical model, and may be problematic for attempts to individualise the programmes.

- There is a tendency in team sports to operate technical and tactical drills through duration (number of minutes) rather than volume of repetitions. This acknowledges the complexity of team drills, a skills-acquisition model that builds on variation, the challenge of controlling the demand/'feed'/environment, and the individualisation of needs. The inescapability of this is that training loads are not pre-determined with any precision.
- In the majority of team sports there is a 'quality of outcome' issue in that performance is relative, in terms of opposition, level of challenge, and player capacity. This provides a measure of difficulty for the coach in evaluating progress.
- A specific issue is the need to integrate the preparation and development needs of the individual in relation to representative team requirements and those of the club. This may be most evident when representative team tournaments are played 'out of season'.
- A number of very practical issues may impact without notice – weather conditions, facility availability, equipment, funding.
- Although this will apply not only to team coaches, the schedule is determined by the fixture list, rather than the player or team's progression and performance readiness. This is perhaps best illustrated in the need to attend to specific rather than general preparation, no matter the players' level of performance.

These factors may seem simply to be a catalogue of potential barriers to the planning process. However, when taken together they point to a planning (and implementation) process that is characterised by constant manipulation of competing demands, a highly contingent set of responses and requirements, a 'performance' that is dependent on a complex aggregation of components, and very individual requirements from players. When this is combined with the immediacy of (and trends in) results, day-to-day interpersonal communication, and the players' and club's emotional reactions to perceived success and failure, the outcome is a highly charged, technically demanding and complex, and coach-dependent environment. In these circumstances, it is possible to understand why the level of 'control' (conceptualised as the management of the process and not the direction of individuals) becomes an issue. The difficulty of implementing a seemingly systematic process and plan may be greeted by a more (seemingly) intuitive, contingent approach, either through design, collective practice, or response to the magnitude of the challenge.

It is partly for these reasons that the delivery stage, that is, the coach's intervention practice becomes so difficult to describe, and why recording and analysing the rugby coaches' experiences has been such a valuable exercise. However, merely from conceptualising intervention practice in relation to the planning process, it is possible to identify a number of features of the coaches' intervention that will impact on planning. These might be couched as action decisions relative to content, scheduling, progression, momentum and coach intervention, and informed by goals, targets, feedback, interaction with players, and continuous evaluation and re-evaluation, in ways that we find difficult to describe. It seems likely that once the meso-cycle plans have been translated into microcycle plans and the weekly microcycle has been translated into a variety of activities (or the session has been arrived at in a less-integrated fashion) these activities will be implemented as planned, unless (a) significant change in the constituent elements (player availability, injury, weather) takes place, (b) the immediate activity within the session provokes a change of plan, or (c) the progress is judged (by players and coach) to be unsatisfactory and necessitates a review. In the 'layer' above this, any threat to the team or individual goals will provoke a review. This is most likely to be linked to match results, but in situations in which the technical model is the driver (for example, in 'academy' sport), a continuous process of comparison to a set of technical expectations may bring about a re-think.

These delivery issues highlight the need for constant monitoring and review, and in intervention terms, the coach's capacity to make appropriate responses to what becomes a messy set of transactions. This description of the planning process has provided a vocabulary for what follows; it has also pointed us in the direction of a number of likely issues:

- The role of the 'plan' as a schedule, a framework, or a stage in the determination of detailed workloads.
- The purpose of the 'plan' as a schedule of delivery units, or an integrated framework of training workloads. The inference might be drawn that the greater the 'skeleton' approach, the greater the reliance on the coach's immediacy of management of the intervention.
- The balance of objectives-led medium-term activity versus short-term responses to prior

performances/results and consequent preparation for the next performance.

- In the light of experience of being subject to highly contingent 'drivers', the coach's reaction may be to reduce the breadth of the planning period to the most manageable proportions.
- It may be difficult for coaches, and players in particular, to cope with constant change. Does this suggest a reliance on routine?

Planning in rugby union

What follows is an analysis of the planning behaviours of rugby union coaches taking part in the coach education programme described earlier. The coaches were asked to submit their planning documentation for the coming season, with sufficient explanation to permit an interpretation of their intentions. The author commented on the documentation and offered some advice on the questions they might ask themselves while reflecting on their implementation of the plans over the season. The student coaches subsequently submitted an analysis of their season's planning, with a reflection on the issues to arise from implementation. Comments were fed back on the quality of the reflection and on the issues that arose. These comments focused on generic planning matters, rather than sport-specific technical content, and as a consequence offer valuable insights into planning more generally.

The coaches varied in their length of coaching experience. The majority were former (many international) players, who were fulfilling roles as head coaches or coaches in the top three divisions of English rugby union. A significant number were coaches within the rugby academies (squads of younger players identified as potentially having the qualities required to become contracted players) of top full-time professional teams. The analysis that follows is derived from that documentation and the author's feedback to the coaches.

The broad picture

All coaches presented season-long planning documents, almost exclusively structured around the competition programme. The principles of periodisation were evident in all plans. Coaches differentiated between the pre-season preparation period(s) and the competition season; with few exceptions, the competition period was further divided into macro- (6–12 weeks) and/or meso-cycles (4–6 weeks). The 'shape' of the plan followed the team sport plans exemplified in Bompa (1994). The general approach to presentation and structure reflects the content of planning elements in coach education, and examples given in relevant materials.

There was mixed practice in the level of detail provided about content priorities. The more sophisticated plans made attempts to describe relative volumes and intensities within cycles. This detail was often absent. Nevertheless, a structured and coordinated pattern of 'rugby elements', often divided into technical and tactical content, demonstrated that the principles of aggregation and reinforcement of rugby-specific content were being adhered to. It was evident in most of the plans that the underlying driver for structuring the plan (other than the competition programme) was the strength and conditioning requirements. We will find later that this was one of the contributory factors leading to limited implementation by many coaches. The physical conditioning content was outlined in such a way that it was clear that good practice training theory principles were being adhered to. The problem of an extended competition season was addressed through periods of lower intensities, revisiting pre-season-type conditioning, and in effect creating double- or triple-periodised seasons.

The comments received from coaches provided evidence that multi-year development and improvement in performance and results was a constant factor, particularly for those teams seeking to move to a higher division or consolidate within that division. However, there was little evidence of this in their plans, and an immediacy of results permeated their implementation and evaluation of the plans. One notable feature of the coaches' implementation behaviour was that there was very limited re-planning. It was often recognised that the original assumptions on which the plans were based had changed. This was most often an awareness that objectives were threatened by results to date, but could also be the impact of new players, players' response to training, rethinking tactics, changes to coaching teams, and so on. The evidence was very strong that such a realisation would lead to a series of short-term measures, almost quick-fix responses, rather than revision of plans in a more comprehensive fashion. A rule of thumb was that objectives were reconsidered after about 6 weeks of the competition season, about which time it became clear that for some teams pre-season objectives were seriously threatened. The comments of the coaches suggest that (almost in spite of the evidence) renewed efforts were made to retrieve these goals rather than set new (perhaps 'lower') goals.

The content itself (description of player activity) was described in terms of different elements of the game (line outs, scrums, defensive lines and so on) and the individuals' performance (tackling, movement, decision choices). There was a good deal of consensus among the coaches in the use of terminology, and it was clear that the sport had promoted such a technical model. The detailed plans were sometimes treated as confidential, but the associated workshop demonstrated that technical and tactical options were widely understood and debated. The coaches' commentaries often focused on issues that impacted on technical development: for example, the interplay between players' physical and technical capabilities, preferred 'ways of playing', what was needed to overcome stronger or equally matched opposition, the extent to which such choices could be stabilised in the time available, and the impact of losing players to injury or weather and other environmental changes.

One question that was rarely addressed well in the coaches' own reflections, but was considered when prompted, was 'how content was devised from the plans'. The common pattern was for coaches to provide an outline plan, to 'flesh out' a monthly schedule, and to devise more detailed content in weekly or microcycle units. The seasonal plan, and even the monthly plan, was used as a guide, but when pressed, coaches seemed to make relatively limited use of these prompts. The mesocycle plans (usually 4 weeks) acted as schedules or organisational prompts with only fairly broad indications of training content. The detail was most often devised on a weekly basis. As the more detailed descriptions of planning behaviour will show, the implementation was highly contingent; that is, a very dynamic set of circumstances required some flexibility in both planning and implementation. The drills and exercises themselves, and the applied knowledge that accompanied them, were a reflection of the coaches' accumulated experience and immersion in the technical aspects of the sport. In practice, implementation behaviour reinforced the apparently intuitive nature of the coach's delivery.

Part-time and full-time coaching

The coaches in the sample were a mix of full-time head coaches, full-time academy coaches, and head coaches of teams that did not consist of full-time professional players, but in which many, if not most, players received some remuneration. The distinguishing feature was that teams trained on a full-time basis, or on (generally) two evenings per week during the season. As might be expected this distinction had a profound impact on the coach's planning. Although not wishing to make any analysis sound negative, a comparison of the non-full-time coaching environments to those offered in a full-time preparation context highlighted their limitations. In 'part-time' planning, there was some doubt about the value of training load determination since there was no real linkage with other sessions in any progressive sense. Indeed, the pressure of time meant that 'content' was squeezed into the time available. It was not unusual for one of the sessions to be devoted to fitness and the other to 'rugby'. In such a context, there was very limited attention to individuals' skills and development.

In the part-time context there was always an accompanying physical conditioning programme, often led by a specialist conditioning coach. However, the coaches admitted that monitoring of this was minimal and players were self-driven in their adherence to the programme. The overall picture was that in-season fitness training was a 'maintenance' programme, with some recognition, perhaps in the middle of the season that some increased attention was warranted (and may on some occasions have been prompted by a negative pattern of results). This placed greater emphasis on the pre-season period, and this was generally more intensive, and planned in greater detail. The pre-season period was reported by the coaches to have 'gone to plan' more often than not. This is perhaps not surprising since there are fewer distractions, fewer injured players, fixtures are (usually) planned in advance, there is less pressure on results, and with fewer games, there is more 'training' time.

Despite some of the differences highlighted here, there were some elements of common practice to emerge. There was value in a review of progress every 4 weeks or so, even where progress was difficult to measure. The process itself requires the coach to engage with the notion of progress markers and performance analysis. The measurement of progress was most often related to the ongoing sequence of results. In the same way, the planning of the week's preparation was informed by performance in the previous game and preparation for the forthcoming game. In addition to any specific focus, there was a continuous reinforcement of key areas; in other words, those fundamental aspects of performance received attention most weeks. The intensity of training was perceived by the coaches to be 'high', perhaps because of a 'cramming' caused by limited training time.

Academy coaching

Rugby Union Academies consist of squads of younger players whom the (particularly full-time) clubs have identified as potentially having the qualities required to become contracted players. They vary in age, ranging from schoolboys who attend during vacation periods and several evenings per week, to university students, and pre-contract professionals, who may attend on a full-time or almost full-time basis. One of the key features of many of these squads is that the players play for different teams. Many will play for school teams and regional representative sides; others may play for the club's second or 'A' team if one exists. The impact for planning, as reported by the coaches in their self-reflections, is that training becomes less about game preparation and more about individual skill and personal development.

Academy coaches who submitted plans tended to be detailed in their scheduling and ordered in their content progressions. They exhibited what might be termed a 'phased skills progression model', that is, they had identified a skills matrix around which to structure the training programme and the individual's progression. Because of the diversity of teams, it was common for coaches not to observe the players in game action. There was a tendency for the older academy players to be absorbed into the club's first team squad preparations if this was required by the head coach. This may have enhanced the effectiveness of the first team squad preparations, but disrupted the academy players' schedules. Coaches appeared to be less concerned about the disruption than the players being 'used' to limited effect.

Performance indicators

It was common for performance criteria to be identified as markers of progress and evaluation tools. There was also a degree of commonality about these and it seemed that the governing body of the sport had encouraged their use (e.g. through workshops and coach education). However, it was much less clear how they were being used. The criteria reflecting outcomes for the season were often employed as a measure of success (or otherwise), and there was evidence of periodic monitoring against these criteria. Coaches would occasionally provide evidence that the criteria had reinforced a perception of satisfactory or unsatisfactory performance, and this may have influenced their training emphasis.

One factor that emerged was that key performance indicators were rarely differentiated by the quality of the opposition. Average scores were unhelpful, as were scores against the strongest and weakest teams. Most helpful were performance indicators from games against those teams whose results were most likely to impact on the team's objectives (in other words, their closest rivals). It was obviously a challenge to set appropriate targets within the performance indictors. Targets tended to be quite 'difficult' to achieve, and teams promoted into a league had a tendency to be over-ambitious. The performance indicators were generally outcome-related, that is, they referred to a phase in the game (for example, line outs, scrums, gain line progress) in which performance was relative to the opposition's performance execution. This meant that the indicators required some interpretation, were probably 'key' in the sense that they differentiated satisfactory and less-satisfactory performance, but were not integrated into the planning process.

Contingency planning

There was no doubt that the coaches' planning could be described as contingent. This was the most obvious characteristic in the coaches' planning behaviour. At best the documentation acted as a guideline for implementation behaviour. It was difficult to conclude, however, whether this was simply the nature of the planning, and was intentional, or whether there were specific issues in these coaches' contexts that made it more likely to be so. This is at the heart of the analysis of planning practice and we will return to it. It might be argued that such a level of contingency is in fact the normal state of affairs, and the coach's expertise and knowledge is used to make the intervention decisions within this framework. This is certainly how the coach's practice could best be characterised. Nevertheless, it was

also possible to identify specific factors that would impact on both the planning framework (perhaps thought of as the outline shape and content of the training session) and the conduct of the activity itself.

The framework of the preparation was influenced by game results, weather conditions, injury to players, access to facilities, coaches' perceptions of 'spirit' among the players, and the player's physical condition. In discussion, coaches gave examples of training sessions that were altered as a result of these factors. It was also the case that training volumes were rarely specified; it was much more likely that 'duration' would be used as a loading factor for rugby training drills and perceived progress within the activity used to determine whether the activity should continue. The most obvious 'driver' for a week/microcycle plan was the evidence arising from the previous game. Perhaps not surprisingly, any perceived deficit in performance was often accompanied by changes to the programme (for example, additional sessions on defence). This appeared to be most likely when a defeat or poor run of performances/results were unexpected. This often resulted in an impression of 'planning for games gone', rather than for 'games to come', although coaches would be likely to argue that they were redressing generic weaknesses in performance.

It is also necessary to emphasise some of the elements in the overall planning context that made the planning process and delivery very contingent. It seems obvious to say that planning is specific to the sport, but we have to ask which factors emerge to shape the planning behaviour that characterises these coaches:

- An example was given by one coach of his team playing matches on 35 consecutive weeks in the season. This provides particular challenges for physical conditioning, and leads to the season being sub-divided into mesocycles based on anticipated fatigue (length of period, weather/ underfoot conditions) or competition schedules in order to allow regeneration and/or attention to underpinning conditioning factors. The coaches' language makes it clear that the need for these changes in emphasis is recognised. They spoke using terms such as variation, freshness, and changes in intensity.
- Intensity was acknowledged as a factor that could be manipulated by the coach. Although planning documentation often identified intended

variations in intensity throughout the season, the coaches' practice appeared to be driven more by the immediate perceptions of need. This might be occasioned by perceptions of a 'hard game', and psychological tiredness or staleness. In terms of 'rugby content', intensity was most often equated with physical 'hits' (contact drills), and managed in that way.

- In situations where the scheduling of home league fixtures was determined by the home team, the weekly microcycle could range from 5 to 9 days. This was generally identified in advance, and provided some variation. However this could also be perceived as disrupting routine.

- Coaches recognised the 'end of season' period as one in which the relative success of the season could be determined, and there was an acknowledgement of the need to be well prepared for that phase. There were varying levels of satisfaction with attempts to 'peak'. In many cases the circumstances simply overwhelmed the intention. One particular example identified too great a reduction in volume and intensity in preparation by the coach, which left the players under-prepared for the intensity of the game that followed.

- To compound the part-time element, teams with two evenings' training often had an emphasis on physical conditioning on one evening and a more rugby technical element on the other. In these circumstances, time pressures meant that most evenings had a measure of high intensity. This situation raises an issue about the model or form of planning that would most suit these circumstances. On the evidence provided, it seems likely that there would be very limited progression-linkages between sessions.

- The sport also has very distinctive 'positional' requirements within the team. The 'backs' and 'forwards' were often treated as two distinct groups, with different physical conditioning, and often different coaches. This might be made more challenging by coaches' not being sure about the number of players who would be taking part in training sessions, until the sessions began (injury, employment priorities for part-time players, representative squad demands). In many cases this was 'managed' by mixing squad personnel, or using academy players – in each instance the knock-on effect was planning problems for other coaches.

- The team personnel appeared to be in a constant state of flux throughout the season. A significant number of the coaches in the sample had only recently assumed responsibilities, either within their clubs, or by moving to new posts. In addition, recent promotion and relegation history impacted on expectations. It appeared to be difficult to judge appropriate goals when teams had moved from one league division to another.

'Contingency' was a 'state of being' that was recognised by all coaches. Broader goals changed only after evidence of a significant threat to the team's goals, but the changes that impacted on the coach's day-to-day planning generally being evident in time to be 'factored in' to the planning process. Coaches did not react to all incidents or events but tried to respond to patterns of performance or perceived progress. Routine micro-cycle planning was carried out sufficiently close to the implementation for 'contingency' to be taken into account. The coaches were clearly operating to a plan (albeit sometimes operationalised tacitly), but there appeared to be an acceptance that forward planning that was too detailed would be inefficient and unhelpful.

Interpretation and good practice

Insofar as these plans were part of a coach education programme, it was necessary to offer some feedback, and in doing so to form an opinion on the planning process that the coaches' planning documentation represented. These plans and the accompanying reflections provided exemplars of extremely diverse coaching practice. For some there was an element of over-planning, that is, a level of pre-determination of content and emphasis that was unlikely to be implemented as planned. For others, there was an overall guideline or framework approach that could easily be interpreted as being ignored in the immediacy of the week-by-week preparation. For the majority of coaches in this case, planning might be portrayed as a statement of intention, derived from a mix of principle and experience. The extent to which future activity could be pre-determined with some accuracy appeared to depend on full-time/part-time distinctions, and the coaches' approach to the coaching intervention. There were several coaches who were not in a Head Coach position within a club who reported a negative impact from the more idiosyncratic, less-predetermined, and often crisis management of senior coaches.

Perhaps unsurprisingly given the physical nature of the sport, the strength and conditioning programme was invariably periodised and training loads were identified in detail, although the measure of individualisation was variable. There were many examples of interesting, perhaps innovative, planning practice: for example, building in 'gap weeks' in each half of the season, creating 'rotation of skills' sessions, creating weekly routines, or devising motivating self-monitoring procedures. There was a development of rugby content from pre-season into the competition season, but the rugby content was less obviously differentiated between cycles within the competition season. The competition matches themselves were generally videoed and analysed by sophisticated software or coach review on the basis of KPI-related markers. The extent to which this led to individualised programmes was dependent on the full-time/part-time context. From this it can be suggested that coaches clearly intended their attention and feedback to be specific to individual players' needs, and this could be seen to varying extents through the plans for individual skill and team unit practices.

The coaches in this case acknowledged that continuity within the intervention programme was both the goal and the potential problem in implementation. This was a function of the specificity of game preparation, the time available for individual improvement, injury and availability. For academy players the individualisation and skills matrices seen in the plans were an indication of the 'improvement/development' agenda. However despite this, the overriding priorities during the season (perhaps more particularly for the part-time teams) were to ensure that the team played as closely as possible to its 'potential' (as well as it might be expected to) given the circumstances within the team/club and the opposition. For the part-time teams, there was a good deal of reinforcement and rehearsal within the training content. Although continuity and progression were overarching goals, there were several factors that militated against this. The sheer scale or range of individual skills, phases of play, tactical options, and the many contingency factors identified previously led to an 'optimising of performance in preparation for games'. The full-time context allowed a more systematic approach. There were also examples of coaches recognising that the momentum of the season had been disrupted, and

'sensing' that a 're-energising' was required. This was often an intuition or feeling by the coach, and was expressed as a need to re-focus, particularly if the problems were perceived not to be 'physical'.

From this process it could not be assumed that coaches were already reflecting adequately on their existing practice. It may have been the case that the demands of the exercise prompted a level of accountability and scrutiny of their practice, rather than provided new planning skills. For many of the coaches, their planning practice was subject to the prevailing practices within their clubs, and it was certainly the case that first team planning determined the priorities of other coaches. However, the response of coaches to the planning and reflection exercise was almost universally positive. At Academy level particularly, the bringing of schedules and 'order' to the programme was valued. For many others the required attention to detail 'resulted in the undertaking of a more robust planning process than previously'. In this case there were many examples of good practice in collective planning and reflection. Most coaches met with assistants and other support personnel to discuss the previous game(s) and to put detail to the next phase (even if solely for one week's preparation and game). In one particularly valuable example, the coach described the factors to be reflected upon at a monthly planning meeting: reviewing results, reviewing KPIs, reviewing planning intentions and implementation, strength and conditioning requirements explained, opposition reviewed, injury updates, games time statistics reviewed, themes established for training, broad priorities for game tactics, individual player reviews, and any other contingencies. As a result of this reflection, the next mesocycle (4–6 weeks) was planned in detail. Some coaches indicated that senior players may be involved in this process, but it seemed from the coaches' accounts of their planning practice that this was generally a coach-led exercise.

Summary

A clear message that permeates all of the coaches' responses in this case is that planning is an exercise in preparing for contingencies. This is partly a reflection of the fluid nature of the intervention itself (manipulating training drills and individual and team activity within these). As we have already suggested this partly explains the skeleton or framework approach to determining the progress of the intervention. The details are 'filled in' by the coach, as it is perceived/adjudged that the circumstances demand. These judgements, or action decisions, are dependent on the coach's expertise, and appear intuitive, although most likely to reflect a sophisticated applied knowledge base in experienced coaches. However, there are also contextual, or environmental, factors that impact on the 'skeleton' itself: the immediacy of results and game preparation, the aggregation of performance components and the need to balance preparation across these elements; varied availability of players and positional requirements.

Coaches who perceive themselves to be coping with the contingency appear to be 'planning for the contingency' rather than 'planning the contingency itself'. In other words, it is necessary to have procedures in place to accommodate the need for flexibility and responsiveness, but within the established framework (regular planning meetings, good information/monitoring systems, and good communications; but also a sound technical model, and developed solutions to common problems on which to draw). This is also helped by not over-planning sessional content.

Planning is a microcosm of the coaching behaviour dilemma, which pits a desire for order and control (not to be interpreted as a negative manipulation, but the management of the continuity and progression of the coaching intervention) against the continuously changing and often highly charged coaching environment. The outcome is a constant tension between formal planning and reactive flexibility. This may be experienced by players and coaches as a balance of routine and variety. In performance sport, and in other domains, the level of interaction between players, players and coaches, the management of rewards, the intricacies involved in performance improvement, and the constant threat to goal achievement create a highly charged, technically complex coaching environment. When we talk about the expertise of the coach, it might be most appropriately expressed as 'maintaining the continuity of purpose and performance despite the complexity and messiness of the intervention programme and environment'.

There are levels of planning that are most appropriately interdependent, but which the coaches' experiences demonstrate may often be operationalised independently. Planning takes place at the strategic, medium-term and weekly stages, but the evidence suggests that these stages may be approached in isolation from each other. At the strategic level there is

system management, scheduling, and getting people and resources to the right place and the right time. This happens within a broad strategic (seasonal) framework that identifies a set of physical, technical and tactical priorities. At the mesocycle level (4–6 weeks) there is a more detailed framework or skeleton that has been determined in relation to the known circumstances. This plan becomes a set of guidelines of physical conditioning, individual development, unit development, and specific game preparation. The rugby coaches appeared to use this 'guide' to good effect. The final level is the weekly microcycle. This is planned in detail, partly in order to be responsive to the immediacy of the previous and succeeding games, injuries, and the impact of these and other contingencies on changing priorities. For most coaches this does not result in a very detailed sessional plan, but rather a sketching out of activities, an aide-memoire. The coaches then use their expertise to deliver and manage the activity itself.

The description above has to be filtered through a lens of part-time or full-time coaching. The chapter has been able to establish that it is necessary to understand the development context, the training environment, and the particular goals set by/for the team in order to appreciate the planning approach that has been adopted. The coaches in this case have demonstrated that planning is an important part of their coaching practice. For these relatively experienced coaches their framework or skeleton approach is not unlike the 'simple sequencing of lesson component and content' adopted by experienced teachers (Hall & Smith 2006 p 428). The coaches appear to conjure a 'mental image' of the session, or perhaps even beyond the session. What needs to be considered now is how coaches develop and access the knowledge required to practice in this way. Coaches demonstrate that they plan their coaching interventions in the light of what is known about their players, the training environment, the many sets of goals within which they work, and their resources and expertise. They deliver these plans with a degree of flexibility and contingency that adheres to overall priorities but nevertheless is responsive to the immediate needs of the situation. Given the complexity of the circumstances and the nature of the sport itself, it is hardly surprising that the coach 'manages' the interplay of action, intent, progression and feedback by appearing to draw upon mental models or images of the session and relying on a developed expertise to deliver the intervention.

References

Bompa, T.O., 1994. Theory and methodology of training, third ed. Kendall Hunt, Dubuque Iowa.

Counsilman, J.E., 1968. The science of swimming. Prentice Hall, Englewood Cliffs.

Cushion, C.J., 2007a. Modelling the complexity of the coaching process. International Journal of Sport Science and Coaching 2 (4), 395–401.

Cushion, C.J., 2007b. Modelling the complexity of the coaching process: a response to commentaries. International Journal of Sport Science and Coaching 2 (4), 427–433.

Cushion, C.J., Armour, K.M., Jones, R.L., 2003. Coach education and continuing professional development: experience and learning to coach. Quest 55, 215–230.

Cushion, C.J., Armour, K.M., Jones, R.L., 2006. Locating the coaching process in practice models: models 'for' and 'of' coaching. Physical Education and Sport Pedagogy 11, 83–99.

Dick, F.W., 1997. Sports training principles, third ed. A&C Black, London.

Gould, D., Giannini, J., Krane, K., et al., 1990. Educational needs of elite US national team, Pan American and Olympic coaches. Journal of Teaching Physical Education 9, 332–334.

Hall, T., Smith, M., 2006. Teacher planning, instruction and reflection: what we know about teacher cognitive processes. Quest 58, 424–442.

Jones, R.L., Wallace, M., 2005. Another bad day at the training ground: coping with ambiguity in the coaching context. Sport, Education & Society 10, 119–134.

Lyle, J., 1992. Systematic coaching behaviour: an investigation into the coaching process and the implications of the findings for coach education. In: Williams, T., Almond, A., Sparkes, A. (Eds.), Sport and physical activity: moving towards excellence. E & FN Spon, London, pp. 463–469.

Lyle, J., 2002. Sports coaching concepts: a framework for coaches' behaviour. Routledge, London.

Lyle, J., 2007. Modelling the complexity of the coaching process: a commentary. International Journal of Sports Science & Coaching 2 (4), 407–409.

Schmolinsky, G., 1983. Track and field (Translation from the German), second ed. Sportverlag, Berlin.

Trudel, P., Gilbert, W., 2006. Coaching and coach education. In: Kirk, D., O'sullivan, M., McDonald, M. (Eds.), Handbook of research in physical education. Sage, London, pp. 516–539.

The professionalisation of sports coaching: definitions, challenges and critique

7

Bill Taylor and Dean Garratt

Introduction

In Western industrialised societies, professionals have long been valued and set apart from other workers because of their specialised knowledge and skills. Traditionally, these professional groups have been described in terms of an 'ideal-type'; that is their quintessential characteristics or attributes, including a distinct knowledge base (*a body of knowledge, professional authority and higher education engagement*), organisation (*professional association, monopoly and licensing, and professional autonomy*) and set of ethics that guides professional engagement (*service ideals, codes of practice and career concept*). The models for these, it is argued, can be found in the antecedents and historical structures that have been associated with the classical professional occupations of theology, law, and medicine.

Recently, successive governments in the UK and elsewhere, seeking to influence and mould the occupational landscapes of contemporary society, have imposed a professionalising process on some sectors of employment (Stronach et al 2002). Under the pervasive influence of the ideology of 'new managerialism' – (both as political philosophy and policy doctrine), 'archetype' professions have been joined by new occupations, such as teaching, nursing, and social work. Increasingly, these groups are now finding that their practices, organisational structures, and notions of what counts as legitimate professional knowledge, are being fashioned and controlled by the state. This fracture between the traditional professional and arrival of new interlocutors gives opportunities for critical reflection, as well as producing openings for detailed analysis of the mechanisms employed in the contested discourses of professionalism.

Therefore, this chapter considers how sports coaches and the activity that is termed coaching might best fulfil individual (and collective) ambitions to undergo a process of professionalisation. That is, a process that would lead society towards viewing coaching as having the equivalent status of existing professional occupations. It would also allow coaches to improve their status and benefit from the many economic, social and cultural advantages that becoming a professional would effectively engender. The chapter will chart the position of coaching in its progress and relation towards full professional recognition. In doing so, it will highlight the considerable problems evident in transforming a mainly voluntary structure and workforce, towards one that can provide a sustainable future that serves individual sports, meets government directives and policy, and supports a new breed of sports coaching professionals. An examination of the literature dealing with the professionalisation of sports coaching will be provided, with the intention to indicate the limits of its potency, direction and conceptualisation. This will be supplemented with an examination of the contribution offered outside sport on the evolving nature of professional occupational structures.

In mapping this journey, the chapter will discuss the definitions, conceptualisations and discourses that surround notions of professionalism, professional practice, and professionalisation. It will then provide the theoretical frameworks by which the modern professional occupations have been examined, judged and critiqued. Finally, it offers the authors' own critical perspective, drawing upon research findings of the lead author on the professionalisation of sports coaching in the United Kingdom.

Relevance to the coaching process/coaching practice

The ambition to see coaching transformed into a form of professionally recognised activity only really gained serious momentum when the government's policy on sport began to focus more on the role of coaches, along with the coordinating structures that support their practice. Coaching began to be regarded as an important element in the drive to increase levels of participation in sport within society as a whole and, more specifically, as a means to enhance levels of performance in the international competition arena (Houlihan & Green 2008). With this increased attention placed on coaching, critical questions were raised about the quality of coaches and their practices across different coaching fields, as well as the ability of coaching support structures to meet new demands and competitive aspirations. The activity of coaching, that is, both its practice standards and underlying infrastructure, was seen as essentially 'problematic' due to a number of proposed solutions being contained within political and policy-driven initiatives. The considered opinion was that while the fragmented pattern of existing (organic) coaching provision had served individual sports reasonably well historically, it was neither sufficiently robust, nor of the appropriate scale to meet future ambitions.

Historically, in the United Kingdom, sports' coaching has been largely confined to 'grassroots activity', prospering on the 'good-will' of amateurs and volunteers working from a broad base of voluntary organisations. The vast majority of individuals engaged in coaching do so within the frame of a voluntary ethos, often fitting in time and effort around other social commitments: job, family and individual sporting interests. Indeed, details from the *Sports Coaching in the UK 11 Study* (sports coach UK 2007) suggest that while the number of 'self-reported' coaches increased from 1.2 million to 1.5 million between 2004 and 2006, 70% of those coaches still receive no financial payment for their efforts. Further to this scenario of somewhat temporary and ad hoc engagements, there have been concerns expressed in relation to the quality and content of coach education courses, across individual sports and within the sector

as a whole (DCMS 2002). Up until recently, individual sports had set their own standards, performance levels and terms of reference for coaches. Those with responsibility for the education of coaches were also affected by differing levels of training and varying degrees of knowledge and educational understanding. This rather confused pattern of differing traditions, standards and applications, while serving the immediate needs of each National Governing Body, actually did little to reassure government and its non-governmental sport organisations (NGOs) (such as UK Sport, Sports Councils & sports coach UK).

Movement towards a professional work force that could commit full-time to the development of expert knowledge, that might value and seek professional development and regard coaching as a sustainable career choice, would be crucial to the process of re-branding the coach, as well as re-designating the roles and responsibilities of the emerging new professional. The recent move towards professionalisation can thus be seen as a key element in the process of 'up-skilling' the coaching workforce. It is also crucial if the occupation of coaching is to play a greater part in the upkeep of the health of the nation, by increasing the public's participation in physical activity and contributing to the success of UK international athletes. Another anticipated benefit of the development of coaching into a so-called legitimate profession – (underpinned by accepted standards of practice and sound education, ethical codes of conduct and well-formed career and development pathways), is that it will have a significant influence on all aspects and spheres within sport. Professional coaches should be able to raise levels of performance at the elite level, thus allowing athletes to compete with confidence on the world stage. In this respect, it is argued that professional coaches will be better equipped to inspire and engage young people into a lifetime of physical activity and better health. In addition, they will also be in a stronger position to shape and influence their own occupation as it develops and matures into an established part of Britain's sporting landscape.

Defining professionalism

Scholars of professionalism regularly acknowledge difficulty in providing useful and inclusive definitions of professionalism, or indeed any of its associated terminology: 'professional', 'professionalisation', 'allied professions', or 'the professions'. A number of bodies, including government and sports organisations, have laid claim to developing more inclusive and practical definitions of professionalism. However, matching the types of behaviours that professionals might be expected to exhibit, means that in reality, such rhetoric is beset by challenge, argument and notable exception. The 'problem' of defining professionalism and what is actually entitled has been considered by a number of authors. A sampling of the literature illustrates the point:

> In spite of the growth in the number of studies of particular professionals and the frequent attempts at theoretical evaluations, the very term professional remains elusive … Seldom does a concept remain as slippery as does the concept of "professions".
> (Perrucci & Gerstl 1969 p 6–7)

As Kalber reinforces, 'neither practitioners or academics have precisely defined what acting in a professional manner entails' (1995 p 106). Broadbent et al (1997 p 5) go on to suggest 'ambiguity is present in the very notion of professionalism'. Indeed, Friedson, one of the foremost exponents and supporters of the subject, summarised the futile nature of this quest more than 30 years ago by stating that, 'the use of the word [profession] is highly confused, and its definition for the purpose of scholarship and social accounting [is] a matter of *wearisome* debate' (1973 p 19). While the confusion surrounding the true nature of professionalism seems justified, it does cause some consternation and concern for those within the sports coaching community. For while the term professionalism may deserve its 'slippery' rhetorical reputation, the fact that there is little agreement on what its practice actually entails does nothing to provide guidance for those 'signing up' to the professionalisation process, or, in fact, in being judged against the existing professions. This point is compounded by the inherent lack of clarity surrounding coaching, in terms of its own absence of definition, identity and conceptual boundaries (Taylor & Garratt 2007). In addition, within the sports sector in general, there is often confusion and conceptual misunderstanding around terms like instructor, coach, sports leader, teacher, trainer and so forth.

While at first glance traditional definitions of the professions may seem rather seductive when applied to coaching, they are inevitably beset by problems. First, there are difficulties connected with policy borrowing (Halpin & Troyna 1995) that render any straightforward transfer of professional terms, definitions and ethics, logistically

problematic. Second, unlike some professions, for example medicine, where there is broad and common agreement and understanding, with a shared vocabulary for defining *the* profession (in terms of status, position and formal accreditation), coaching is decidedly more complex and diverse. Indeed, it has an altogether different set of values and traditions, within and across different spaces for sport. As such, ambitions to achieve a single and definitive or universalised set of definitions is at best conceptually challenging and at worst empirically untenable. Although of course there is an obvious need to address such apparently intractable problems in order to mature the process of professionalisation. In this sense, we suggest it might be more useful to conceptualise professionalism as a much broader concept and not as an end point. That is, an evolving ideology that helps mould and guide practice and interaction, and which moves away from being defined by a list of characteristics that fail to do justice to the dynamic nature of the professions, or, indeed, the processes of professionalisation.

In short, the diverse historical and cultural roots of British sports have left us with markedly differing languages, sporting traditions and attitudes towards notions of professionalism. While some, such as golf, tennis and football have long embraced professional coaching within their ranks, other sports have simply struggled to come to terms with the loss of amateurism and the moral position invoked by this void. The journey towards the professionalism of coaching in the UK will neither be unified nor integrated, for most sports start this process from different points of departure. In turn, these different starting points occasion differing degrees of engagement that are mediated through the associated conditions of commercialism, market interaction, and state regulation.

Review of literature

Until the late 1960s and early 1970s, successive governments had what can only be described as an 'at arms' length approach' to sport, its national governing bodies (NGBs) and the coaching practices found therein (Coghlan & Webb 1990, Roche 1993, Houlihan 1997). Individual sports, and by implication their coaches, were seen as self-standing 'experts in the field', and the autonomy and sovereignty that this approach provided was valued and maintained by both sides (Green & Houlihan 2005). The 1970s saw a number of government reports and policy documents which began to draw closer links between sport and the state (for example, 1972 GB Sports Council established, HMSO 1973, House of Lords Report – Sport and Leisure [Cobham Report], 1977 White Paper, A Policy for the Inner Cities). While few of these documents made any explicit reference to the occupation of coaching, they did fundamentally alter the relationship between sport and government. This structured the agenda to employ sport (and by implication its coaches) as a social tool and bring it to the attention of a wider body of policy makers concerned with the welfare state (Brown & Butterfield 1992, Roche 1993). The following decade saw a more explicit focus on coaching. The GB Sports Council strategy – *Sport in the Community: The Next Ten Years* (1982) – provided grants to NGBs for elite coaching and its development. In the mid-1980s the then British Association of Sports Coaches and the National Coaching Foundation agreed to formulate a 'think tank' to consider the future of coaching. Both the Sports Council for Wales (Coaching, Sports Science & Sports Medicine 1987) and the Scottish Sports Council (A National Strategy for Coach Education & Coach Development 1988) produced their own documents with the intention of co-ordinating and outlining the structures to enable coaching to develop.

Coaching Matters (Sports Council 1991) and later, UK Sports Councils' *The Development of Coaching in the United Kingdom: a consultative document* (2001) formalised this call for a more integrated approach and focused direction. Both within this document and more recently, there has been a proliferation of debate concerning the professionalisation of coaching and of establishing a framework for a coaching profession (Sports Council 1991, UK Sport 2001, DCMS 2002). For example, in their *Vision for Coaching*, UK Sport strongly recommended that the standards of coaching be elevated to those of 'a profession acknowledged as central to the development of sport and the fulfilment of individual potential' (UK Sport 2001 p 5). Following the publication of the Government's *Plan for Sport* (2001) came the establishment of a Coaching Task Force, set up to review the role of coaching and to tackle 'the shortage of coaches, both professional and voluntary, and recognise coaching as a profession, with accredited qualifications and a real career development structure' (www.culture. gov.uk/sport/coaching.htm, accessed 18/05/06).

While such deliberative policy moves have been united in their desire for coaching to undergo radical change and modification (and thereby benefit from the host of perceived advantages that professionalism will bring), few have gone as far as offering details on the actual workings of the professionalisation process. This was until the recent publication of the *UK Coaching Framework* (sports coach UK 2008). It would be fair to say that until this point, questions surrounding the 'professionalisation of coaching', 'coaching as a profession', and 'notions of what it means to be a professional coach' had been given scant regard by most researchers and commentators working in the field of sports science and its related, allied disciplines.

The early academic papers on the professionalisation of coaching (Chelladurai 1986, Lyle 1986, Woodman 1993), for example, tended to deal with the subject in a more limited, traditional and rationalistic manner, concentrating on the features that a profession would have to acquire in its efforts to gain acceptance and credibility (see Lawson 2004 for a general discussion). Chelladurai (1986) strikes a note of caution concerning the development of coaching as a bona fide profession. Comparing coaching with the archetypal established professions of law and medicine, he suggests that society is unlikely to bestow on coaching any notion of professional equivalence, or indeed the status and authority it effectively seeks. For Chelladurai, the fact that coaching is often judged by the measurement of performance-based outcomes and not by the nature of the process itself, and that it is generally regarded less significant than the practice of other established professions, like law and medicine, means that public acceptance and wider community endorsement remain highly improbable. Chelladurai suggests the way forward is for coaching to focus on internal developments that operate as a precursor to wider acceptance and professional status. In the early 1980s, a number of countries (Canada, Australia, France and Great Britain) were beginning to establish generic forms of coach education that would go some way to underpinning the development of coaching as professional practice (Campbell 1993).

For Woodman (1993), the professionalisation of coaching – *'an emerging profession'* – was thought to emanate from the adoption and application of knowledge of the sciences. In this commonly cited paper, the author celebrates the increasing practice of basing coaching programmes, systems and decision making on a foundation of biophysical scientific knowledge. Woodman sees the rationalisation of the process of coaching along scientific lines, as evidence of a discourse of an emerging profession. Of course, this claim was further enhanced by the adoption of certain types of knowledge already accepted within other sports-science-related occupations, such as biomechanics, sports psychology and performance physiology. In considering the traits and characteristics of what a new coaching profession might look like, the paper deals with the issues in a factual and rather uncritical manner. Woodman reflects upon the nature of professionalisation and professional practice in a somewhat simplistic and fragmented fashion. Through a 'deficit model', the nature of coaching, coaching theory, the knowledge base for coaching, possible employment, deployment, and other associated elements are all dealt with separately. It is suggested that all coaching needs to do to achieve professional status, is address the shortcomings within these elements. Doing so will naturally produce occupational maturity and will automatically lead to a state of professionalisation and professionalism. This resonates with other work, in which the sub-issues of coaching are treated separately and independently, and without further reference to the social, political and cultural processes that are critical to any professionalisation movement. Those very processes, in fact, are particular to the structure of British sports coaching, operating along the lines of voluntarism and community action.

It is additionally interesting to note that the somewhat isolated calls made within this period by Petlichkoff (1993), Dyer (1992) and Sullivan and Wilson (1993), to educate coaches in sociological and social psychological forms of knowledge, vital to producing an effective coach–athlete relationship, have generally gone unanswered. Indeed, it was not until recently through the emergence of Jones (2000, 2006), Jones et al (2004), Jones and Armour (2000), Jones and Wallace (2005) that these issues have re-emerged as important points of discussion, for much of the early work on the coaching profession was wholly descriptive in nature.

Adopting a rationalistic and functionalist perspective, much of the literature tried, with varying degrees of success, to benchmark where the occupation was within the professionalisation process and made further suggestions to enable the profession to move forward. Much of the discussion revolved around the occupation developing a common set of aims and outcomes, cutting across national and international boundaries. Yet at no time was any conceptual understanding shown of the cultural,

historical and situational complexities engendered within the individual sports systems of different countries. Nor was any level of awareness demonstrated towards the individual and unique position of coaches in terms of their professional development. This dual preoccupation with 'policy borrowing' (where policy is imported from other countries on the assumption of a natural cultural 'fit') and benchmarking (particular grades of coaching in a predetermined march towards professional status), disregarded both the complexity and nuanced nature of NGBs, as well as the culturally rich heritage of British coaching as a whole. In fact, these assumptions served to divert attention away from a form of organic development that would have allowed coaches and their sports an opportunity to move beyond the limiting structures of volunteerism and towards something of an emerging occupation. That is, one that was mindful of it own history and location(s), yet which intended to bring the ambitions of practising coaches to the forefront in its own efforts to fashion professional definitions, understandings and occupational boundaries.

Lyle (2002) returns to the professionalisation process in his book *Sports Coaching Concepts: A Framework for Coaches' Behaviour*. In this later writing, he considers wider issues that relate to the social status of coaching, both in terms of 'ascribed status' (the status given to an occupational group by virtue of their inherent characteristics) and 'achieved status' (gained through achievement, association, and success in the performance-coaching arena). He also suggests that 'achieved statuses' could be gained by the acquisition of certified qualifications. Citing the Office for National Statistics (2000), Lyle notes that sports coaching is now classified as an associated professional group and suggests that this position could be due to the 'increasing scientification of practice and the value placed on sport itself' (2002 p 200). Within this, he alludes to the lack of macro- and theoretical analysis of sports coaching and the inclusion of the professional status of coaching, by suggesting much critical commentary and empirical research has been 'issues focused'. Consequently, Lyle has failed to contextualise key professional concerns, or indeed shed light on the tensions that are manifest within the wider social and occupational dynamics of sports coaching.

Other authors, namely Trevor Slack (who based much of his work on the North American experience) and Geoff Nichols (working within a British and European context), have approached the issue of professionalisation from the changing perspective of the role of National Governing Bodies (NGBs) within sport. These have been central players in the development of new structures to support the education and promotion of coaches and coaching in the UK. Thus, to discuss the professionalisation of sports coaching and its individual practice, without paying due attention to these organisations is at the same time failing to give appropriate consideration to their importance in the future development of the professionalisation movement.

Nichols et al in their comprehensive paper *Pressures on the UK Voluntary Sport Sector* (2005) begin to deal with this shortcoming. In so doing, they detail the shift in government policy to force NGBs away from a culture of 'mutual aid' towards one of 'service provision'. Convincingly, the authors argue that the government's agenda (and resulting pressure) to professionalise NGB services and operations, will force them to compete for membership and patronage in an increasingly competitive leisure market. The UK government has already allocated monies under the 'NGB modernisation programme' in order to provide additional support to this process and further develop commercial structures and business practices in the internal structure of individual NGBs.

Adopting a critical stance in their analysis, Nichols et al (2005) conclude that central directives and agendas are changing the very fabric and status of once-independent organisations. In addition, the continued linkage between the monies that NGBs can draw down from government funding agents and their ability to meet the government's agenda has in some cases resulted in feelings of anger and resentment, a loss of autonomy and confusion of identity. In our own work on the professionalisation of coaching and the changing nature of coaches' engagement (Taylor & Garratt 2007, in press), these feelings of disquiet and uncertainty have been articulated and expressed in a number of field interviews with practising coaches and NGB officers responsible for coach education or coaching structures.

A local football coach (level 2) commented when asked about the recent changes:

> There is an assumption by government that professionalisation will mean a change in my behaviour. Well, I just don't buy that. Just because I turn out each Sunday for the love of the game, and not for the money, and I haven't got time to go on all these new courses, doesn't mean I am not professional. No one came down to see me coach before making those assumptions.

A British Canoe Union officer and level 5 coach who holds a regional post added:

> Sometimes it is difficult to keep up to date with all the new material … it is not just the rate of change but … but I mean … what it all means. We have to submit documentation with QCA-speak [sic] in it or we will get knocked back.

Later on in the same interview they said:

> I have concerns … yes, many concerns about what we do … I mean do we [the NGB] represent our members or are we here to carry out government bidding. It's like I have got two masters, one that voted for me in this position, the other funds the organisation [NGB] [laughs and shakes head].

Thus, while they (Nichols et al 2005) only allude to the effect these pressures are having on the occupation of coaching and coaches, working under the direction of NGBs, there must, in fact, be a relationship between the degree of support the NGB is able to provide to its own coaches while under pressure to modernise and align its internal structures and practices to a centrally imposed professional ideal.

Christine Nash (2001) in her study of volunteerism in Tayside, Scotland, considers the pressure on voluntary sports coaches, highlighting some of the inherent contradictions in government policy that focus on the value of volunteering (in terms of developing notions of community and citizenship), whilst also seeking to encourage certification within the field. This small-scale study suggests that voluntary coaches are less likely to accede to this subtle pressure, for reasons relating to the payment of fees, administrative processes and limited reimbursement of course costs. The issue of professional development of coaches is addressed by Jones et al (2004) in a study of elite coaches. They suggest that in a critical number of cases coach education courses were found to be of little direct benefit to the professional development of different areas of sports coaching. The suggestion is that in the past UK NGB coach education courses have tended to focus primarily on the technical issues of coaching, whilst ignoring the importance of the development of coaches' pedagogical and conceptual knowledge and understanding. The inherent failure to intellectualise the process in this way has effectively undermined coaching in its claim to possess a theoretical body of occupational knowledge.

Turning to the influence of wider literature on professionalism, much of the debate within other occupations has been on how contemporary professional identities have been formed. These aspects relate particularly to the transitions within coaching which are likely to create plural identities, emergent cultures and traditions and/or locations that are situated potentially 'in-between' (Anzaldua 1987, Bhabha 1996). This theoretical concern is compounded by debates concerning the nature of 'professionalism' rehearsed elsewhere, and beliefs concerning how the possession of more specialised forms of knowledge can lead to greater efficiency and improved performance within particular designate professions. General debates around the topic (Downie 1990, Eraut 1994, Locke 2001) are illustrated with numerous exemplars from teaching and teacher education (Guskey & Huberman 1995, Day & Hadfield 1996, Sachs 2001, Day 2002, Bates 2004), higher education (Middlehurst 1995, Nixon et al 2001), nursing (Trnobranski 1997, Humphreys 2000, Stronach et al 2002), law (Moorhead, 2001, Boon et al 2005), the arts (Arts Council England 2005) and professional sport (Smith & Stewart 1999, Williams 2002).

How does coaching measure up?

Earlier in this chapter, we argued that any characterisation of sports coaching through a simple list of traits and attributes has considerable methodological flaws. However, adopting such an approach does have a number of significant advantages. First, it provides a benchmark by which the current position of sports coaching can be measured against other established professions. Second, it allows sports and policy-making bodies to identify 'the gaps in the picture' which, in turn, encourages these organisations to direct attention and resources to deal with the shortfall. Third, such a methodology resonates with the wider policy-making community, as well as with other professions. So how does sports coaching measure up in any benchmarking process? And what are the attributes in need of particular consideration and/or specific remedial action?

A body of knowledge

Professionals by most conventional definitions are regarded as 'knowledgeable others'; as such, professionals 'profess'. Although this statement may seem obvious or even tautological, few authors writing on sports coaching and/or the nature of coaching knowledge have given any serious attention to this basic prerequisite: that the epistemology and practice (or praxis) of coaching involves being knowledgeable or expert in the chosen field. One exception to this apparent lack of attention can be found in the work of Potrac and Cassidy (2006). However, while the authors suggest a theoretical framework through which coaches might actively convey their knowledge, they do inadequately not deal with the thorny question of whether in fact there is a distinct body of knowledge to confer pass on? And yet, tellingly, the concept of a specialist body of knowledge is one of the central claims to authority of any professional, as it serves to define the jurisdiction within their chosen occupation. Without such a claim to rarefied knowledge, what is there to separate the professional coach from the merely novice 'other'? While most sports can lay claim to a distinct body of sports-specific, technical knowledge, few are as confident when it comes to identifying a coherent base of knowledge that is deeply embedded in coaching practice.

There are no doubt excellent examples of professional-level coaching to be found among a number of sports. Those of sailing, skiing, golf, tennis, top-level soccer, and athletics have generated models of 'best practice' in coaching. But these have tended to be developed at the higher ends of performance where coaches are in full-time professional engagement. In addition, these 'pools of excellence' are rarely the products of a systematic and effective coach education process; it is more often the case that such coaches are generated by more exceptional mentors working either alone or in small isolated clusters.

In other locations and sports, there is something of a deep suspicion surrounding professionally generated knowledge, and a marked anti-intellectualism that has hindered the process of importing best practice from other disciplines and educational sectors. Taking sport as a whole, one of the patterns to emerge is that coaching practices and standards continue to remain unequal. They are often localised and have been seldom generated and inspired by productive NGB coach education systems (Jones et al 2004). In the UK, World Class Performance Programmes (WCPP) funded by the state, have allowed a number of NGBs to employ high-level coaches from overseas. The employment of these coaches has, in turn, witnessed the import of expert and specialised forms of external knowledge. These coaches, a number of them from ex-Eastern Block countries, are often products of mature,

state-funded university-based coach education systems (Naul & Hardman 2002, Houlihan & Green
2008). These are systems that are often based on a
lengthy and theoretically involved framework of
training, combining sports science with pedagogical
theory. Unfortunately, the process of importing
coaching experts to work with elite performers in
the UK, has failed to percolate down due to the presence of ring-fenced WCPP funding and the isolated
nature of their work.

Among other occupations the development of
expert knowledge has been closely associated with
the engagement of higher education. Indeed, many
professionals in Europe and North America, such
as teachers, nurses, and doctors, are educated to at
least degree level. In fact, in some of the more
established occupations, the professions themselves
are responsible for regulating and tightly controlling
the education and training of new professionals,
with associations often taking on the roles of awarding body, university staffing and standards regulator.
So, if coaches do have a claim to expertise where
does this come from? In many sports, the coaching
workforce has emerged directly from the field of
current and ex-performers. Indeed, this relationship
has been legitimised by a number of official (via
state or sports organisations sponsorship) programmes that have 'fast-tracked' elite performers
in to senior coaching roles. The assumption here is
that because ex-performers have 'been there and
done it' this 'experience' alone provides the adequate know-how and legitimacy required to work
with, and coach other elite performers. It is argued
that ex-performers are in a unique place to guide
and advise others, particularly those in the arena of
elite performance and competition. While this
model may be justified under certain conditions, it
does nothing to advance coaching's claim to be mir-
roring the professional education processes of other
allied occupations (Lyle 2002). It could also be
argued, for example, that the assumptions upon
which this movement is based serve to devalue the
importance of developing pedagogical skills over
time, as well as the experience gained from their
application in the field. The model is premised on
the assumption that 'knowledge of how to do' is
easily transferred to 'knowledge on how to coach,
how to do', in the absence of any educational experience on the part of the neophyte coach. Such
schemes seem to have an almost mesmerising
attraction to policy-makers, who actively work to
privilege and promote ex-athletes in order to allow

them to remain in the sport at any cost. However,
such fast-tracking schemes can have the effect of
devaluing coaching; educational processes should
be more properly based on professional reflection
and development over time, with emphasis on
learning the craft in the context of practice. We
do not fast track doctors merely because they were
continually ill as children, so why coaches just
because they once happened to be athletes?

The direct engagement of universities in the education of coaches and coaching in the UK has also
been marginal. In fact, until the mid 1990s there
were very few higher-education degrees explicitly
dealing with the pedagogical fundamentals of coaching. Those that covered the subject did so under the
dominance and guise of the biophysical sports
sciences, where the skills required for successful
coaching were often confused and conflated with
notions of practical achievement and/or the distant
application of psychology and physiology, as well
as other biomedical approaches. In recent years,
however, named coaching degrees have emerged
across the higher-education sector. Bush (2007),
for example, reported that in 2006 there were 192
undergraduate degree courses in the UK concentrating on coaching, representing 11% of all sports-
related degrees. While these developments are to
be welcomed there remain some concerns regarding
the centrality of coaching pedagogy, and its theoretical underpinnings, within specific coaching degrees.
One area, in which universities have made a valid
contribution to the field, is in the generation of
research and propagation of theoretical understandings around the coaching process.

Since the 1990s, there has been significant
growth in the publication of academic journal articles that deal with the practice and delivery of
coaching, as well as a number of other texts that
have successfully added to the body of subject
knowledge. In addition to writings that deal directly
with coaching, there has been an emerging realisation that other bodies of social and educational theory have much to offer coaching, in terms of
conceptual understandings and the ability to situate
coaching as a social, cultural and inter-personal act.
The consideration and 'reading' of cultural studies,
educational theory, relationship and group studies,
chaos/complexity theory and social anthropology
can help provide us with a more enlightened perspective, or set of theoretical 'lenses' through which
to study coaching. Thus, it should be seen as a social
and culturally embedded *educational* activity, and

not perhaps in terms of any traditional application of management, leadership and/or organisation theory, which have haunted and held back the development of effective coaching theory. Interestingly, what has yet to be established within the field is the degree to which advancements within academia have impacted on the practice of individual coaches operating in different areas of sport. While it is surely the intention of many authors to do this, it may be disingenuous to suggest that the readership of much academic writing has extended beyond the academic and policy-making communities (a small collective). This separation and slippage between theory and practice in the UK has been identified by scUK, which is, in turn, making efforts to bridge the divide by organising forums and seminars where interested parties can meet and exchange ideas. So does coaching have an identified body of knowledge that serves to define its parameters and set it apart from other similar occupations? Somewhat tentatively, the answer is probably: 'yes, an emerging one'.

Nevertheless, the emergent body of knowledge continues to suffer from an inherent lack of maturity. At its core, it lacks constructive relationships between theory and practice and still has no designated organisation, or 'home', that is responsible for the dissemination and regulation of knowledge. On a more positive note, however, there is a strong indication that collective action is beginning to take place. There is an intellectualisation of coaching knowledge and more individuals are attempting to theorise and marry the complexities of the technical with aspects of practical delivery. Most importantly perhaps, there is a realisation of need for a distinct body of knowledge: a legitimate, credible and well-practised body that can help establish coaching as a respected profession. Yet what remains to be discovered is if alternative theories and readings of coaching – the emergence of a sort of counter-orthodoxy – will be encouraged and embraced by the organs of the state? Lessons from the field of nursing and teaching would suggest that the delivery systems of state-sponsored education are reluctant to countenance the values of researchers and practitioners operating as part of any counter culture that would seek to challenge the status quo (Stronach et al 2002). If the body of accumulated (coaching) knowledge is to continue to mature and grow increasingly sophisticated in order to influence both structural change and practice within the field, then all epistemologies and methodological stances must be given equal value, and the relationship between theoretical development and evidence-based practice must be strengthened.

Organisation

At the core of most archetype professions lies a key organisation or centrally inspired body that takes responsibility for controlling the quality of delivery, standards of provision, membership requirements and definition of issues of strategic importance and common interest. Typically, this will constitute an expression of unity and group consciousness, borne of members' common vocational experience, values, aims and interests. Entwined in this notion of self-regulation and professional autonomy is the recognition that an association of professionals operates as a legitimate body to protect the autonomy of members, while upholding standards and protecting the public from forms of so-called un-professional conduct. As Larson notes, 'their broader purpose is to strengthen and elevate the professions' status' (1977 p 30). Hitherto, the field of sports coaching in the UK is devoid of such a body. The organisation, certification and management of coaching has, with varying degrees of success, been mainly the responsibility of the NGBs of individual sports. Other bodies in the UK, such as the Central Council for Physical Recreation (CCPR) and the National Qualification Council (NQC) have generally offered a portfolio of low-level, generic sports leadership awards that have included the teaching of basic coaching competencies. Within this disparate and fragmented structure, the notion of establishing a set of universal organisational standards has been difficult, if not impossible, to achieve in practice.

Only since the advent of the United Kingdom Coaching Certificate (UKCC) has any form of directed regulation actually emerged. While in some sports settings coaches have managed to organise their own representative groups (The Association of Mountaineering Instructors; The Swimming Teachers' Association, and the Professional Golfers' Association Professional Coach, being some examples), with the aim of providing a focal point for coaches to exchange shared interests and benefit from collective membership, the vast majority of coaching (both voluntary and professional) carried out in the UK occurs outside of any such formal framework.

An early attempt to bring coaches together under one organisation was made by The British Institute of Sports Coaches (BISC), which combined with the National Coaching Foundation (NCF, sports coach UK's predecessor) in 1993 to form the National Coaches Association (NCA). This organisation offered both membership services and insurance for coaches across all sports, but then later faded away due to a lack of resources and capacity to deliver services across the full spectrum of UK sports. This fractured and atomistic picture of sports coaching has meant that the occupation of coaching as a whole has been unable to take any unified action to foster developments, nurture a collective identity or, indeed, regulate the activities of coaches. These issues are exacerbated by the fact that only 50% of active coaches in the UK hold any coaching qualification that is recognised by a governing body. So while this figure is noticeably up from 38% in 2004 (sports coach UK 2007), it nonetheless serves to illustrate the scale of the problem in bringing together coaches; that is, coaches with a limited requirement to belong to any sports-specific coaching scheme, let alone a national group whose ambition is to represent the interests of all coaches.

This shortfall in organisational structure has been identified by a number of governmental bodies; indeed sports coach UK, in *the UK Framework for Coaching* (sports coach UK 2008), effectively targeted the licensing and registration of coaches as one of its key policy priorities. While the final format of this policy is still under consideration, it is evident that the licensing of any occupational membership is a key component of professional status. What remains unanswered is if the registration and licensing of coaches is to be left to the NGBs, will it then become part of the remit and responsibility of a government organisation, such as sports coach UK? Both scenarios thus remain problematic. If NGBs are themselves left to structure the formalities of registration and licensing, then there will be obvious consequences for developing a united professional body, with the practice of coaching remaining fragmented and sport-specific. The occupation of coaching will then be relegated to a series of relatively muted and powerless positions, where notions of more organically inspired growth will at best be unlikely, and at worst actively discouraged. If the registration and licensing responsibilities are taken on by government via centrally organised sports agencies, then coaching may fail to convince other professional groups, as well as the public at large, that it has managed to secure true independence.

However, the registration and licensing of its membership is but one feature in a broadening constellation of attributes that serve to define the role of a professional organising body. Thus, to convince the public of its true legitimacy, any professionally representative group must be seen to stand apart from, and actively resist, government interference, while at the same time attempting to serve the publics' best interest. Compounding this is the issue that while a sizable proportion of coaches continue to operate as volunteers there is little to attract new individuals to a single organisation, or indeed convince them of the supposed advantages that collective membership would bring. While technically, NGBs continue to represent the home of coaching in the UK their operation is nevertheless isolated. Increasingly, they are also impacted by centrally imposed forms of standardised policy, not just in the realm of coaching but also in being accountable to areas of funding and management practices. These external pressures are compounded by an increasingly expectant public: one in which higher levels of provision, with better access and improved delivery, within coaching are now naturally expected. In addition, media attention seems to range from a search for the 'feel good factor' that success in international sport readily brings, to ironically blaming sports in their failure to engage the interest of unhealthy youngsters. However, while these situations bring some commonality to the position that is occupied by NGBs, disparate sports have yet to organise a coherent and collective body that can represent a unified voice; a voice that can challenge the hegemony of a centrally imposed policy discourse.

Not surprisingly, sports coaches are often impeded by similar restrictive policy issues and logistical barriers. On the whole, it can be argued that coaches have a relatively limited collective consciousness in which they have few opportunities to realise their shared identities, similarities and common interests across different spaces for sport, or practical levels of coaching engagement. The very idea of a single, independent organisation being able to connect the essentially disparate practice of coaching in the UK is currently highly unlikely. In the first place, that role has to fall to central government via one of its sports agencies, such as sports coach UK, but therein lays the contradiction. If coaching is to reposition itself as a recognised profession, allowing practitioners to become full-time and genuinely professional, then it is imperative that it should be represented by an independent body that is able to mitigate government pressure, protect its own membership, convince the public of its independent standing and bring internal governance and autonomy to the occupation. Any government agency taking the lead to unify coaching as an occupation under one umbrella organisation, must as its central aim make a firm commitment to extend full responsibility for the running and management of the organisation to the coaching community.

Ethic of professional service

The analysis of the twin concepts of 'professional ethics' and 'service ideals', coupled with a detailed discussion of their centrality to the notion of being professional, could itself merit a separate chapter. Indeed, both of these terms, as with many others in the field, are typically problematic in terms of their contested terrain and definition, which is subject to individual application and situated judgements. If asked, most coaches would defend their actions as being both principled and ethical, and ultimately guided by a sense of 'best practice'. If questioned further as to what the constituents of these principles and practices might be, then we are likely to get a range of answers depending of the level of coaching, the sport under consideration and the intended outcomes of the particular type of coaching engagement. While most NGBs in the UK have a 'code of ethics' and corporate statements committing themselves to inclusiveness and open practice, the manner in which these statements serve to guide coaches in their day-to-day delivery is open to conjecture and debate. But to what degree is this really a problem, in the sense of any ethical commitment being localised and sport-specific? And to what extent does it undermine coaching in its aspirations to mature and achieve professional status?

However construed, the notion of professional ethics is historically embedded in the cultural constructs of the very concept of professionalism. The relationship of the archetype professions (such as law and medicine), with society at large is based on the idea of placing the needs of the client first, since very often the client is vulnerable (if not entirely powerless) in coming into contact with the qualified professional. In terms of practical mastery, in these situations the individual is often not sufficiently informed to judge the appropriateness of the advice or intervention given. Therefore, the commitment to uphold professional ethics helps protect the uninformed client and serves to maintain the public's trust in the profession, where professionals are seen as guardians and protectors of professional

judgement and practice. Yet does this picture adequately capture and describe coaches' actions in their relationships with athletes and performers? Certainly, coaches working with young performers at the level of performance and talent development have considerable power, knowledge and influence. So much so, in fact, that in some cases there is a substantial imbalance in power between coaches and their clients, where coaches are in total control to decide upon the format and content of training, competition and performance targets.

However, in contrast there are other scenarios in which the coach has considerably less power. Elite professional golf and tennis players, for example, can switch coaches, as and when they please. Also, talented performers in other sports can, and do change clubs and coaches, especially in cases where the relationship is not working to the client's best advantage. But these situations are relatively limited, for in the majority of coaching contexts the coach is able to structure and steer the various processes of practical engagement, including programmes of learning and competition. Coaching relationships are thus more generally affirmed on an imbalance of power and knowledge. As a consequence, we argue that a supporting framework of ethical 'codes' is required to guide behaviour and other forms of coaching engagement. However, having already noted that individual sports each have their own code of ethics, any move to introduce a unifying code to regulate practice (via CCPR and sports coach UK) is at best only likely to add to the mélange of incongruous forms. In the process it may also serve to dilute the ethos of coaching within individual sports. Consequently, in the absence of a universal set of principles to guide the relationship between coaches and their athletes in sports coaching in the UK, there remain difficulties in reassuring the public that important relationships are being properly informed by fair and morally reputable forms of practice.

While criticised for being overly romantic, the notion that professionals are 'called' to a particular occupation through personal obligation to help others and 'give service', continues to remain a common ideal in the landscape of contemporary professionalism. Similar to the way in which principles are embedded in professional ethics, 'the service ideal' (Lawson 2004) serves to support and actively maintain the atmosphere of trust between the public and their so-called serving professionals. Such notions of trust represent the ethical cornerstone of professional practice in its relationship with the wider public. The 'service ideal' is thus based on a mix of altruism, obligation and professional responsibility, the elements of which can be seen to resonate strongly with the reasons given by coaches as to why they entered the field. This concept of 'giving back to the sport', a sport that once gave them many years of enjoyment, friendship and identity as an athlete, is not uncommon. Within the critical mass of voluntary coaches, the notion of community betterment and social welfare also resonates strongly in the wider ideals of volunteerism and community action (Nash 2001).

During research on the nature of the volunteer and the professionalisation process, the authors of this chapter interviewed a number of community-based coaches about their club-based experiences, out of which emerged a set of notions around the idea of social obligation and belief in the value of a collective good. A tennis coach (unqualified) emphasised this implicit social contract:

> They call me coach sometimes ... it's a bit of a piss take really; I also collect the match fees and set the nets on a Tuesday night before practice. I coach the beginners and the young people when they want, now my knee won't let me complete. We all muck in ... if there is a job that needs doing ... people usually step forward; it keeps us going as a club really ... it's important you know ... the idea that we all chip in, without that attitude we're all buggered

This sense of moral action with the volunteer coach giving back to the sports community is noted in this comment:

> As soon as coaches start taking money for the job ... the whole nature of what they do, changes. Not only will they think differently, but so will the kids and the parents. Being a volunteer in some way protects you ... if you do it for the love ... it means something more. I give back to the sport because it gave to me ... and not for the 20-quid a-bloody-hour I might earn'
> (Community-based Football Coach, Level 1).

This is not to suggest that all voluntary coaches are driven by this 'service ideal' or that it is manifested equally across all practices and spaces for sport. However, the concept of the coach and his/her participants, being both producers and consumers of their own experiences, serves to bind them together in a relationship of trust and mutual aid (Taylor & Garratt 2007). Within the psyche of British sport there is a deep commitment to wider notions of sport as community welfare and, indeed, of sporting engagement as a valued form of social practice. If these positions can be seen to represent an accurate description of the mainly voluntary activity that constitutes sports coaching in the UK, and additionally held up as an identifiable 'service ideal', then any discussion on the future professionalisation of sports coaching must address a number of fundamental questions:

- If a closer relationship with the marketplace is an important co-requisite of the processes of professionalisation, will this serve to attack and undermine the fundamentals of voluntary coaching involvement; namely, community betterment and mutual aid?
- Can the voluntary commitment shown by the majority of coaches be effectively transformed to a professional 'service relationship', without jeopardising the trust and support of participants, athletes and the public?
- Will the future of the professional bring with it the additional complexities of commercialisation, commodification and an increased focus on outcomes at the expense of coaching processes?

Where is coaching on the professionalisation journey?

We have so far suggested that the practice of coaching is a long way from being considered truly professional in any authentic or traditional sense. Indeed, as Lyle (2002) argues, no matter what set of benchmarks are employed to assess its actual position, it remains the case that against most putative criteria coaching continues to exhibit a relatively weak condition; for while such criteria are likely to produce a degree of permanency within the field, the social, political, cultural and economic conditions that serve to encourage or restrict its growth are considerably more fluid and open to change. As we have stated before '...benchmarks are relatively fixed, in so far as they derive from first principles as "matrixed" standards, enablers and barriers, in contrast ... [enablers, barriers and social conditions] can be regarded as transient and dynamic, and, therefore, subject to the vagaries of supply and demand, as well as other external influences and conditions' (Taylor & Garratt 2007 p 31).

Therefore, any process of professionalisation is transitionary and ongoing, and inevitably subject to the radical effects of commercialisation, globalisation and commodification of knowledge within the subject. Within these shifting environs it is important to recognize that the vision held by the state, and that of its agencies, of coaching becoming a profession of the future, might never be fully realized. The development of any professional pathway is neither linear nor is it one that can be simply plotted along some form of binary continuum, from voluntary to full-time, or indeed amateur to professional.

For some (Humphreys 2000, Johnson 1984, Nixon et al 2001), the development of a sustainable and committed profession has more to do with the emergence of a culture and philosophy that is organic and democratic than anything externally constructed or otherwise centrally imposed. The ambition of UK government to see ' . . . by 2012, the practice of coaching in the UK . . . be elevated to a profession . . .' (UK Sport 2001 p 5) should not be seen as an all or nothing scenario. The 'professionalisation of coaching practice' is not merely restricted to those in full-time coaching employment. Nor is it rigidly bound to any stated code of professional ethics, with the aim to provide exclusive guidance to professional contexts. On the contrary, most voluntary coaches would seek to defend their practice as being intrinsically 'professional', especially in terms of passion, commitment and responsibility to what they do. Over a period of four years (2004–2008), the lead author interviewed over 50 coaches in the process of collecting data for a number of related research projects. Most of the subjects had coached and/or continue to coach part-time on a volunteer basis. One of the few commonalities to emerge across the range - (irrespective of qualifications, sport or level of engagement), was a firm commitment to coaching on the understanding of its fundamental value, social and educational, and perceived collective benefits. Yet in real terms, it remains the case that if coaching is to be regarded equally alongside other established professions, and similarly successful in securing sustainable funding streams from the state, it will need to meet externally imposed criteria. Accordingly, we now turn to analyze the role of the state in this process, by offering a more critical perspective on the emergence of new professions and the pervasive influence of managerialist policies within government.

Critical reflections of the professionalisation process

From a research perspective, little is known about the professionalisation of sports coaching in the United Kingdom; still less is actually understood in relation to the perceptions of coaches working across different spaces for sport. Within the number of centrally-driven and government sponsored reports that are currently circulating the discourse of the 'professionalisation of sport coaching', the voice of multiple disparate coaching communities has remained largely muted. Evidence collected from semi-structured interviews with grass roots coaches (Taylor & Garratt 2007) seems to suggest that while generally NGBs have been consulted, the voice of many practising coaches has fallen silent, as one coach put it:

> Yes, of course I am sure that the Governing Body [NGB name of sport omitted] has been in talks about this and that. But their job is to run the sport . . . coaching is just one part of it. Nobody asked me or any of the coaches in the club what they wanted. The Governing Body just put forward what's best for the sport' (Coach working for a Local Authority).

While it should not be too surprising that NGBs have been identified as the representatives of coaches and individual sports practices, the extent to which coaches have any degree of influence within particular sports differs markedly across the field. Historically, in some sports - (notably swimming, athletics and other technical sports) coaches have occupied a central position, while in others the more marginal position of the coach has meant they have been less able to influence and affect policy. In addition, policy initiatives that have directly involved coaching have often been tied up with wider sporting objectives of social and health promotion, administration governance and the building of sports systems. On the whole, what is best for UK sport (and by association specific sports) has often been taken to operate co-terminously with what is best for the process of coaching. Thus, the construction of a discourse of professionalisation and parallel agenda for change within coaching has not emerged from the interests of volunteer coaches, participants and/or administrators; rather it has developed almost exclusively from the aims and interests of the state.

The mechanisms of twentieth century state intervention have attracted a number of critical positions including feminism, post-structuralism and critical theory. In their different ways, these have often conceptualised the state's power and interest over new and emerging professional groups as part of the hegemony of neo-liberal discourse and philosophy of new managerialism (Travers 2007). That is, a political philosophy whose principal concern involves tighter forms of regulation, auditing and rationalisation. Emerging professions, like coaching, are not only subject to these insidious conditions, but also perhaps more menacingly the fact that they operate to construct what counts as legitimate – (both ontologically and epistemologically), within those very occupations. The pervasive influence of the new managerialism and its associated cannons has not only threatened particular conceptions of professional knowledge but simultaneously introduced new forms of bureaucratisation. That is, a form of reductionism that seeks to 'control consumption [and] fractures the dominant cultural and aesthetic values' (Boon et al. 2005: 474), consequently revolutionizing the acquisition and classification of professional practice, from the 'outside in' (Dawson 1994).

The imposition of external constructs and definitions of professionalism on coaching not only serve to redefine existing forms of practice but effectively devalue and marginalize the voice of those who are keen to maintain 'old practices'. More than this, however, new forms of bureaucratisation are instrumental in unsettling and reshaping the landscape of professional identity[ies] (Beck & Young 2005, Bernstein 2000), creating an elision and conflation between the construction of the 'professional subject' and the classification and framing of professional knowledge (Bernstein 1971). Consequently, imposed forms of regulation that seek to control what counts as knowledge can engender an erosion of the status and legitimacy of professions as organic and relatively autonomous professional 'fields' (Bourdieu 1988), which is particularly true for those where power is already significantly constrained or otherwise muted.

The latter is especially pertinent to the professionalisation of coaching in sport across the UK, for the aim to universalise standards, according to particular benchmarks, presents a technically rational conception of professionalism (Eraut 1994), which glosses over differences in tradition, culture and practice in different areas of sports coaching. Indeed, such professional 'employments' are constituted by particular social and cultural antecedents, riven with the values and interests of the *habitus* (Bourdieu & Passeron 1977), which are specific to individual areas of sports coaching. Given the ambition to develop a coaching profession with enduring qualities that extend beyond the 2012 Olympic Games, there is a growing imperative to examine how different sectors of coaching are managing newly imposed standards and to evaluate the impact on coaches operating between the boundaries of voluntary and 'professional' practice.

Our own writing picks up on this critical perspective, using Bourdieu's concepts (1977, 1986, 1988) (Taylor & Garratt in press) as a means to examine the professionalisation of sports coaching. Bourdieu - a French philosopher and social anthropologist, has left us with a rich vein of theory with which to study individual agency and the structural conditions that regulate society. Within the arena of sports coaching there has been little direct application of his work; indeed, Cushion's & Jones' (2006) paper on symbolic violence within a football club is a unique and notable exception.

Central to any Bourdieurian application of social and cultural theory is the linked notions of habitus, capital, and field. While Bourdieu's work extends far beyond the limitations of these concepts, due to a lack of space here the reader is referred to the work of Jarvie & Maguire (1994) for a more comprehensive but accessible, introductory account. In essence, Bourdieu (1986) links agency (practice) with structure (via capital and field) through the process of 'habitus'. For him, our social practices – (those such a sports coaching), are the result of various habitual schemas and personal dispositions. When these social behaviours (habitus) are combined with resources (capital) they are actualised and played out in certain social terrains (fields). These terrains or fields, such as those found within sports coaching, both modify and reproduce forms of capital and allow individuals and groups to exhibit their cultural predispositions and social behaviours: 'habitus'. Individuals develop habitus from their cultural and situated antecedents and social learnings, leading to a set of evolving dispositions that become as much a part of who they are, as they, in turn, become intrinsically a part of them. Bourdieu concludes in his famous quotation: '. . . when habitus encounter a social world of which it is a product, it is like a 'fish in water'... it takes the world about itself for granted' (cited in Wainwright & Turner 2008).

An individual or group brings particular forms of capital to each field. For Bourdieu (1986), capital is a representation of the resources that carry currency and influence. Some capital has symbolic power such as the status gained by a coach from being a successful ex-performer. Extensive knowledge of advanced tactics or technical aspects in sport may afford coaches significant cultural power, while social capital is imbued in significant positions of status and authority: for example, a coach heading team selection. For Bourdieu (1986), economic capital is pre-eminent, for it is the most robust and significant form of capital that is associated with money and other financial resources. He maintains that while symbolic capital would not necessarily transfer from one putative field to another, economic capital - in its ability to provide access to other resources, is far more dominant across terrains, allowing those who possess it to preserve their privilege in differing fields and locations. However, not all forms of capital are so easily reassigned.

The government's desire to professionalise sports coaching can be seen as a deliberate attack on the value of symbolic capital linked with the concept of volunteerism, which has been part of British sport for at least 150 years. It can also be regarded as a coordinated attempt to redefine the field by privileging certain forms of knowledge and regulated practice over more 'organic' and locally-inspired forms of coaching. Again, Bourdieu (1977) argued that within particular fields, certain types of capital have hierarchical power: high-status and lower-status. New forms of occupational structure and professional knowledge, endorsed and legitimated by the state, may challenge existing forms of capital, with the effect of relegating traditional types that lack currency and status. However, when interviewed one coach offered some resistance to this argument,

> They [meaning scUK] seem to take delight in complicating simple things . . . they have all this new jargon, you know fancy words, about what to coach and how they want it done. Well we do a pretty good job down at [name of club omitted] we will go on coaching the way we have always done it . . . well I will, it's our club . . . I don't hear any of the kids complaining (Local Football Coach, Level 2).

We would argue that as a technically rational approach to the constitution and development of professionalism and professional knowledge is further advanced, the currency of more traditional types of capital will continue to be challenged. With the increased emphasis on longer periods of coach education, which are, in turn, likely to lead to increased costs to the trainee; the position of economic capital will be positively enhanced. Equally, knowledge and understanding that corresponds to the new forms and complexities of coach education (UKCC), will serve to produce valuable forms of cultural capital, especially for those who are able to take up new opportunities. The net result is one in which existing coaches are likely to feel threatened and unsure of their position, value and identity. Indeed, this increased cost of initial training and continuous professional development (CPD) may well attract individuals who see a positive future in the new profession and with this an opportunity to forge a serious career.

However, during this period of shifting values and conceptual redefinition we would expect to see a number of existing coaches drop out of the system – maybe because their sense of value has been diminished, or otherwise that their voices are unheard. If, in its ambition to professionalise the structures of coaching and coaches across Britain's sporting landscape the state fails to take account of the contractions inherent in a technocratic model of professional delivery, then we may well be left with a suitably schooled body of coaches who are incapable of exercising (due to a lack of confidence and/or occupational freedoms) professional judgements on what is best for the individual athlete and sport, in general. While the evolving dynamic of professionalisation is being played out, it is essential that we understand the changes that are occurring at the level of delivery. That is, where the fundamental relationship between coach and participant is presently being redefined and radically re-structured. Failure to do so is likely to result in yet further alienation and disengagement.

A few final words. . .

There is little doubt that coaching and the structures that support it are entering a stage of unprecedented funding from within sport and by the UK government. Organisations such as scUK have been extremely successful in bringing about this new focus and elevating the practice of coaching to one worthy of serious consideration. But what are the real social and cultural costs of this new and forceful movement? To what degree has real consultation taken place with the existing army of volunteer coaches; and, is the vision of the coach as a professional who is central to any athletic endeavour, really one that local clubs and communities can recognise and engage with?

We remain unconvinced that the envisaged model of the coach as a professional, is one where the coach is valued as an independent intellectual, in which coaching is fundamentally seen as a cognitive activity that has, at its heart, educational intentions. The transmogrification of coaching from a somewhat sophisticated to a banal and rudimentary practice is typical of what Furedi (2004) might refer to as part of the trivialisation of contemporary culture. This is where policy typically operates to 'dumb-down' the quality of educational experience, and where it inflicts on the imagination of the public (or in this case coaches) a process of 'infantilization', 'expressing a pessimistic and anti-democratic account of people' (2004 p 145). Therefore, there is a risk that the newly conceived 'docile' coach will become a technocrat who has been limited by a narrow curriculum whereby autonomy and problem solving skills have given way to routine, structure and fragmentation (Macdonald & Tinning 1995). In order to address this missed opportunity and path towards the death of the coach as intellectual, we argue that education and pedagogical theory needs to be at the forefront of any progressive coach education philosophy.

We would also argue that although consultation has taken place when formulating and formatting policy, most of it has been done with NGBs both individually and collectively. However, their remit is to represent their particular sport as a whole, and coaching is just one of their priorities. The pace and nature of these proposed changes has been so rapid that few NGBs have had the time or effective machinery in place to engage fully and consult with their communities of coaches. Most sports have somewhat ponderous and complex communication systems, whereby policy consultation from central organisations to local activist and back again is both slow and beset by thorny problems. Without the explicit approval and signing up of the community volunteer, any change could be perceived as an unwarranted imposition and thus, ultimately, resisted. One of the abiding features of British sport and, by implication, its coaching practice, is the rich and diverse socio-cultural heritage. Without a grasp and deep appreciation of these key characteristics, any attempt to homogenise practices or education would ultimately fail to do service to each sport and those individuals delivering on poolside, pitch, court and sports hall up and down the UK.

Invitation to further study

Within the process of professionalisation there are a number of unanswered questions that need to be critically addressed. Since the transformation from mainly voluntary engagement to a situation of fully-paid professional employment is an unlikely scenario in UK sports coaching – (one for which there is no extant model or previous experience as a guide to new practice), we must be prudent only to engage in tentative speculation. Until quite recently, the professionalisation of sports coaching has been largely overlooked and ignored by academics. While in one

sense disappointing, in another this absence of attention creates a welcome opportunity to develop a number of critical and methodological approaches to the social and educational study of sports coaching. Since social interaction is centrally positioned in the coaching process (Jones et al 2004), we contend that research should be principally concerned with identifying better ways of understanding coaching cultures, notions of professionalism and the relationships existing between voluntary coaches, sports industry professionals, adult participants, administrators and National Governing Bodies, as collective and individual 'orchestrators of culture'.

There is little doubt that coaching in the UK is going through a period of unparalleled change. No longer are coaches and the structures that support them the forgotten cousins of the modern sporting landscape. The government's vision for coaches is one in which they are implicated as central actors in a broad range of social purposes: increasing physical activity participation rates; contributing to sustained international medal success; enhancing the ever-widening role of sport as a tool of social welfare. Thus, at the cornerstone of the professionalisation agenda (of coaches and coaching) is the ambition to address a variety of social aims and purposes, which further implies the possibility of a radical shift in culture, along with significant structural change. However, in this, our contention is that the government (and its sports organisations) has failed to account for the inherently conservative nature of NGBs, the desire of many coaches to hang on to notions of community action rooted in volunteering and the resistance of many others towards the criticism that their practice was deemed 'unprofessional'. Any sustained bid towards the professionalisation of (coaching) practice requires, at its heart, an organic commitment to change. This is because any anticipated benefits will automatically accrue to the individuals involved in those particular sports. An externally driven agenda will therefore only succeed if the individuals on the touchline feel valued and considered and are duly consulted and invested in.

The following research questions are not intended to be exhaustive. Nor do they represent a comprehensive list of priorities for further social inquiry. Rather, they are meant as much to stimulate consideration and discussion, as to provide a broad and critical agenda. They hopefully go some way in enabling us to learn more on how to navigate through one of the most significant contemporary challenges to face the activity of coaching in sport.

Addressing the impact of professionalism on coaching performance

- How does sports-coach UK's Action Plan impact on individual coaches and in doing so operate to construct and manage their professional performance?
- How does the professionalisation of sports coaching impact on the motivation of in-coming coaches/volunteers?
- How are tensions expressed and/or resolved by professionals in relation to their vocational responsibilities and effectiveness, within sports coaching?

Addressing the impact of professionalism on coaching relationships

- What are the implications for general accountability in sports coaching if the notion of 'professional' is to be sustained?

- How will traditional relationships between athletes and voluntary coaches be changed by the implicit 'commercialisation' of coaching or 'business model' that professionalism brings?
- What implicit models of professionalism can be seen to emerge from coaching relationships and how do these models locate with other identified professions?

Assessing the movement towards the professionalisation of sports coaching on an international scale

- What are the issues in establishing an international brand for the professionalisation of the sports coach?
- Is there a place for policy borrowing across countries? Or are practices so diverse that the transfer of policy between nations will inevitably fail to acknowledge individual differences?
- What lessons are to be learnt from the high-level, global coach trading across sporting, cultural and international boundaries?

References

Anzaldua, G., 1987. Borderlands /La frontera: The new Mestiz. Aunt Lute Books, New York.

Arts Council England, 2005. Arts Council England - Report of the Peer Review. Arts Council England/ Department for Culture. Media and Sport, London.

Bates, R., 2004. Regulation and autonomy in teacher education: Government, community or democracy? Journal of Education for Teaching 30 (2), 117–130.

Beck, J., Young, M.F.D., 2005. The assault on the professions and the restructuring of academic and professional identities: a Bernsteinian analysis. British Journal of Sociology of Education 26 (2), 183–197.

Bernstein, B., 1971. Class, codes and control. Volume 1: Theoretical studies towards a sociology of language. Routledge, London.

Bernstein, B., 2000. Pedagogy symbolic control and identity. Rowman Littlefield, London.

Bhabha, H.K., 1996. Culture's in-between. In: Hall, S., du Gay, P. (Eds.), Questions of cultural identity. Sage, London, pp. 55–61.

Boon, A., Flood, J., Webb, J., 2005. Postmodern professions? The fragmentation of legal education and the legal profession. Journal of Law and Society 32 (3), 473–492.

Bourdieu, P., 1977. Outline of theory and practice. Cambridge University Press, Cambridge.

Bourdieu, P., 1986. Distinction: A social critique of the judgement of taste. Routledge, London.

Bourdieu, P., 1988. Homo academicus. Polity, Cambridge.

Bourdieu, P., Passeron, D., 1977. Reproduction in education, society and culture. Sage, London.

Broadbent, J., Dietrich, M., Roberts, J., 1997. The end of the professions:

the restructuring of professional work. Routledge, London.

Brown, B., Butterfield, S.A., 1992. Coaches: a missing link in the health care system. Am. J. Dis. Child. 146 (2), 211–217.

Bush, A., 2007. What is coaching? In: Denison, J. (Ed.), Coaching knowledge: understanding the dynamics of sports performance. A C Black, London.

Campbell, S., 1993. Coach Education around the world. Sports Science Review 2 (2), 62–74.

Chelladurai, P., 1986. Professional development of coaches: Coach education preparation for a profession. In: Proceedings from the VIII Commonwealth and International Conference on Sport, Physical Education, Dance, Recreation. E & F N Spon, London, pp. 139–150.

Coghlan, J., Webb, I.M., 1990. Sport and British politics since 1960. Falmer, London.

Cushion, C.J., Jones, R.L., 2006. Power, discourse and symbolic violence in professional youth soccer: The case of Albion Football Club. Sociology of Sport Journal 23, 142–161.

Dawson, A., 1994. Professional codes of practice and ethical conduct. J. Appl. Philos. 11 (2), 145–153.

Day, C., 2002. School reform and transitions in teacher professionalism and identity. International Journal of Educational Research 37 (8), 677–692.

Day, C., Hadfield, M., 1996. Metaphors for movement: accounts of professional development. In: Kompf, T., Boak, T., Bond, R.W. et al. (Eds.), Changing research and practice: teachers' professionalism, identities and knowledge. Falmer Press, London.

Department for Culture Media and Sport (DCMS), 2002. The coaching task force – final report. Department for Culture Media and Sport, London.

Downie, R.S., 1990. Professions and professionalism. Journal of Philosophy of Education 24 (2), 147–159.

Dyer, W., 1992. Real Magic. Harper-Collins, New York.

Eraut, M., 1994. Developing professional knowledge and competence. Routledge, London.

Friedson, E., 1973. Professionalism and the occupational principle. In: Friedson, E. (Ed.), The professions and their prospect. Sage, Beverly Hills CA, pp. 19–37.

Furedi, F., 2004. Where have all the intellectuals gone? Confronting 21st century philistinism. Continuum, London.

Green, M., Houlihan, B., 2005. Elite sport development: policy learning and political priorities. Routledge, London.

Guskey, T.R., Huberman, M., 1995. Professional development in education – new paradigms and practices. Teachers College Press, New York.

Halpin, D., Troyna, B., 1995. The Politics of Education Policy Borrowing. Comparative Education 31 (3), 303–310.

Hargreaves, A., 2000. Four ages of professionalism and professional learning. Teachers and teaching. Theory and Practice 6 (2), 151–182.

HMSO, 1973. House of Lords Report, Sport and Leisure (Cobham Report). HMSO, London.

Houlihan, B., 1997. Sport, policy and the politics. Routledge, London.

Houlihan, B., Green, M., 2008. Comparative elite sports development: system, structures and public policy. Butterworth-Heinemann, Oxford.

Humphreys, J., 2000. Education and the professionalisation of nursing: non-collective action and the erosion of the labour-market control. Journal of Education Policy 15 (3), 263–279.

Jarvie, G., Maguire, J., 1994. Fields of power, habitus and distinction. In: Jarvie, J., Maguire, J. (Eds.), Sport and leisure in social thought. Routledge, London.

Johnson, T.J., 1984. Professionalism: occupation politics or ideology. In: Goodlad, S. (Ed.), Education for the professionals: quis custodiet? SRHE & NFER, Nelson.

Jones, R., 2000. Developing an integrated coach education programme; the case for problem based learning'. 2000 Pre-Olympic Congress, Sports Medicine & Physical Education International Congress. Sports Science Abstracts. Online. Available www.ausport.gov.au./fulltext/2000/preoly/ 20 July 2006.

Jones, R.L., 2006. The sports coach as educator: Re- conceptualising sports coaching. Routledge, London.

Jones, R.L., Armour, K., 2000. Sociology of sport theory and practice. Longman Pearson, London.

Jones, R.L., Armour, K., Potrac, P., 2004. Sport coaching cultures: from theory to practice. Routledge, London.

Jones, R., Wallace, M., 2005. Another bad day at the training ground: coping with ambiguity in the coaching context. Sport, Education and Society 10 (1), 119–134.

Kalber, L.P., 1995. Professionalism and its consequences: a study of internal audits. Audit: Journal of Practice and Theory 14 (1), 64–86.

Larson, M.S., 1977. The rise of the professional: a sociological analysis. University of California Press, Berkeley CA.

Lawson, W., 2004. Professionalism: The Golden Years. Journal of Professional

Issues in Engineering Education and Practice 130 (1), 26–36.

Locke, T., 2001. Questions of professionalism: Erosion and reclamation. Change: Transformations in Education 4 (2), 30–50.

Lyle, J., 1986. Coach education: preparation for a profession. In: Proceedings from the VIII Commonwealth and international Conference on Sport, Physical Education, Dance, & Recreation. E & F N Spon, London, pp. 1–25.

Lyle, J., 2002. Sport coaching concepts: a framework for coaches' behaviour. Routledge, London.

Lyotard, J.F., 1984. The postmodern condition. Manchester University Press, Manchester.

Macdonald, D., Tinning, R., 1995. Physical education teacher education and the trend to proletarianisation: a case study. Journal of Teaching in Physical Education 15, 98–118.

Middlehurst, R., 1995. Professionals, professionalism and higher education for tomorrow's world. In: Paper presented at the Higher Education in a Learning Society Conference, St Edmund Hall, Oxford.

Moorhead, R., 2001. Third way regulation? Community legal service partnerships. The Modern Law Review 64 (4), 543–562.

Nash, C., 2001. Volunteerism in sports coaching: A Tayside study. In: Graham, M., Foley, M. (Eds.), Leisure volunteering: marginal or inclusive. University of Brighton/LSA Publications, Brighton.

Naul, R., Hardman, K., 2002. Sport and physical education in Germany. Routledge, London.

Nichols, G., Taylor, P., James, M., et al., 2005. Pressures on the UK Voluntary Sport Sector. Voluntas 16 (1), 33–50.

Nixon, J., Marks, A., Rowland, S., et al., 2001. Towards a new academic professionalism: a manifesto of hope. British Journal of Sociology of Education 22 (2), 227–244.

Perucci, R., Gerstl, J., 1969. Professional without community: engineers in America. Ramdon House, New York.

Petlichkoff, L.M., 1993. Coaching children: understanding the motivational process. Sport Science Review 2, 48–61.

Potrac, P., Cassidy, T., 2006. The coach 'as a more capable other. In: Jones, R.L. (Ed.), The sports coach as educator. Routledge, London, pp. 39–50.

Roche, M., 1993. Sport and community: rhetoric and reality in the development of British sports policy. In: Binfield, J.C., Stevenson, J. (Eds.), Sports, culture and politics. Sheffield Academic Press, Sheffield.

Sachs, J., 2001. Teacher professional identity: competing discourses, competing outcomes. Journal of Education Policy 16 (2), 149–161.

Smith, A., Stewart, B., 1999. Sports management: a guide to professional practice. Allen Unwin, London.

sports coach UK, 2007. Sports Coaching in the UK II. scUK, Leeds. Online. Available: http://www.sportscoachuk.org/research/Research+Publications/Sports+Coaching+in+the+UK+II.htm 8th Sept 2008.

sports coach UK, 2008. UK Coaching Framework. scUK, Leeds. Online. Available: http://www.sportscoachuk.org/The+UK+Coaching+Framework/ 8th Sept 2008.

Sports Council, 1982. Sport in the community: the next ten years. Sports Council, London.

Sports Council, 1991. Coaching matters: A review of coaching and coach education in the United Kingdom. Sports Council, London.

Strathern, M., 2000. Audit cultures: Anthropological studies in accountability, ethics and the academy. Routledge, London.

Stronach, I., Corbin, B., McNamara, O., et al., 2002. Towards a uncertain politics of professionalism: teacher and nurse identities in flux. Journal of Education Policy 17 (1), 109–138.

Sullivan, P.A., Wilson, D.J., 1993. The coach's role. In: Cohen, G.L. (Ed.), Women in sport: issues and controversies. Sage, Newbury Park CA.

Taylor, W., 2007. The professionalisation of sports coaches. Paper presented at the LSA Annual Conference, University of Brighton, 6–9th July 2007.

Taylor, W., Garratt, D., 2007. The professionalisation of sports coaching in the UK: issues and conceptualisation. scUK, Leeds. Online. Available: http://www.sportscoachuk.org/Resources/SCUK/Documents/Research/Professionalisation%20Report.pdf 28th Sept 2008.

Taylor, W., Garratt, D., in press. The professionalisation of sports coaching: relations of power, resistance and compliance, Sport, Education and Society.

Travers, M., 2007. The new bureaucracy: quality assurance and its critics. Policy Press, Bristol.

Trnobranski, P.H., 1997. Power and vested interests – tacit influences on the construction of nursing curricula? J. Adv. Nurs. 25, 1084–1088.

U.K. Sport, 2001. The UK vision for coaching. UK Sport, London.

Wainwright, S.P., Turner, B.S., 2008. Reflections on embodiment and vulnerability. Medical Humanities on line 29, 4–7.

Williams, P., 2002. Battle lines on three fronts: The RFU and the lost war against professionalism. The International Journal of the History of Sport 19 (4), 114–136.

Woodman, L., 1993. Coaching: A science, an art, an emerging profession. Sports Science Review 2 (2), 1–13.

Becoming a high-performance coach: pathways and communities

8

Clifford J. Mallett

Introduction

Elite sport in many Western countries (and increasingly in developing countries) is a culturally significant activity that captures the attention of the public, and especially the written and visual media. Coaches who work in high-profile sports in these countries attract and often assume a controversial position within the public domain because they are charged with the responsibility of producing successful (winning) results.

Coaching work at the elite level in sport (Olympic and professional sports) is a dynamic, complex and challenging vocation. The work of high-performance coaches has evolved over the past few decades and, reflecting transformations in society and sport itself, has become increasingly more demanding and complex. The increased commercialisation of sport has resulted in increasing demands on coaches in elite sport to deliver 'cutting edge' advice and direction to athletes and this has differentially impacted upon the work of coaches. Recent research (Jones & Wallace 2005, Bowes & Jones 2006) has highlighted the organised chaos associated with coaching, especially in high-performance sport; however, the degree of coaching complexity is context-dependent (Trudel & Gilbert 2006). In other words, high-performance coaching work is often idiosyncratic and usually relies upon the coaches' individual interpretation of their role (Mallett et al 2008). Furthermore, with the perceived failure of coach education/accreditation to cater for the learning needs of high-performance coaches (e.g. Dickson 2001, Lyle 2002), an important question is, how do high-performance coaches learn

their craft? For these reasons, coaching scholars and aspiring coaches are interested in the backgrounds and practices of high-performance coaches.

This chapter will introduce what we know (and don't know) about the pathways to becoming a high-performance coach and then consider the influence of others in how coaches of elite athletes, squads and teams learn their craft. The chapter is organised in three sections: (a) an understanding of high-performance coaching; (b) the pathways to becoming a high-performance coach; and (c) supporting theory and research conducted on situated learning in elite sports coaching environments – with a focus on communities of practice. Key themes foregrounded in this chapter include: problematising high-performance coaching; acknowledgement of the variability in playing and coaching experiences in developing high-performance coaching expertise; and a critique of the concepts of *communities of practice* and other social networks in developing coach expertise within the highly contested environment of high-performance coaching.

What is high-performance coaching?

In understanding high-performance coaching we might consider the work performed by coaches in elite sporting environments in comparison to work performed by coaches in other contexts (e.g. junior sport). Lyle (2002) distinguished between different forms of coaching (participation, sport teacher, performance, representative team) highlighting the context-specific nature of coaches' work. Trudel and Gilbert (2006) categorised coaching into three major forms – recreational, developmental, and elite sport coaching. Nevertheless, recent research (Mallett et al 2008) has shown significant variation in what coaches do both within the same team (club) and between teams. Despite these variations, high-performance coaching would appear to be characterised by several features (Lyle 2002, Trudel & Gilbert 2006). The work of high-performance coaches is typically orga- nised, systematic, deliberate, but highly fluid and dynamic (Woodman 1993). High-performance coa- ches undertake a range of tasks related to producing winning performances in elite international competi- tion, which involves the highest levels of commitment by the coach and athlete/s to achieve public perfor- mance goals (e.g. Grand Final, Olympic medals) through participation in intensive planning, training and competition (Côté et al 1995, Lyle 2002, Trudel & Gilbert 2006). High-performance coaches usually engage in highly complex decision-making tasks involving extensive data collection, analysis and man- agement, and extensive interaction with a range of per- sonnel (e.g. players, assistant coaches and ancillary staff). Furthermore, this highly structured and forma- lised environment increasingly requires that high-per- formance coaches work preferably on a full-time basis.

The extent to which coaches engage in high-per- formance coaching is dependent upon the satisfac- tion of eight key criteria for full engagement in the coaching process (Lyle 2002).

- Stability of personnel – e.g. stable coach–athlete– scientist relationship;
- Continuity of engagement – engagement in multiple training sessions each week, every week;
- Extended time period – stable coach–athlete engagement preferably over several years;
- Intensity of engagement – sufficient duration of engagement in weekly training sessions and competitions;
- Commitment to goal-orientated instrumental relationship – relationship seeks to achieve longer-term goal/s usually associated with performance outcomes;
- Control of variables – coach seeks to control performance variables (e.g., lifestyle factors, recovery) to enhance performance outcomes;
- Planned progression – detailed planning and monitoring of training and competition performances; and
- Individualisation – personal development.

Athletes and players involved in professional, semi- professional, and Olympic sports are typically engaged in coach–athlete relationships that satisfy most if not all of the above criteria proposed by Lyle (2002). For example a high-performance coach in athletics might be involved in the following key interrelated tasks:

- Planning and implementation of daily, weekly, monthly, annual, and perhaps 4-year training and competition plans;
- Negotiating (international-level) goals with athletes – performance, key performance indicators (power, speed, endurance performance tests), skill development (advanced technique), psychological development (performance routines, mental skills);
- Monitoring (data collection and analysis) and regulating training and competition on the basis of shifts in physical, social, psychological and/or emotional well-being;
- Recruiting and scouting players and staff;
- Leading and managing other personnel (e.g., sport medicine and scientists);
- Liaising with stakeholder organisations responsible for funding and governance (e.g. Athletics Australia, Australian Sports Commission); and
- Seeking and negotiating personal funding and sponsorship for athlete/s.

Although there have been attempts to categorise different forms of coaching (see above), the bound- aries between the various forms are not distinct. Even within the category of (elite or high-) perfor- mance coaching there is significant variation in what coaches do. For example, the five Head Coaches of the Australian Rugby team (Wallabies) over the past two decades have adopted different approaches to the coaching process – some have contributed with a more hands-on approach (direct intervention using Lyle's [2002] terminology) and others had more of a focus on a managerial role and used their assistant coaches to undertake the more direct intervention tasks. The head coaches are likely to have based their interpretation of their role and their emphasis within the coaching process on num- ber of factors, for example, their perceptions of the key work tasks of the Wallabies head coach position, their perceived strengths and weaknesses, and access to other expertise. Increased professionalisa- tion has been accompanied by increased demands on coaches' ability to manage human resources.

Importantly however, over the last 10 years, the demands made of senior (head) and assistant coaches have necessitated changes in the roles undertaken by them. For example, in the Australian Football League (AFL) there have been dramatic changes (Mallett et al 2007). These changes have seen an increase in coaching staff from around 2–4 to 5–7 coaches at each club over that same period. Furthermore, ancillary (support) staff has increased such that overall many senior coaches in the AFL in 2008 were responsible for between 10 and 25 (mostly full-time) staff.

Central to high-performance coaching is the need for the coach to assume leadership and management of the coaching process. As previously stated the extent to which the high-performance coach takes direct responsibility for delivering all the above tasks is dependent on the environment in which they operate, and their expertise and confidence in relation to the perceived demands of their role (including the competency of the coach in all aspects of coaching; availability and access to other expertise; and funding). Coaches may manage a multidisciplinary team of para-professionals (e.g. sports medicine, psychologist, strength & conditioning expert, tactical analyst) who work directly with the athletes/players or alternatively, a team of para-professionals may directly support the coaches and therefore work indirectly with the athletes/players. There are several models of how the coach interacts in the workplace with other personnel to deliver high-performance coaching (see Cavalheiro et al 2005), however, all models require the high-performance coach to exercise a leadership and management role.

The main aim of high-performance coaching is the purposeful leadership and management of competition sport performance, which is achieved through a planned programme of preparation, training and competition, usually within a unique environment (Côté et al 1995, Cross & Lyle 1999). Although coaches engage in sophisticated, structured, and serially designed coaching plans, coaching is none-the-less time- and context-bound and therefore dynamic, complex, and uncertain (Saury & Durand 1998), prompting Cushion et al (2003) to consider coaching as 'structured improvisation'. Although high-performance coaches attempt to control as many variables as possible, in reality the coach still needs to be responsive to a dynamic environment in which there is, at times, limited control. 'Structured improvisation' captures the 'complexity of coaching arguing that

coaching is in fact largely uncontrollable, incomprehensible and imbued with contradictory values' (Cushion 2007 p 397). Based on the work of Fenwick and Rubenson (2005), Mallett (2008) described (high-performance) coaching as

> a complex, social, and dynamic activity that is not easily represented as a set of tangible and predictable processes ... and might be considered within a broader set of relations: the interdependence between (a) the coaching tasks undertaken by coaches, (b) coaches' relations with other people (e.g., athletes, other coaches, parents), and (c) the coaching situation and context in which they operate. The agentic engagement of coaches in a situated coaching practice makes the coaching process highly idiosyncratic ... (2008 p 419).

The fluid nature of high-performance coaching, which requires constant cycles of planning, monitoring, action, and reviewing, contributes to the dynamism and complexity inherent in coaching (Bowes & Jones 2006). This problematised view of coaching reflects the 'muddiness' or 'turbulence' in which coaches operate, especially in elite sport, and influences what and how coaches learn. Nevertheless, it is proposed that the head coach attempts to bring order to this 'chaos'. Bringing some order to this 'messiness' is central to effective leadership and management of the coaching process.

The pathways to becoming a high-performance coach

How did you become a high-performance (elite) coach? This is a frequently asked question of coaches in elite sport. The life histories of coaches are quite fascinating and seem to be of interest to people both inside and outside of sport. Importantly, the life histories of coaches are likely to impact on what and how they learn. Coaches' life histories have been found to influence the development of coaching knowledge (e.g. Salmela 1996, Gilbert & Trudel 2001, Gilbert et al 2006), which subsequently contributes to their developing identities as coaches that, in turn, influence their personal agency (individual action). It is this relationship between coaches' personal histories, their agency, and their subsequent engagement with social experiences that makes research into the backgrounds of high-performance coaches so useful in understanding and informing the coach development process.

Quantitative (e.g. Gilbert et al 2006, Lynch & Mallett 2006) and qualitative (e.g. Schinke et al 1995, Rynne 2008) research methods have been used to examine the pathways to becoming a high-performance coach. For instance, quantitative data have provided some guidance into the amount of investment required to become a successful high-performance coach. To complement the quantitative research, information from interviews (qualitative research) has provided some rich data about coaches' perceptions of the utility of various activities to coach development. Both quantitative and qualitative research methods should be valued for the unique and complementary contributions they can make to our enhanced understanding of the high-performance coach development process. The following section highlights some of the major quantitative and qualitative research undertaken that has examined the pathways to becoming high-performance coaches.

Data on the life (pre-mediate) experiences of successful high-performance coaches can only be collected retrospectively. Whilst there may be some concerns with accuracy of recall, steps to minimise this problem can be taken (Gilbert et al 2006). In addressing this issue, Gilbert and colleagues developed a retrospective interview protocol and schedule based on research on the coaching process (Côté et al 1995), coaches' learning (Trudel & Gilbert 2006), and an adaptation of the interview procedure described by Côté et al (2005). This 2-hour face-to-face structured interview using a questionnaire enables the collection of quantitative data that identify important developmental profiles of activities (pre-mediate experiences). The data collected in their interview schedule can be checked against public records and by accessing other coaches, athletes and employers (Côté et al 2005). The face-to-face questionnaire was designed to facilitate coaches' recall of events rather than inferences and reconstructions (Côté et al 2005, Gilbert et al 2006). Furthermore, Côté et al refer to a number of studies highlighting high test–retest reliability of past sporting activities.

Through their structured interview schedule, researchers such as Gilbert, Côté, Mallett and colleagues have captured data on major aspects of coach development. These include: sport participation experience, coaching experience, and formal education.

Sport participation experience

It makes sense that coaches are likely to coach in a sport with which they have significant playing experience. Trudel and Gilbert (2006) reported that over 90% of 'elite sport' coaches were competitive athletes in the sport they coach. A background in playing the sport they now coach seems likely to contribute to understanding the technical and tactical aspects, as well as the 'culture' of the sport (Jones et al 2003, Mallett et al 2007).

Several studies of high-performance coaches, using the Gilbert et al (2006) interview schedule, have shown their history of engagement in extensive hours of training and competing in the sport they now coach. For example, several Australian studies have shown that, typically, high-performance coaches (n = 55) averaged between 10 and 20 years of playing the sport they now coach (Lynch & Mallett 2006, Mallett & Rynne unpublished work 2008, Rynne 2008). Furthermore, the Australian data suggest that it is more likely that team sport coaches played their sport for longer than individual sport coaches. Erickson et al (2007) who interviewed 19 individual and team high-performance sport coaches from Canada found they had played on average for 5 and 8 years, respectively. Of note was the significant variation in duration of sport participation in both the Australian and Canadian samples. Nevertheless, all studies reported that coaches had a minimum of 5 years playing experience in the sport they now coach, which might suggest that this engagement is a prerequisite for high-performance coaching in that sport.

The development of some base knowledge and understanding of the sport from early sport participation is not unexpected. Experience as an athlete has been extensively reported as an important source of coaching knowledge and practice (Sage 1989, Bloom et al 1998, Cushion et al 2003, Irwin et al 2004). For example, most of the coaches interviewed in the Mallett et al (2007) study reported a background in observing matches (live, video replays), which seemed to lay some foundation in analytical skills for coaches in the AFL. Studies by Bloom et al (1998) and Cushion et al (2003) suggested that coaches develop some of their initial conceptions of what and how to coach from when they were athletes. These pre-mediate experiences as an athlete can assist knowledge construction that can be drawn on in later years as a coach.

What makes some players (and not others) become coaches? Coaches often report continuing association with their sport as a reason for entering the vocation (Mallett et al 2007). Could the notion of 'identity' be key to deciding to become a high-performance coach; perhaps dissatisfaction in one's playing career influences one to become a coach; the strong influence of a coach on one's personal development may be important; perhaps an interest in helping others could be a deciding factor; possibly some key experiences (proto-coaching or technical immersion) might be a factor? We need answers to these questions, and they suggest an obvious research agenda.

Is success as a player a prerequisite for a successful career in high-performance coaching? Mallett et al (2007) found that high-performance Australian Football League (AFL) coaches reported an extensive playing background in Australian football. However, not all coaches in the AFL had playing experience in the AFL (highest competition level). This finding indicated a slight shift away from the line of thinking that playing at the highest level was essential to a coaching career in the AFL. The majority of high-performance coaches report that they were generally above-average players among their peers (around 7–8 out of 10) (Gilbert et al 2006, Mallett et al 2007, Rynne 2008). A playing background in the sport they coach probably assists in the early stages of a career by enabling the coach to get a 'foot in the door'; after which, the coaching record of a coach becomes more pertinent to future employment opportunities (Mallett et al 2007). A limitation of the research that asks participants to rate their sport ability has been the clear identification of the frame of reference for that judgement. For example, when reporting on athletic ability do participants base their judgement in relation to their peers on: the best performers in the world, the players in the league in which they play, or their team mates?

The evidence suggests that in becoming high-performance coaches, experience in playing the sport they coach is probably advantageous, but success at the highest levels is not essential (e.g. Irwin et al 2004, Lynch & Mallett 2006, Erickson et al 2007, Mallett et al 2007, Rynne 2008). Having played the sport they coach probably helps the coaches in several ways:

- Knowledge of skills, rules, strategies and tactics (at an appropriate level);
- Understanding the culture of the sport;

- Self-efficacy in knowing about the sport (and perhaps gaining some credibility); and
- Perceived identity (sense of belonging) within the sport. Nevertheless, previous experience in playing the sport may contribute to the reproduction of inappropriate coaching practices.

Coaching experience

Experiential learning (e.g. coaching work) has been identified as the primary source of coaching knowledge in the development of expertise (Salmela 1996, Saury & Durand 1998, Gilbert & Trudel 2001, Lyle 2002, Jones et al 2003, Mallett et al 2008, Rynne 2008). Simon and Chase (1973) proposed a '10-year rule' for developing expertise. Moreover, extensive coaching experience in developing expert knowledge is consistent with Ericsson et al's (1993) notion of 'deliberate practice' – focused effort on improving performance through structured practice. Ericsson et al (1993) concluded from their research that to achieve an expert level of performance, approximately 10 000 hours of deliberate practice was required.

Erickson et al (2007) found support for Simon and Chase's (1973) '10-year rule' and partial support for Ericsson et al's (1993) notion of 10 000 hours of deliberate practice. Australian data also support Simon and Chase's '10-year' rule (Lynch & Mallett 2006, Mallett & Rynne unpublished work, 2008, Rynne 2008). Many of the Australian coaches sampled had coached for around 10 years prior to engagement in high-performance coaching. Again, this was not consistent across sports and even within sports there was significant variation. Netball coaches typically coached for almost 20 years prior to working at the national level whereas basketball coaches had coached for around 10 years before securing a high-performance coaching position (Mallett & Rynne unpublished work, 2008). The data from Australian coaches also revealed that individual sport coaches coached more hours on average than their team sport counterparts. This is not surprising considering the number of contact hours in multiple weekly training sessions in which athletes in individual sports engage. Overall, it appears that most high-performance coaches typically engaged in between 5 and 10 years' coaching experience prior to commencement of their elite coaching careers.

Some coaches had limited experience coaching prior to engagement in elite sport coaching whereas others had extensive experience at the developmental level. Some former elite athletes in Australia commenced their high performance coaching careers almost immediately post retirement. Trudel and Gilbert (2006) reported research that suggested most elite coaches 'have five or more years of assistant coaching experience before assuming a head coach position' (p 538). High-performance coaches are most likely to develop their craft from early experience as a developmental coach rather than from extensive experience at the recreational level (Lynch & Mallett 2006, Mallett & Rynne unpublished work 2008, Rynne 2008). This finding was supported by Canadian research (Erickson et al 2007).

Nevertheless, extensive work experience alone is insufficient to develop high-performance coaching expertise (Eraut 2004, Lynch & Mallett 2006). The importance of self-reflection in making one's experiences meaningful and subsequently developing one's coaching knowledge and refining coaching practices has been extensively reported (Gilbert & Trudel 2001, Cushion et al 2003, Irwin et al 2004, Mallett 2004, Trudel & Gilbert 2006). The work of Donald Schön (1983) has contributed much to our understanding of experiential learning and the significance of 'reflection-in-action' and 'reflection-on-action' in sports coaching. Key to the transformation of experience into coaching knowledge is 'reflection-in-action' (during coaching work), 'reflection-on-action' (post coaching work) and 'retrospective reflection-on-action' (after the season) (Gilbert & Trudel 2001, Trudel & Gilbert 2006).

Formal education

Trudel and Gilbert (2006) reported that most elite sport coaches in North America are tertiary educated and around two-thirds of elite developmental coaches completed postgraduate study. Unsurprisingly, most tertiary-educated coaches majored in physical education. Nevertheless, much of the research reported by Trudel and Gilbert from North America is from the U.S. Collegiate system, which varies in the degree to which coaches can be considered high performance. Trudel and Gilbert (2006) also reported research that showed that 56–84% of elite coaches in Europe, Asia, and South Africa held undergraduate degrees. In Australia, research from several studies (Lynch & Mallett 2006, Mallett & Rynne unpublished work, 2008, Rynne 2008) has shown that around 65% of coaches surveyed (n = 55) were tertiary-educated predominately in the fields of physical education and/or sports science. Again there was significant variation between sports and studies.

In the quest for improving their coaching knowledge and practice elite coaches in many Western countries have completed accredited coach education courses. Although coaches may initially complete these courses with a motive of self-improvement and personal satisfaction, the higher levels of coach accreditation are often seen as a 'ticket' to the big stage (Dickson 2001, Rynne 2008). That is, the highest level of coach accreditation is perceived as a prerequisite for elite coaching positions and credibility within the sporting community. In Australia coach accreditation is synonymous with coach education. Dickson (2001), in reviewing coach accreditation programs in Australia, reported that successful completion of courses was valued because they provided improved vocational opportunities and advancement. However, they did not afford authentic context-specific information necessary for learning to become a high-performance coach. Coach accreditation is accordingly viewed as a low-impact activity, terms of allocated time, in the development of elite coaches (e.g. Dickson 2001, Lyle 2002, Cushion et al 2003, Rynne 2008). Nevertheless, it can serve to affirm coaching knowledge and practices as well as providing a catalyst for challenging the thinking of coaches. Therefore, caution is warranted in thinking that coach accreditation is not useful for some coaches in their development.

Much of the data collected from high-performance coaches (e.g. Erickson et al 2007, Rynne 2008) on formal education (coach accreditation and tertiary education) shows the significantly lower amounts of time invested compared with coaching itself, which is not surprising. The extensive time involved in coaching practice far exceeds what is possible in formal coach education activities. Of greater importance to developing coaching expertise is the quality of the experience and its subsequent contribution to coach development. High-performance coaches appear to make up for perceived limitations in knowledge by accessing and aggregating other sources (Mallett et al 2007, Rynne 2008). Importantly, it is the complementarity of these varied experiences that contributes to individual high-performance coach development.

Influence of pre-mediate experiences on high-performance coaching

Research reveals that there is significant variation in the range of experiences prior to becoming a high-performance coach (Erickson et al 2007, Rynne 2008). However, much of the retrospective data collected on high-performance coaches does not report the varying influence of pre-mediate experiences in developing high-performance coaches' expertise. Rynne (2008) asked 24 high-performance individual and team sport coaches to rate the value of contribution of a variety of coach development activities at three stages of their coaching career: (a) first 2 years, (b) middle 2 years, and (c) last 2 years. The high-performance coaches in his study rated 'on the job experience' as the most valued coach development activity during all three stages of their careers. Personal reflection and discussions with colleagues were also highly valued by the participants in the study, although, interestingly, these were more valued as the coaches developed their craft. The importance of reflection in coach development was discussed earlier in this chapter (e.g. Gilbert & Trudel 2001, Cushion et al 2003, Irwin et al 2004, Trudel & Gilbert, 2006). Discussions with colleagues (and observing other coaches) were also valued. Tertiary study was not rated highly, but it should be noted that only one-third of coaches in Rynne's study were tertiary educated. Those who had actually completed tertiary study valued highly their university education, especially in the middle and latter stages of their career. Salmela and Moraes (2003) also found their coaches highly valued tertiary education. Overall, Rynne's data suggested that as high-performance coaches developed they seemed to value a greater variety of sources for developing their craft. That finding might be linked to an increase in self-efficacy (Eraut 2004) and increased access to learning opportunities (e.g. working with other colleagues). In some cases the increase in access might be connected with a move from voluntary and/or part-time to full-time coach employment.

A stage-based model of high-performance coach development

Several researchers (Salmela 1995, Schinke et al 1995, Erickson et al 2007) have proposed stage-based models of coach development. Recently, Erickson et al (2007) proposed a developmental model of sports coaches, which sought to identify what experiences were necessary to reach high performance. Their model was considered similar to the Developmental Model of Sport Participation (DMSP) (Côté 1999, Côté & Fraser-Thomas 2007).

Stage 1 – Diversified Early Sport Participation (age 6–12 years)

- Participate in many different recreational team and individual sports

Stage 2 – Competitive Sport Participation (age 13–18 years)

- Participate in at least one competitive sport
- Play several sports, but focus on one sport eventually coaching
- Leadership opportunities (for team sport coaches) occur in this stage

Stage 3 – Highly Competitive Sport Participation/Introduction to Coaching (age 19–23 years)

- Participate in the sport they coach at a highly competitive level (e.g. university/premier grade)
- Entry into coaching

Stage 4 – Part-time Early Coaching (age 24–28 years)

- Retired as an athlete at a highly competitive level
- Engaged in major non-coaching activities (e.g. job, university studies)
- Coaching part-time at developmental level and/or as an assistant coach at the elite level
- Most interaction with mentor coaches occurs during this stage

Stage 5 – High Performance Head Coaching (age 29+ years)

- First position as a high-performance head coach (see Erickson et al 2007).

The five-stage model of high-performance coach development (Erickson et al 2007) provides a generic chronological template of learning opportunities that can contribute to coach development. As a model it is only a guide. The research on high-performance coaches shows significant variation in pathways. Therefore, further research on Erickson et al's (2007) five-stage model of coach development is necessary before more definitive conclusions can be made about the validity of the model. To what degree the model best represents high-performance coach development is yet to be examined. In particular some cross-cultural research would be useful in identifying similarities and differences. Moreover, it is an empirical model representing what may have gone before rather than an idealistic model (a model 'for') on which to base future coach development programs (i.e. it is a model of what has worked rather than what might work best). In proposing the model some key questions might be: (i) How essential is participation in a range of sports for developing high-performance coaching expertise?; (ii) How important are the first three stages to developing high-performance coaching expertise?; and (iii) Specifically, does coach expertise in sports such as gymnastics require a sampling or early specialisation background as pre-requisite for the latter stages of the model?

Summary

In summary, several key points emerge from the research on high-performance coach pathways. First, an important finding is that there seems to be significant variability in playing and coaching experiences (Erickson et al 2007, Mallett & Rynne unpublished work, 2008, Rynne 2008). Some coaches who have less experience as high-performing players appear to engage in more hands-on coaching activities, and conversely successful players who become coaches probably rely less on their 'delivery skills' on the field (Mallett et al 2007). Coaching work at the elite level is dynamic and has undergone significant transformation in recent years, which prompts the question – is it possible that in 10 years' time most high-performance coaches will have comparatively less elite playing experience in the sport they coach and more extensive background in coaching science (including leadership and management training) than the current cohort? Second, accumulated hours from coaching experiences seem to contribute most to coach development. Early sport participation, especially in the sport they now coach, also provides some opportunities for learning how and what to coach as well some knowledge of the culture of the sport. Formal learning opportunities (tertiary education and coach accreditation) are generally perceived as providing the least contribution to coach development, but in some circumstances it is highly valued. Despite these findings, more focused research examining the specific nature of the contributions of playing and coaching activities (e.g. critical incidents) to developing coach expertise would progress understanding and potentially inform the development of high-performance coaches. Finally, it is the capacity (and agency) of the coach to integrate those pre-mediate experiences that will contribute most effectively to professional development. How the individual coach engages with opportunities for learning (e.g. conversations with coaching peers), as well as progression opportunities, will most likely determine their career pathway as a high-performance coach. Of interest is how these learning opportunities facilitate high-performance coaching knowledge and practices.

Coaching communities in high-performance coach development: theory and research

The field of workplace learning (see Billett 2006), which has roots in Vygotsky's work, has been generative in understanding high-performance coach development (Rynne et al 2006). Prominent within the workplace learning literature is the focus on relations of the individual and the social. Consistent with this situated notion of learning is the concept of social networks such as communities of practice. As described earlier, high-performance coaches learn primarily through participation in coaching work (Mallett et al 2007). Accordingly, in order to understand better the nature of coaches' work and how they learn their craft, it is useful to consider the notion of social networks, such as 'communities of practice' (CoP). Community of practice is a popular concept within the research on coaches' learning (e.g. Culver & Trudel 2006, Galipeau & Trudel 2006, Trudel & Gilbert 2006); however, the concept of CoP is relatively under-theorised. What follows is an explanation of CoP and other concepts of social networks.

In recent years the terms 'communities' and 'communities of practice' have become synonymous with vocational learning. The concept of communities of practice (CoP), which was developed by Jean Lave and Etienne Wenger, has been given considerable attention in the areas of management and education. The evolution of the concept of CoP comes from Scribner and Cole's (1981) initial work on the literacy of the Vai community. They found cognitive theories of learning were unable to account fully for their data and subsequently drew upon anthropology to complement cognitive accounts of learning (Barton & Tusting 2005). This resulted in a greater acknowledgement of the social contributions to learning. In this evolution process, cognitive models of learning were gradually intertwined with the social (e.g. Rogoff & Lave 1984) and eventually the development of a theory of learning that foregrounded the social (Wenger 1998). It is noteworthy that the early works of Scribner and Cole (1981) and Rogoff and Lave (1984) were psychological accounts of learning rooted in the Vygotskian tradition. Lave sought to develop a theory of learning that would accord legitimacy to different knowledges (e.g. such as that found in coaching workplaces) in an attempt to understand individual differences in learning (Creese 2005). After studying apprenticeship as a model of learning, Lave and Wenger (1991) shifted their thinking to notions of 'situated learning' and 'communities of practice'. Apprenticeships, which sought to develop specific vocational knowledge and practices, involved a particular type of learning for specialised purposes. In this context, learning for (coaching) work might be considered different to more formal learning through institutions such as universities.

The idea of learning as social practice has origins in the work of 20th century Russian psychologist, Lev Vygotsky (1896–1934), who believed that learning was a social activity and that knowledge was something that existed among people, as a function of language and communication, rather than existing in isolation within the heads of individuals (Vygotsky 1978). More broadly constructivist views of learning emphasise the active role of the learner in the process of learning. Furthermore, learners construct their own understandings by making sense of information and building personal meaning (McInerney & McInerney 2002). There are several forms of constructivism (e.g., personal, social, information-processing). However social constructivism is more central to the notion of communities of practice.

Social constructivism focuses on the construction of shared knowledge in social contexts. Vygotsky's social constructivist theory of cognitive development, which is also referred to as socio-cultural theory or cultural-historical theory, emphasises the larger social, cultural and historical influences in which learning is embedded (McInerney & McInerney 2002). Learners (in this case coaches) become cultivated into the 'knowledge and symbols of their society', which emphasises the importance of ongoing interaction between the learner and their social environment (including others) in order to facilitate learning (McInerney & McInerney 2002 p 4). If learning is essentially social in nature then the role of knowledgeable others (e.g. experienced coaches) 'becomes one of negotiation and provision of guidance through shared social experience' (Christensen 2001 p 69). Through this sharing of information there is an interdependent relationship (Billett 2006) between the learners and the community. The appropriation of culturally relevant knowledge by the learner (Kozulin & Presseisen 1995) facilitates learners (coaches) increasingly becoming part of the (coaching) community and the community becoming part of the learner's; 'individuals are therefore both part of, and the product of, this collective culture' (McInerney & McInerney 2002 p 45). Reciprocity is a feature of these communities in which the group evolves through the actions of the members and conversely the learner within the collective. Learners are immersed in a culture that is represented by these tools, social structures and language, which directs the potential for learning.

Vygostky viewed cognitive development as a social, historical, and cultural process. The use of tools or cultural artefacts, social structures and language assist the learner in the appropriation of knowledge through the enculturation process. Tools (e.g. computers, video cameras, pens) facilitate extension of knowledge by scaffolding opportunities for learning. Social structures are represented by family, social groups (e.g. sport), and work organisations (e.g. football teams/clubs). Within these social structures learning is mediated by knowledgeable others (co-construction of knowledge). Vygotsky considered language as perhaps the most important tool of and for learning. Language (e.g. verbal, maths, music) is the means by which learning is both developed and transmitted (Vygotsky 1986).

Situated learning (Lave & Wenger 1991), which is consistent with social constructivism, focuses on the contexts (social structures) that construct and constitute learning. A central discussion regarding situated approaches to learning that emerged in response to Lave's critiques of traditional notions of cognition and pedagogy relates to the concept of 'community of practice' (CoP). The concept of CoP stems from a rejection of the idea that learning 'is an individual process, that it has a beginning and an end, that it is best separated from the rest of our activities, and that it is the result of teaching' (Wenger 1998 p 3). Central to this critique of conventional understandings about learning is the notion that we learn through our lived experiences from participation in everyday life. That is, participation in communities of practice facilitates 'situated' learning. In his introduction to their book, William F. Hanks explained, 'Rather than asking what kinds of cognitive processes and conceptual structures are involved, they ask what kinds of social engagements provide the proper context for learning to take place' (Lave & Wenger 1991 p 14). It is not so much that learners acquire structures or models to understand the world but that they participate in frameworks that have structure. Learning (in and though coaching work) is thus 'an evolving, continuously renewed set of relations' (Lave & Wenger 1991 p. 50). Learning exists among people and it is socialisation into communities of learning that facilitates knowledge construction.

Legitimate peripheral participation is a term that was coined by Lave and Wenger (1991). The term provides a theoretical explanation of the way that novices (e.g. assistant basketball coaches) become experienced members of a community of practice (e.g. head basketball coaches). Essentially, novices become experienced members by taking part in small, simple, low-risk tasks, which may be superficial but nevertheless are productive and integral (i.e., legitimate) to the purposes and practices of the community. It is through this peripheral participation that new members develop familiarity with the language, processes, and codes of the (coaching) community. Lave and Wenger theorised that it is important for peripheral players to be able to see how their small contributions fit with those activities and goals of the more expert members of the community. Thus, it is important for novices (e.g. early career coaches) to have social and practical access to (coaching) experts as part of their socialisation into the community. Lave and Wenger (1991) proposed that legitimacy was gained by being accepted and gaining informal authority through consensus within the group. This notion often sits uncomfortably with the more formal view of groups where simple domain knowledge or rank due to organisational hierarchy is seen as a source of authority.

Communities of practice

Lave and Wenger (1991) defined a CoP as 'a set of relations among persons, activity, and world, over time and in relation with other tangential and overlapping communities of practice' (p 98). That is,

CoP are groups of people (coaches) who share an interest in some activity (e.g. coaching) and who learn how to do it better through regular interaction (Lave & Wenger 1991). In more recent conceptions of CoP, there has been something of a shift in thinking. For example, Wenger (1998) drew upon a broader theoretical background, including anthropology and social theory, and CoP became a central concept in a social theory of learning. Wenger (1998) elaborated the theory of situated learning and extended the concept of community of practice. In this work, Wenger moved away from the notion of legitimate peripheral participation, suggesting that the structure/agency divide implicit in this concept was perhaps misleading. Instead he developed the concept of community of practice to become a central aspect of a social theory of learning and its links with other interrelated concepts: practice, meaning and identity. Specifically, Wenger articulated the coherence between (coaching) practice and the (coaching) community (Creese 2005). It is important to note that while this definition allows for agency (intentionality), it does not assume it. That is to say that in a CoP, learning can be an 'incidental outcome' rather than the expressed purpose of the members' intentions. Therefore, a strength of this social theory of learning is its capacity to account for incidental learning, which has support in the coaching literature (e.g. Mallett et al 2007). Wenger (1998) proposed that we could belong to more than one (coaching) community at the same time. Furthermore, people are likely to move in and out of CoP as well as becoming central in some and more peripheral in others (Wenger et al 2002).

The concept of CoP considers learning from outside formal learning situations (e.g. schools), and in particular in workplaces (e.g. high-performance sporting organisations). It also takes into account adult learning. Furthermore, CoP has proved useful as a theoretical concept and has been of value in practice (Barton & Tusting 2005). There are three special features, which must exist in a community, for it to be considered a CoP; a joint enterprise, mutual engagement, and a shared repertoire.

A joint enterprise, which is the result of a collective process of situated negotiation, is concerned with what the community is about; that is, they share a common purpose or goal for participation in the community. The members must interact in activities and discussions such that they share information and actively and extensively assist each other to pursue common goals. A head coach and two assistant coaches actively working together in a Premier League football team over several years to produce an outstanding team is an example of a joint enterprise in high-performance sports coaching.

Mutual engagement in which participants are engaged in actions with others in the community's work and whose meanings they negotiate with one another is a defining feature; 'practice resides in a community of people and the relations of mutual engagement by which they can do whatever they do' (Wenger 1998 p 73). For instance, a group of coaches from a sports high school working on developing a long-term athlete development program for elite youth athletes might demonstrate mutual engagement. A sporting team may or may not be a CoP, depending on whether or not those within the team community have a shared commitment as well as shared competence.

A shared repertoire produces resources and artefacts (e.g. routines, tools, vocabulary) that belong to the community and identify members of that community. Importantly, this resource-building does not need to be the result of conscious agentive action. A shared repertoire of concepts, cases, and stories can be the by-product of ongoing conversations rather than the intended result of interaction. Communal resources such as the language used to communicate about the team's strategies and tactics is an example of a shared repertoire. That language allows the members of the CoP to communicate with each other (and develop their collective sense of identity) and can differentiate them from other CoP.

A CoP is relatively autonomous in the sense that it establishes its own set of understandings about its specialty and applications, and it establishes and regulates its own membership boundaries and hierarchies. Wenger et al (2002) contends that the development of each of these three characteristics simultaneously is the way to cultivate a community of practice by enhancing its coherence (i.e. production of a fully functioning CoP).

Coaches' community of practice

The concept of CoP has been adopted in many vocational fields, especially management and education, which is understandable if we recognise that the concept of a community of practice privileges a social view of learning that acknowledges informal

groups (social networks) (Barton & Tusting 2005). Recently, Trudel and colleagues (e.g. Culver & Trudel 2006, Galipeau & Trudel 2006) examined the concept of CoP within developmental coaching contexts and proposed the notion of a coaches' community of practice (CCoP) (Galipeau & Trudel 2006). Culver amd Trudel (2006) defined a CCoP as 'a group of people (coaches) who share a common concern, set of problems, or a passion about a topic, and who deepen their knowledge and expertise in this area by interacting in an ongoing basis' (p 98). Moreover, they argued that interaction alone between coaches is insufficient to support the view that a CCoP was operational. In their investigation, Culver and Trudel found that within teams there was evidence of a CCoP, especially through the mutual engagement of personnel (coaches, ancillary staff) and a shared repertoire. Nevertheless, they proposed that a fully operational CCoP was less likely to be found within a team because of the lack of a joint enterprise and suggested that in highly contested teams there is more likely to be an individual enterprise. They concluded that a fully functioning CCoP was less likely to be found operating between teams and within the national and international governing bodies. They proposed that there were opportunities for other social networks to be operational in broader levels of governance but as expected these were dependent on the people in leadership positions. In attempting to understand the 'web' of social relations formed by coaches in developing their craft, Galipeau and Trudel (2006) proposed that coaches learn from others through alternative modes of social networks. Moreover, Wright et al (2007) found that youth ice hockey coaches sought information to develop their practice from sources (social networks) external to their CCoP.

Limitations of the concept of 'community of practice'

It is important to consider some of the limitations of the concept of CoP, especially those that might relate to high-performance coaches' learning. Overall, the concept of community of practice is relatively under-theorised. It seems to be a concept that is derived from a range of observed social phenomena based on research into apprenticeship and vocational activity. In Wenger's (1998) concept of

CoP, the individual is marginalised and as a consequence individual difference is generally unaccounted for. To not acknowledge the individual in a substantive way in theories of learning denies the significant contribution of the learner (coach) to the learning process. Moreover, issues of power, conflict, value and morality are marginalised in writings on CoP (e.g. Lave & Wenger 1991, Wenger 1998). In work organisations, such as elite sporting teams, it is important to recognise that they are complex, interpersonal, political and hierarchical spaces in which there is status difference, all amidst the need for collaboration (Watkins 1991, Boud & Garrick 1999). High-performance coaches often work in a highly contested and volatile work environment, which seems in contrast to the notions of apprenticeship upon which CoP was initially developed. In the traditional apprenticeship models developed over the past 2000 years or more it is likely that the context of the community was less competitive. It is assumed that the master would be proud (and recognised) for producing outstanding tradespeople. Repeated success in producing quality tradespeople probably reflected positively upon the master. In an environment in which masters are supportive of apprentices' learning it is expected that what and how they learn will be promoted. In contrast, high-performance coaching environments are highly contested with power dynamics and fights for survival, which characterise an environment that provides differential access to a community's knowledge and resources. Although Wenger (1998) suggested that CoP were not always benign environments, some of the literature espousing the promotion of CoP has viewed them as unproblematic; exceptions in the coaching literature include Jones et al (2002), Cushion et al (2003), Bowes and Jones (2006), and Culver and Trudel (2008). Furthermore, in the CoP literature little attention is given to the ways in which the accumulation of resources (and the trading of resources within a system of valuing) differentially distributes relations of advantage and disadvantage. Further discussion on the notion of social networks (communities) and high-performance coaches' learning will be discussed later in this chapter.

There are further limitations to the concept of CoP. Elkjaer (2005) proposed that when applying the CoP model in research, the 'how' of learning seemed to be lost in the broader concept of 'learning as participation'. Eraut (2002) criticises CoP on the basis that communities change but Lave and Wenger (1991) and Wenger (1998) do not comment on how they change and the subsequent impact of those changes on learning. Our understanding of the notion of CoP would improve if some analysis of the types of knowledge that CoP research privileges and those that it fails to recognise were examined. In addition, CoP focuses on what social, cultural, material and institutional resources are developed but further theorising about why or how they have come about would develop our understanding of CoP.

Notwithstanding these limitations, the notion of situated learning and some aspects of CoP do provide a useful framework for developing a better understanding of how high-performance coaches' learn their craft through their participation in the actual work of coaching. High-performance coaches learn primarily through participation in coaching work (e.g. Mallett et al 2007). Consistent with Vygotsky's notion of the co-construction of knowledge, Mallett and colleagues found that coaches prefer to learn from interacting with others in developing their craft. This interdependent relationship between the coaches (learners) and the community (including others) helps the coach to become more immersed in the culture of high-performance coaching. Of interest is an enhanced understanding of the nature of the social relations that promote high-performance coaches' learning. How do high-performance coaches interact with others in developing their coaching knowledge and practices? Some recent research has examined the concept of CoP and other social networks in coaching and is discussed next.

Other concepts of social networks (for learning)

Galipeau and Trudel (2006) reported that coaches of youth sport learn from others through many social networks, including CCoP, informal knowledge networks (IKN) (Allee 2000) and networks of practice (NoP) (Nichani & Hung 2002). Culver and Trudel (2006) propose that coaches' engagement in different types of social interactions influences the quality of coaching experiences and the subsequent development of practice. Coaches interact with others but the nature of these interactions can both facilitate and inhibit learning and therefore some further understanding of these social relations is underscored. As with CoP, a key concern with conceptions of other social networks is that they are under-theorised. Scholars describe some aspects of the relationships between members but do not comprehensively provide a deeper insight into the nature of these relationships and more importantly how people learn through these interpersonal relations. This lack of insight is more evident with the conceptions of IKN and NoP, which limit accurate representations of what the original authors meant by such terms. Nevertheless, I will describe what is known about IKN and NoP.

In an *informal knowledge network* the relationships between members are loose. The notion of IKN according to Allee (2000) differs from a CoP in the sense that there is no joint enterprise that binds them together because the main aim is to exchange information. IKNs operate when coaches generally know each other and informally interact to share information. For example, communication with a sport psychologist about a challenging player and/or a fitness advisor about issues with concurrent training might be considered an IKN. However, the nature of these relationships seems somewhat superficial – they are just 'a set of relationships' (Allee 2000 p 8). Trudel and Gilbert (2006) noted that the high school coaches in Sage's (1989) study showed the existence of an IKN and that it was central to the development as a coach. Sage reported that the coaches in his study who were fortunate in commencing their coaching careers as an assistant coach learnt much from observing the more experienced head coaches. The description of learning mostly through observations of more senior coaches in their team suggests a passive transmission of information and the sense that the learner was less agentic in directing what they learned. Those participant coaches who commenced their coaching careers as a head coach learned through trial and error; they reported little or no guidance from others.

In a *network of practice* (NoP) (Nichani & Hung 2002), typically members (coaches) are less familiar with other members, they come from multiple organisations, and regular interactions are more likely to be conducted through communication technologies such as the Internet (Nichani & Hung 2002). The only connection between members in a NoP is the indirect and explicit flow of information. Furthermore, reciprocity is not generally a feature of communication within NoP (Brown & Duguid 2000). Nichani and Hung (2002) use the expressions 'learning to be' and 'learning about' to distinguish between CoP and NoP. In a CoP, 'learning

to be ... is about 'knowing how' by application and practice' that promotes enculturation within the community (Nichani & Hung 2002 p 50). In contrast, unfamiliar members of a NoP seek factual information concerned with 'learning about' something. Internet chat sites, in which the participants are less familiar and information is exchanged, are opportunities for a NoP.

In several recent studies (Mallett et al 2008, Occhino et al 2008, Rynne 2008), Mallett and colleagues examined how professional high-performance coaches in Australia learn for and during coaching work. Essentially, they have found that coaches prefer to learn from significant others (often other experienced coaches) and agentically seek people (confidantes) whom they trust and respect. Although the influence of others on their learning was dominant, the use of CCoP, NoP, and to a lesser extent an IKN, were not strongly reported. Instead, the participant coaches in three separate studies consistently reported (what has subsequently been termed) a *dynamic social network* (DSN) that most influenced their learning. This is not to deny some existence of partially functioning CCoP, IKN, and/or NoP in their development, but those social networks were not primary sources of learning. The dynamic social networks reported by high-performance coaches in Australia evolved over time, and in many cases took some time (several years) to unfold. Their social networks were dynamic because as coaches developed their craft they sought others to assist in their problem-solving. Although, theoretically, a fully functioning CCoP might be an ideal pursuit, the realities of the highly contested nature of high-performance sport generally inhibit the development of such social networks. That is not to say that there are no examples in elite sport of well-functioning CCoP; they are the exception rather than the rule. Even though a CCoP might be a utopian ideal, it should not deter coaches from taking up the challenge of attempting to create such a productive environment for learning, especially within teams and squads.

In summary, any attempts to facilitate coaches' learning through social networks should be encouraged. Like other workplaces, high-performance sporting teams and squads are characterised by cultural practices, competition, group affiliations and hierarchies, which impact on differential opportunities to access guidance and engage in regular and novel work activities (Billett 2001). Trudel and Gilbert (2004) found the contested nature of youth hockey leagues tended to thwart CCoP, therefore it is not surprising that CCoP do not function effectively in high-performance sport. It is unsurprising that coaches view others in sport 'more as opponents than collaborators' (Culver & Trudel 2008 p 5) when you consider that 'typically over 90% of elite sport coaches are former competitive athletes' (Trudel & Gilbert 2006 p 538). The enculturation of high-performance coaches from an early age into the highly contested nature of sport in which winning is essential to survival makes collaboration seem improbable.

One of the key issues that emerged from the research on high-performance coaches' learning is that there is a general perception by the sport administrators and the public at large that employed coaches are already experts and know what they need to know (Mallett et al 2007). This line of thinking further inhibits the development of social networks such as a CCoP. In coach learning environments that are thwarted by coaches' insecurities about 'secret information' that gives them an edge on their opponents, coaches are likely to be limited in developing a network of confidantes, whom they trust and respect. However, coaches should be encouraged to develop their own social (coaching) network to complement other sources of information for learning and developing their craft (Mallett et al 2007).

Summary

This chapter provided an overview of the work of high-performance coaches, which was followed by what we know about the pathways to becoming a high-performance coach. The work of high-performance coaches is multifaceted and complex. Coaches of elite athletes and teams operate in a turbulent and dynamic environment, which makes preparing for such a vocation challenging. Variability in the contributions to high-performance coach development was highlighted, although it was evident that coaching work was the most highly valued experience. Nevertheless, extensive coaching work alone did not facilitate coach development. The capacity of coaches to meaningfully engage in coaching work relies on their ability to reflect upon their work. Moreover, engagement of 'people of influence' to mediate high-performance coaches' learning (through reflection) was foregrounded. The literature on workplace learning was briefly introduced as a novel lens through which to examine high-performance coach development. A key focus within the workplace learning framework is the situated nature of learning. The concept of community of practice, which is consistent with situated learning, was to some extent generative in understanding how high-performance coaches learn their vocation; however theoretical and practical limitations of the concept of CoP (and other social networks) were highlighted. The highly competitive nature of high-performance coaching can limit the effectiveness of social networks, such as CoP, in developing coaching expertise. Australian high-performance coaches reported the importance of confidantes they respected and trusted in developing their knowledge, but the development of this small and continually changing group evolved over a long time. The concept of dynamic social networks (people of influence) was introduced as another potential way of understanding the web of social relations in high-performance coaches' learning. There are many gaps in our knowledge of high-performance coach development (in part, due to the under-theorising of concepts of social networks); however, further systematic research into social networks can be generative in developing these concepts. How and what high-performance coaches learn is an important area of research that over time can inform the coach development process.

References

Allee, V., 2000. Knowledge networks and communities of practice. Journal of Organization Development Network (OD Practitioner) 32 (4), 4–13.

Barton, D., Tusting, K., 2005. Beyond communities of practice: language, power, and social context. Cambridge University Press, Cambridge.

Billett, S., 2001. Co-Participation: affordance and engagement at work. New Directions for Adult and Continuing Education 92, 63–72.

Billett, S., 2006. Relational interdependence between social and individual agency in work and working life. Mind, Culture and Activity 13 (1), 53–69.

Bloom, G.A., Durand-Bush, N., Schinke, R.J., et al., 1998. The importance of mentoring in the development of coaches and athletes. International Journal of Sports Psychology 33, 410–430.

Boud, D., Garrick, J., 1999. Understandings of workplace learning. In: Boud, D., Garrick, J.

(Eds.), Understanding learning at work. Routledge, London, pp. 1–12.

Bowes, I., Jones, R.L., 2006. Working at the edge of chaos: understanding coaching as a complex, interpersonal system. The Sport Psychologist 20, 235–245.

Brown, J.S., Duguid, P., 2000. The social life of information. Harvard Business School, Boston, MA.

Cavalheiro, C.A., Soter da Silveira, P.C., Palermo, P.C.G., 2005. Multidisciplinary training: the orbital model. New Studies in Athletics 20 (4), 7–18.

Christensen, C., 2001. Transforming classrooms: educational psychology for teaching and learning. Post Pressed, Flaxton, Queensland.

Côté, J., 1999. The influence of family in the development of talent in sport. The Sport Psychologist 13 (4), 395–417.

Côté, J., Fraser-Thomas, J., 2007. The health and developmental benefits of youth sport participation. In: Croker, P. (Ed.), Sport psychology: a Canadian perspective. Pearson, Toronto, pp. 266–294.

Côté, J., Salmela, J., Trudel, P., et al., 1995. The coaching model: a grounded assessment of expert gymnastic coaches' knowledge. Journal of Sport & Exercise Psychology 17 (1), 1–17.

Côté, J., Ericsson, K.A., Law, M.P., 2005. Tracing the development of athletes using retrospective interview methods: a proposed interview and validation procedure for reported information. Journal of Applied Sport Psychology 17, 1–19.

Creese, A., 2005. Mediating allegations of racism in a multiethnic London school: what speech communities and communities of practice can tell us about discourse and power. In: Barton, K., Tusting, K. (Eds.), Beyond communities of practice: language, power, and social context. Cambridge University Press, Cambridge, pp. 55–76.

Cross, N., Lyle, J., 1999. The coaching process: principles and practice for sport. Butterworth-Heinemann, Oxford.

Culver, D., Trudel, P., 2006. Cultivating coaches' communities of practice: developing the potential for learning through interactions. In: Jones, R.L. (Ed.), The sports coach as educator: re-conceptualising sports coaching. Routledge, London, pp. 97–112.

Culver, D., Trudel, P., 2008. Clarifying the concept of communities of practice in sport. International Journal of Sport Science and Coaching 3 (1), 1–10.

Cushion, C.J., 2007. Modelling the complexity of the coaching process. International Journal of Sport Science and Coaching 2 (4), 395–401.

Cushion, C.J., Armour, K.M., Jones, R.L., 2003. Coach education and continuing professional development: experience and learning to coach. Quest 55, 215–230.

Dickson, S., 2001. A preliminary investigation into the effectiveness of the National Coach Accreditation Scheme. Australian Sports Commission Report, Canberra.

Elkjaer, B., 2005. Stupid organisation: how will you ever learn? In: 4th International Conference on Researching Work and Learning. University of Technology, Sydney.

Eraut, M., 2002. Conceptual analysis and research questions: do the concepts of 'learning community' and 'community of practice' provide added value? Paper presented at the Annual Meeting of the American Educational Research Association, New Orleans, LA.

Eraut, M., 2004. Informal learning in the workplace. Studies in Continuing Education 26 (2), 247–273.

Ericsson, K.A., Krampe, R.T., Tesch-Römer, C., 1993. The role of deliberate practice in the acquisition of expert performance. Psychol. Rev. 100 (3), 363–406.

Erickson, K., Côté, J., Fraser-Thomas, J., 2007. Sport experiences, milestones, and educational activities associated with high performance coaches' development. The Sport Psychologist 21, 302–316.

Fenwick, T., Rubenson, K., 2005. Taking stock: a review of research on learning in work 1999–2004. In: 4th International Conference on Researching Work and Learning. University of Technology, Sydney.

Galipeau, J., Trudel, P., 2006. Athlete learning in a community of practice: is there a role for the coach? In: Jones, R.L. (Ed.), The sports coach as educator: reconceptualising sports coaching. Routledge, London, pp. 77–94.

Gilbert, W., Trudel, P., 2001. Learning to coach through experience: reflection in model youth sport coaches. Journal of Teaching in Physical Education 21 (1), 16–34.

Gilbert, W., Côté, J., Mallett, C., 2006. Developmental paths and activities of successful sport coaches. International Journal of Sport Science and Coaching 1 (1), 69–76.

Irwin, G., Hanton, S., Kerwin, D.G., 2004. Reflective practice and the origins of elite coaching knowledge. Reflective Practice 5 (3), 425–442.

Jones, R., Wallace, M., 2005. Another bad day at the training ground: coping with ambiguity in the coaching context. Sport, Education, and Society 10 (1), 119–134.

Jones, R.L., Armour, K.M., Potrac, P., 2002. Understanding the coaching process: a framework for social analysis. Quest 54, 34–48.

Jones, R.L., Armour, K.M., Potrac, P., 2003. Constructing expert knowledge: a case study of a top-level professional soccer coach. Sport, Education and Society 8 (2), 213–229.

Kozulin, A., Presseisen, B.Z., 1995. Mediated learning experience and psychological tools: Vygotsky's and Feuerstein's perspectives in a study of student learning. Educational Psychologist 30, 67–75.

Lave, J., Wenger, E., 1991. Situated learning: legitimate peripheral participation. Cambridge University Press, Cambridge.

Lyle, J., 2002. Sports coaching concepts: a framework for coaches' behaviour. Routledge, London.

Lynch, M., Mallett, C., 2006. Becoming a successful high performance track and field coach. Modern Athlete and Coach 22 (2), 15–20.

Mallett, C.J., 2004. Reflective practices in teaching and coaching: using reflective journals to enhance performance. In: Wright, J., Macdonald, L., Burrows, L. (Eds.), Critical inquiry and problem-solving in physical education. Routledge, Sydney, pp. 147–158.

Mallett, C., 2008. Modelling the complexity of the coaching process: a commentary. International Journal of Sport Science and Coaching 2 (4), 419–421.

Mallett, C.J., Rynne, S., 2008. Developmental paths and activities of Australian high performance coaches. Unpublished manuscript.

Mallett, C., Rossi, T., Tinning, R., 2007. Coaching knowledge, learning and mentoring in the AFL. Report to the Australian Football League Research Board, Melbourne.

Mallett, C., Rossi, T., Tinning, R., 2008. Knowledge networks and Australian Football League coach development: people of influence. In: Association Internationale des Ecoles Superieures d'Education Physique Conference Proceedings. Sapporo, Japan.

McInerney, D.M., McInerney, V., 2002. Educational Psychology: constructing learning. Pearson Education Australia, Frenchs Forest, NSW.

Nichani, M., Hung, D., 2002. Can a community of practice exist online? Educational Technology 42 (4), 49–54.

Occhino, J., Mallett, C., McCuaig, L., 2008. Mentoring and other networks in high performance football coaching. In: Association Internationale des Ecoles Superieures d'Education Physique Conference Proceedings. Sapporo, Japan.

Rogoff, B., Lave, J., 1984. Everyday cognition: its development in social context. Harvard University Press, Cambridge, MA.

Rynne, S., 2008. Opportunities and engagement: coach learning at the Queensland Academy of Sport. The University of Queensland, Unpublished Doctoral thesis. Australia.

Rynne, S., Mallett, C., Tinning, R., 2006. High performance sport coaching: institutes of sport as sites for learning. International Journal of Sport Science and Coaching 1, 223–234.

Sage, G.H., 1989. Becoming a high school coach: from playing sports to coaching. Res. Q. Exerc. Sport 60 (1), 81–92.

Salmela, J., 1995. Learning from the development of expert coaches. Coaching and Sport Science Journal 1 (2), 3–13.

Salmela, J., 1996. Great job coach: getting the edge from proven winners. Potentium, Ottawa.

Salmela, J.H., Moraes, L.C., 2003. Development of expertise: what do experienced athletes remember? In: Starkes, J.L., Ericsson, K.A. (Eds.), Expert performance in sports: advances in research on sport expertise. Human Kinetics, South Australia, pp. 275–294.

Saury, J., Durand, M., 1998. Practical knowledge in expert coaches: on site study of coaching in sailing. Res. Q. Exerc. Sport 69 (3), 254–266.

Schinke, R.J., Bloom, G.A., Salmela, J.H., 1995. The career stages of elite Canadian basketball coaches. AVANTE 1 (1), 48–52.

Schön, D.A., 1983. The Reflective Practitioner: how professionals think in action. Basic Books, New York.

Scribner, S., Cole, M., 1981. The psychology of literacy. Harvard University Press, Cambridge, MA.

Simon, H.A., Chase, W.G., 1973. Skill in chess. American Scientist 61, 394–403.

Trudel, P., Gilbert, W., 2004. Communities of practice as an approach to foster ice hockey coach development. Safety in Ice Hockey 4, 165–179.

Trudel, P., Gilbert, W., 2006. Coaching and coach education. In: Kirk, D., O'sullivan, D., Macdonald, D. (Eds.), Handbook of physical education. Sage, London, pp. 531–554.

Vygotsky, L., 1978. Mind in society: the development of higher psychological processes. Harvard University, Cambridge, MA.

Vygotsky, L., 1986. Thought and language. MIT, Cambridge, MA.

Watkins, K.E., 1991. Facilitating learning in the workplace. Deakin University Press, Victoria.

Wenger, E., 1998. Communities of practice: learning, meaning and identity. Cambridge University Press, Cambridge.

Wenger, E., McDermott, R., Snyder, W.M., 2002. Cultivating communities of practice: a guide to managing knowledge. Harvard Business School Press, Boston MA.

Woodman, L., 1993. Coaching: a science, an art, an emerging profession. Sport Science Review 2 (2), 1–13.

Wright, T., Trudel, P., Culver, D., 2007. Learning how to coach: the different learning situations reported by youth ice hockey coaches. Physical Education and Sport Pedagogy 12 (2), 127–144.

Coach education effectiveness

9

Pierre Trudel, Wade Gilbert and Penny Werthner

Introduction

This chapter on coach education effectiveness is divided into five sections. First we highlight events indicating that coach education has recently received special attention from sport stakeholders as well as members of the coaching research community. In the second section, we present an overview of studies that have assessed coach education program effectiveness. This analysis of the literature shows a scarcity of studies on this topic and, more disturbingly, the scientific evidence that does exist suggests that coach education training programs have no long-term significant impact on actual coaching practice. The next two sections are used to argue that this apparent shortcoming must be nuanced. In the third section we explain why using a human learning approach can help to understand coach education better, and then we provide definitions of a number of specific concepts among which is the notion of lifelong learning. In the fourth section we discuss the implications of considering the human learning approach and the notion of lifelong learning for measuring coach education effectiveness. We conclude the chapter by providing some recommendations to national sport governing bodies.

A new interest toward coach education

Perhaps more than ever the effectiveness of coach education is being questioned as an influx of resources into the training of coaches and coaching science around the world has brought with it a heightened level of accountability. Major coach education initiatives are taking place at both international and national levels. The *International Council for Coach Education* hosts international conferences and is in the process of developing a global coach network (International Council for Coach Education n d, J. Bales, personal communication 2008). Individual countries have also invested heavily in re-organising coach education, including the United Kingdom with its UK Coaching Certificate initiative (Nelson & Cushion 2006, sports coach UK n d), Canada with its National Coaching Certification Program (Coaching Association of Canada n d, Trudel & Gilbert 2006), the United States with the recent creation of the National Council for the Accreditation of Coach Education (National Association for Sport and Physical Education [NASPE] n d), and Australia with its Australian Institutes and Academies (Rynne et al 2006). These government and sport organisation initiatives are taking place concurrently with a much-increased expansion of coaching science. Since 2006 three new scientific journals have been created – *International Journal of Sports Science & Coaching, International Journal of Coaching Science*, and the *Journal of Coaching Education*. Further evidence of this rapid interest in coach education and coaching science can be seen in the recent publication of extensive scientific reviews (Gilbert & Trudel 2004, Trudel & Gilbert 2006), comprehensive data-based texts on coaching and coach education (Lyle 2002, Cassidy et al 2004, Jones et al 2004, Jones 2006, Bloom 2007) and a special issue of *The Sport Psychologist* dedicated to coach education (Gilbert 2006). A consequence of all these initiatives is an increasingly pluralistic and inconsistent worldview of answers to questions such as, how do coaches learn to coach? and, how can we measure coach education effectiveness? This is not surprising given that the field still continues to debate vigorously the very nature of the coaching process itself (Lyle 2002, Abraham et al 2006, Cushion 2007, Côté & Gilbert 2009).

Research on coach education program effectiveness

We have limited our review of the literature on coach education program effectiveness to studies published in English language journals in the last 10 years (1998–2007). These studies can be divided into three categories; small-scale coach education training programs (four studies), university-based coach education programs (four studies), and large-scale coach education training programs (six studies). An overview of these studies is presented in Tables 9.1–9.3. We strongly recommend the reader consult each article for a deeper understanding of the methodologies used and the limits of each study.

Small-scale coach education training programs

Over the past 30 years, two researchers from the United States, Ronald Smith and Frank Smoll, with various colleagues, have conducted an impressive line of research on the effects of a cognitive-behavioural approach to coach training. Given that their research is unique and continues to evolve today, a brief overview of their intervention program and their findings is presented.

Initially, two studies were completed to establish a baseline of coaching behaviours and athlete attitudes and perceptions. The two studies were completed in the late 1970s and early 1980s with youth baseball (n= 51) and basketball (n = 31) male coaches of boy's teams (n = 724 athletes) ranging in age from 8–15 years old (Smith & Smoll 1990, Smith et al 1978, 1983). Coaches' behaviours were coded during at least two games (range 2–5 games) using the Coaching Behavior Assessment System (CBAS), and in the first study the coaches also completed a coaching philosophy questionnaire. Athlete perceptions, attitudes, and self-esteem

Table 9.1 Small-scale coach training program studies 1998–2007

Authors	Context	Participants	Intervention	Results
Smith et al (2007); Smoll et al (2007)	Basketball	37 coaches 216 athletes	Mastery Approach to Coaching (MAC) 75 minute workshop	Athletes who played for MAC trained coaches perceived coaches to be more mastery-oriented (as opposed to ego-oriented), increased their mastery goal orientation scores, lowered their ego orientation scores, and exhibited decreases in anxiety from preseason to late season
Coatsworth & Conroy (2006); Conroy & Coatsworth (2004)	Swimming	7 coaches 135 athletes	Adaptation of Coach Effectiveness Training (CET) 2 hour workshop	No significant effects on youth fear of failure, a general tendency to increase positive self-esteem over the season – particularly for girls, moderate or no change in coaching behaviours
Trudel et al (2000)	Ice hockey	28 coaches	Body checking and injury prevention 2 hour workshop	Coaches reported improved knowledge on body checking instruction, satisfied with material and would use again, no change in number of minor aggressive penalties or number of athlete injuries
Cassidy et al (2006)	Rugby	8 coaches	Rugby Coach Development (CoDe) 28 hours of meetings across 6 months	Coaches became more aware of the learning preferences of their athletes and changed how they coached, and they valued structured opportunities to discuss and share ideas

were assessed at the end of the season using two questionnaires, one of which eventually became known as the Washington Self-Description Questionnaire (WSDQ). Although the specific results varied between the two studies, the findings showed that coach behaviours strongly influence athlete attitudes toward their coach, as well as their perceptions of themselves, their coaches, and the actual sport experience. The results were most striking for young participants with low self-esteem, showing that this group of athletes responded most positively to coaches high in reinforcing and encouragement behaviours. Coaches scoring low on support and high on punishment were least liked by their athletes. The results also showed a large discrepancy between coaches' perceptions of their behaviours and their actual behaviours. These studies laid the foundation for the creation of the Coach Effectiveness Training (CET) program. The CET is a brief (2.5 hours) workshop designed to promote principles of positive control, to help coaches conceptualise winning as giving maximum effort, and to nurture self-awareness and self-monitoring in coaches.

The effectiveness of the CET program has subsequently been tested in four separate studies. The first study was conducted with 31 baseball male coaches and 325 athletes who were 10–15 years of age (Smith et al 1979). A multi-method approach was used to provide the coach training. At the end of a 2-hour workshop, coaches were given a manual with behavioural guidelines and a personal behavioural profile based on observation (using the CBAS) of two games at the beginning of the season with norms for comparison. Coaches were also asked to complete self-monitoring forms after the first ten games of the season and reminder phone calls were made periodically. Athletes' perceptions, attitudes, and self-esteem were assessed with questionnaires. Results indicated that compared to the untrained coaches, coaches in the experimental group provided greater amounts of reinforcement to their athletes. Athletes of the experimental group coaches evaluated both their coach and their team's interpersonal climate more positively. Trained coaches were perceived to be more reinforcing, more encouraging, more technically instructive, and less punitive in response to mistakes. It was also found that the low-self-esteem athletes were the group of athletes who exhibited the greatest positive change in attitudes toward their coaches.

The results of the second intervention study are reported across three publications (Barnett et al 1992, Smoll et al 1993, Smith et al 1995). The intervention was tested with 18 male baseball coaches and 152 athletes 10–12 years of age. The researchers did not collect data on the coaches' behaviours but asked the athletes to answer a questionnaire on their perceptions of the coaches' behaviours, and on their attitudes toward the coaches and other aspects of participation. Athletes also completed three tests on self-esteem (WSDQ) and anxiety (Sport Anxiety Scale [SAS] and Sport Competition Anxiety Test [SCAT]) immediately before and after the season. Athletes of trained coaches perceived their coaches to engage more frequently in desirable behaviours, liked their coaches and teammates more, rated their coaches as better teachers, and had more fun than players of untrained coaches. In terms of anxiety and self-esteem, athletes of trained coaches showed a decrease in anxiety over the course of the season but no general self-esteem trend was evident. However, there were significant increases in self-esteem for the sub-sample of boys who started the season with low self-esteem. Lastly, only 5% of the boys who played for trained coaches did not return the following season, compared to 26% of the boys who played for untrained coaches.

Smith, Smoll and colleagues revised their coach training protocol in their most recent study (see Table 9.1, Smith et al 2007, Smoll et al 2007). The CET program was modified and is now referred to as MAC (Mastery Approach to Coaching). It is briefer in duration (75 minutes) and the content is delivered through a lecture approach rather than a discussion. The MAC intervention is based upon two major themes: (a) positive coaching behaviours and (b) defining success as giving maximum effort. A 28-page researcher-designed coaching manual (Smoll & Smith 2005) and a self-monitoring form are still provided to the coaches. Using a quasi-experimental design, the MAC was tested with 37 community-based basketball coaches and 216 athletes (mean age = 11.5, SD = 1.63), which for the first time included girls (n = 99). The athletes completed four different measurement instruments (anxiety, motivational climate, achievement goal for sport, and academic achievement goal) at the beginning and at the end of the sport season (12 weeks later). Athletes who played for MAC-trained coaches perceived their coaches to be more mastery-oriented (as opposed to ego-oriented), increased their mastery goal orientation scores, lowered their ego orientation scores, and exhibited decreases in anxiety from preseason to late season. No changes were found for the control group athletes. These group differences were noted equally for boys and for girls.

To our knowledge, only one study has been completed on Smith and Smoll's coach education interventions by someone other than the original authors. David Conroy and J. Douglas Coatsworth (Coatsworth & Conroy 2006, Conroy & Coatsworth 2004) tested the effectiveness of the CET intervention with seven early-career swimming coaches (mean years of coaching experience = 2.43 years) and 135 swimmers (52 boys and 83 girls, mean age = 11.4, SD = 2.23, range = 7–18). They deliberately selected a sample very different from those used in the Smith and Smoll line of research in an attempt to explore the effectiveness of the CET intervention in diverse youth sport settings. Four coaches received the CET intervention and three coaches received a control training program consisting of 2 hours on injury prevention and emergency first aid. The intervention group coaches received a 2-hour workshop based on the CET, and were given a copy of Smoll and Smith's coaching manual. Coaching behaviours were coded in two 1-hour practices for each coach using the CBAS and the athletes completed a self-esteem scale and a performance failure appraisal (Performance Failure Appraisal Inventory) three times across a 7-week swim season (beginning, middle, and end). The results, published in two separate articles, indicated no significant effects on the participants' fear of failure, a general tendency to increase positive self-esteem over the season – particularly for girls, and only moderate or no change in coaching behaviours. This is the first published study showing very limited or no significant impact, either for coaches or their athletes, following participation in a CET-based workshop. These findings were partially attributed to several methodological limitations noted both by Conroy and Coatsworth themselves and by Smith and Smoll (Smith et al 2007). These limitations include a small sample size (only seven coaches), suitability of the fear of failure instrument for this age group, insufficient data points for the coaching behaviours, homogeneous sample for race and SES, and the relatively brief nature of the workshop. As Conroy and Coatsworth concluded, how realistic is it to expect ingrained coaching behaviours to change a few weeks after exposure to a 2-hour workshop?

Similar to the studies presented so far, Trudel et al (2000) developed an intervention strategy that focused on a specific coaching element. Their intervention strategy was developed especially for ice hockey coaches and applied to 28 coaches and their players (14–15 years old) in competitive leagues. The three-part intervention research started with a 2-hour individual meeting with each coach. Using specially made video recordings, the meeting sought to (a) make coaches aware of the problem of injuries and penalties, (b) demonstrate the importance of teaching body checking, (c) furnish teaching materials, and (d) present the concept of self-supervision and how to use this technique during the season. Coaches also had to present a video montage to their players explaining the importance of making legal body checks and the techniques involved. Finally, the coach had to teach body checking during at least four on-ice training sessions at the start of the season. The hypothesis was that if coaches applied the principles of self-supervision and used the teaching materials provided, they would be able to help players use body checks correctly, and fewer minor aggression penalties and injuries would be noted. When the researchers compared the data collected during that hockey season with the data of the previous season, no significant differences were found. To the question 'how do we explain that the intervention strategy pleased coaches but did not produce the desired results?' the authors stressed the fact that it is almost impossible to control all variables when research is conducted in the sporting milieu and no pressure, other than what was said during the workshop, is put on the coaches to be compliant. For example, some coaches admitted that they had not completely followed the intervention strategy, giving reasons such as the lack of time, and coach and player changes during the season. The authors concluded that, 'considering that minor league hockey exists with the participation of many individuals (organizers, officials, parents, coaches, players) it is probably unrealistic to believe that a short term intervention implicating only the coach, will suffice to reduce violence' (p 246).

The study by Cassidy et al (2006) with eight rugby coaches in a developmental sport context is very different from the studies presented so far because the researchers did not try to measure the effectiveness of a behavioural approach. Using a qualitative methodology, they examined the effectiveness of a theory-based coach education program (CoDe) that can be qualified 'as a boutique, community-orientated, short-term (28 hours over 6 months), classroom based, theoretical, educational/personal development coaching program with no assessment component that was offered free of charge to the volunteer coaches' (p 148). Once the program was completed, in-depth semi-structured interviews were conducted with each coach to collect data on their perceptions of participating in the CoDe. Results indicated that coaches appreciated the fact that, contrary to training courses they had attended in the past that focused on technical sport components, CoDe helped them to see the complexities associated with the coaching process and critically reflect upon their own approach. This was achieved mainly through formalised opportunities where the coach educator facilitated discussion, interaction, and negotiation of meaning among the coaches instead of lecturing and prescribing coaching and theoretical principles.

From this brief overview of studies published on small-scale coach education training programs it is important to highlight a number of issues. First, it is extremely difficult to determine the effect of a coach education training program even when the researchers (a) have full control of the intervention content, (b) can select a trained researcher as facilitator to conduct the workshop, (c) decide the sport and competitive context, and (d) separate coaches into control and experimental conditions. For example, Trudel et al (2000) found no significant differences even if coaches said they appreciated the intervention strategy. Second, studies such as those conducted by Smith and Smoll can sometimes show significant differences in favour of the trained coaches but are these differences large enough to be meaningful, and can these results be generalised to all coaches and athletes? For example, on 12 behaviours measured by the CBAS, trained coaches scored better than the untrained coaches only on the reinforcement behaviour (Smith et al 1979). For athletes the biggest difference reported on their perception of the sport context was just over one-half of a point on a 7-point scale (trained coaches M = 5.59, untrained coaches M = 4.95) for the question, 'do you like your manager/head coach more or less than you did at the beginning of the season? (Smith et al 1995 p 134). For the Mastery

climate, trained coaches scored on average 26.23 (SE = 0.36) and the untrained coaches 25.08 (SE = 0.48) on a maximum of 30 (Smith et al p 50). We also do not have any data on the long-term impact of these training programs. Will the few, relatively small, changes found still be evident in following years when coaches do not have self-monitoring forms to complete, do not receive reminder phone calls, and their athletes are not assessed on the research variables? Third, studies on small-scale coach education training programs have provided information on only a very limited segment of youth sport; generally competitive team sports.

Our conclusion is that, at the moment, there is no substantial body of evidence to support the widespread or long-term effectiveness of coach education training programs, even in highly controlled and small-scale quasi-experimental settings. After nearly three decades of sophisticated research on the CET/MAC, Smoll et al (2007) concluded that, because of the lack of a true experimental design, or comparison to alternative coach education interventions, 'we cannot rule out the possibility that simply receiving an intervention (regardless of its content or nature) helped change the coaches' behaviour' (p 40). We might also wonder if we should strive to find the 'best' model (i.e., best practices). The search for such a model may be futile as 'coach training programs are clearly not equally effective in all situations' (Conroy & Coatsworth 2004 p 211).

University-based coach education programs

Contrary to the studies presented in Table 9.1, studies on university-based coach education programs (a) do not focus on a specific sport, (b) the duration of the intervention is longer, (c) there are fewer participants, and (d) the focus (Cassidy et al 2006 being the exception) is not to change certain specific coaching behaviours but, to use Jones and Turner's (2006) expression, to 'help coaches acquire the "quality of mind" necessary to deal with, and excel at, the dynamic nature of their work' (p 185).

In the first example, Demers et al (2006) discuss the development of their university undergraduate coach education program designed to develop reflective practitioners. For them, there is a 'need for a professional education program that could reach beyond the many limitations that a community-based program must accommodate, such as cost, time involved in training, as well as assessment requirement for coaches to demonstrate competency' (p 164). The researchers reported that to develop and implement their curriculum based on competency-based and problem-based learning (PBL) approaches, faculty members have to work together and time might become a barrier. It was also stressed that students might have difficulties transferring the knowledge presented in courses to their practice (internship). It was suggested that one way to help students link the concepts to their coaching practice is to create specific assignments that require students to complete critical reflection reports.

For Jones and Turner (2006) coaching must be 'intellectualised'. This requires 'developing theory related to its complexity, while appreciating the need to grow the aforementioned "quality of mind"

in coaches through habits of reflection, problem-solving, and critique; elements that are integral to PBL' (p 183). These researchers introduced the principles of PBL during the final year of a Bachelor of Arts degree (Coach Education and Sport Development). Results showed that students had begun to think differently about coaching but the process itself was extremely challenging. For example, tutors need to be well trained in order to provide a balance between allowing student discussion time and intervening to make sure that important learning issues are raised. Students not familiar with a PBL approach might be somewhat antagonistic to this approach and therefore will need additional support and clear information and expectations. The problematic scenarios have to be selected carefully and support from a resource technician (e.g., a librarian) is important to help direct students to the relevant information. Finally, in a PBL approach,

Table 9.2 University-based coach education program studies 1998–2007

Authors	Context	Participants	Intervention	Results
Demers et al (2006)	Non-sport specific	Undergraduate college students	Baccalaureate in Sport Intervention (BIS) 3-year undergraduate program	Competency-based/problem-based learning approach requires constant faculty member collaboration, focused assignments are needed to help students make connections between course concepts and coaching practice
Jones & Turner (2006)	Non-sport specific	Undergraduate college students (n = 11)	12-week problem-based learning (PBL) curriculum	Problem-based learning approach is often novel to students, will require training in PBL approach, clearly define problems along with time and resources to find solutions, students gain better understanding of coaching complexity but evaluation process is challenging
Knowles et al (2001)	4 sports	Undergraduate college students (n = 8)	1 year (60 hours) of reflective practice coursework	Most coaches believed program was beneficial to coach development and generally growth in reflection skills was noted, coaches recommended early and mandatory support workshops, facilitator role is difficult and multi-faceted which may require counselling skills, reflective journal writing is time-consuming and requires clear structure, must set aside workshop time for reflective writing, assessment of reflection skills is problematic
Knowles et al (2006)	3 sports	Coaching science degree graduates (n = 6)	1 year (60 hours) of reflective practice coursework	No evidence of reflecting at critical or practical level, coaches tended to reflect primarily on coaching problems, although coaches acknowledged that written reflection was important in reflective process, none of them made time for reflective writing (reflection was limited to mental notes and peer discussion)

participants often must work in small groups, and therefore finding enough time to meet could become a significant barrier to consider.

Two studies have reported on the impact of a program to develop and assess reflective skills among students of a Bachelor of Science (Honours) coaching science degree (Knowles et al 2001, 2006). During the first semester of their second academic year, students (coaches) attended theoretical lectures that focused on conceptual and practical issues associated with reflective practice. In the second semester, students were engaged in 60-hour coaching placements and also had to participate in five workshop sessions to discuss coaching topics, keep a reflective journal, and complete an academic year (annual) report. Results showed that, for some coaches, the workshop sessions allowed collective discussion and the generation of action plans while other coaches felt the sessions were not useful, as they preferred to work alone. It was also found that students needed extra support during the early stages of their placement, and the role of the workshop facilitator is complex and multi-faceted. For example, the facilitator often had to conduct one-on-one sessions with the participants to address fully certain coaching issues. This highlights the potential need for workshop facilitators to not only have sport science, pedagogy, and reflection skills, but also effective interpersonal skills. The coaching placements differed in terms of their potential to impact the development of reflective practice. Assessment of the level of reflection is a daunting task because students typically will vary in their writing skills. The authors concluded, 'coach educators cannot therefore assume that development of reflective skills will be a naturally occurring phenomenon that runs parallel to increasing coaching experience' (p 204). In an attempt to better assess the effectiveness of their program Knowles and colleagues later studied how graduates of this coaching science degree deployed reflective processes in their coaching practice. Using interviews with six graduates, no evidence was found of reflecting at a critical or a practical level. When coaches did report reflection, they tended to reflect primarily on coaching problems. Although the coaches acknowledged that written reflection was important in the reflective process, none of them made time for reflective writing. Reflection was limited to mental notes and peer discussion. One possible reason for these findings is that in the field, coaches often work in isolation. This situation is in stark contrast to what

they experienced when they were undergraduate students working in an environment with skilled tutors and reflective workshops. In their conclusion, the authors made reference to the difference between the academic experience and actual coaching practice: 'In summary, the in-built reflective rigour present in the undergraduate program is at variance with the post-graduation reality of sports coach employment' (p 176).

These four studies share the common objective of developing reflective coaches who will increase their capacity for creating effective solutions to their coaching issues. As shown by the results of these studies, it is not easy to teach or assess the reflective process. Participants were university students involved full time in coaching programs delivered by accredited institutions. Even under these intensive and controlled conditions, very little evidence of growth in coach reflection skills was noted, and even less evidence was found for use of reflection post-graduation. There seem to be challenges both for those who deliver the program and for the participants. In a program aimed at preparing reflective practitioners (coaches) the instructor has to be well prepared to use non-traditional approaches like problem-based learning. For the student-coaches the challenge might be to adapt to a new teaching/learning approach in which the evaluation criteria are less specific and require them to share orally or in writing their thoughts about coaching issues and possible solutions. These four studies, when viewed in conjunction with the Knowles et al (2005) review of national governing bodies' coach education program inclusion of reflective skills, paint a dismal portrait of coach education's ability to develop reflective practitioners. Knowles et al (2005) found that none of the programs directly taught or nurtured reflection in their curriculum. Clearly much work is required if reflection is expected to become a primary characteristic of coaches who complete episodes of coach education. We think it is important to also note that very few university-based coach education programs focus on developing reflective coaches. A review of university-based coach education programs in the United States shows a very traditional, and uniform, curriculum (McMillin & Reffner 1999). All programs include a mix of coaching theory, sport science sub-disciplines (i.e., biomechanics, sport psychology) and some form of coaching practicum. This trend is also evident in a review of online coach education curriculum descriptions at universities that have established coach education programs (e.g., Boston University, Concordia University, Georgia Southern University, University of Bath, University of Essex). Unfortunately, no studies on the effectiveness of these types of traditional programs were found while preparing this chapter.

Large-scale coach education training programs

The results of six studies that have examined the impact of large-scale coach education training programs are presented in Table 9.3. Three of the six studies focused on coaching efficacy as a dependent variable. Coaching efficacy is 'defined as the extent to which coaches believe they have the capacity to affect the learning and performance of their athletes [and the concept] comprised four dimensions: game strategy, motivation, technique and character building efficacy' (Malete & Feltz 2000 p 410). In the study by Campbell and Sullivan (2005), Canadian coaches completed the Coaching Efficacy Scale (CES) before and after participation in Level 1 of the National Coaching Certification Program (NCCP). The results showed a significant increase for each of the four dimensions, and also significant differences in favour of women coaches with respect to character building and motivating their athletes. Lee et al (2002) conducted their study with coaches in Singapore. CES results of untrained coaches were compared with CES results for a group of coaches trained at Level 1 or 2 of the National Coaching Accreditation Program (NCAP). Significantly higher coaching efficacy scores were found on two dimensions; game strategy and teaching technique. The only gender difference found was a weak effect on the game strategy dimension; male coaches scored higher. The third study of this kind was completed by Malete and Feltz (2000) with two groups of American coaches. One group of coaches participated in the Program for Athletic Coaches Education (PACE) and the other group did not. Both groups completed the CES before and after the PACE. Results of the study showed that there were significant differences on all four dimensions of the CES but these differences were minor (less than 1 point on a 9-point scale).

The impact of participation in Canada's National Coaching Certification Program (NCCP) on coaches'

encouragement of imagery use among their athletes was the focus of a study by Hall et al (2007). An imagery-use questionnaire (The Coaches' Encouragement of Athletes' Imagery Use Questionnaire [CEAIUQ]) was given to 291 coaches (215 male and 76 female) from 26 different sports. Two hundred and two of these coaches had completed at least one of the NCCP's five levels of coach education training programs. The other 89 coaches had not completed any of the NCCP coach education training programs. Results showed that coaches who had completed NCCP training were significantly more likely to encourage imagery use among their athletes. However, there was no significant difference among coaches based on the level of NCCP training that was completed.

McCullick et al (2005) conducted a study to understand what components of the Ladies Professional Golf Association – National Education Program (LPGA – NEP) (a) women coaches perceived to be the most beneficial to their development and (b) teacher educators perceived to be most beneficial to the preparation of certified golf coaches. Data were collected from interviews, participant journals, and field notes. The participants appreciated the program structure because they enjoyed the progression of the curriculum and the balance between time in the class and outside on the practice tee, as well as on-site feedback. Participants also stressed the importance of learning pedagogical knowledge, as well as being taught by credible teacher educators. The integration of research into the program curriculum was well received because it showed that teaching golf should be based on a sound body of knowledge, not on speculation or tradition.

Gilbert and Trudel (1999) developed an evaluation strategy for large-scale coach education training programs and applied the strategy with one coach. A multiple method context-dependent approach was considered the most reliable way of accessing the complexity of the coaching process. Data were collected using different instruments (participant observation, interviews, knowledge test, and systematic analysis of videos) in three phases: (a) baseline (three games and two practices), (b) intervention (level 2 course), and (c) post-intervention (three games and two practices). The results showed that the course was not delivered as designed, no new knowledge was gained, and both the use and non-use of course-related knowledge was evident in the field.

Table 9.3 Large-scale coach education program studies 1998–2007

Authors	Context	Participants	Intervention	Results
Campbell & Sullivan (2005)	Multiple sports	213 coaches	National Coaching Certification Program (NCCP) Level 1 16 hour workshop	All dimensions of coaching efficacy (game strategy, teaching technique, motivation, and character building) increased significantly, women more confident on motivation and character building
Lee et al (2002)	Multiple sports	235 coaches	National Coaching Accreditation Program (NCAP) Level 1 or 2	Participation in NCAP improved two of the four dimensions of coaching efficacy - game strategy and teaching technique, a weak effect for male coaches was found on the dimension of game strategy efficacy
Malete & Feltz (2000)	Multiple sports	51 coaches	Program for Athletic Coaches Education (PACE) 12 hour workshop	Participation in PACE improved two dimensions of coaching efficacy - game strategy and teaching technique, all coaches had high coaching efficacy scores prior to the course, and some coaches indicated that the course simply confirmed their current coaching practice
Hall et al (2007)	Multiple sports	291 coaches	National Coaching Certification Program (NCCP) Levels 1–5	NCCP trained coaches encouraged imagery use significantly more than untrained coaches, level of certification was not a significant factor in coaches' encouragement of imagery use
McCullick et al (2005)	Golf	5 coach educators 26 coaches	Ladies Professional Golf Association – National Education Program (LPGE – NEP) 10 day workshop	Women coaches said the program needs to be well structured, taught by knowledgeable teachers, and integration of research must be part of the program
Gilbert & Trudel (1999)	Ice hockey	1 coach	National Coaching Certification Program (NCCP) Level 2 22 hour workshop	Multiple method evaluation approach shows course was not delivered as designed, no change in coach's knowledge, and very little change in coach's instructional behaviours

These six studies show two different strategies for measuring the effectiveness of large-scale coach education training programs. One strategy consists of using a questionnaire to measure coaching beliefs (efficacy) or behaviours (imagery encouragement). A benefit of this strategy is that information from a large sample of coaches can be obtained relatively quickly and economically. However, in terms of coaching behaviour it is not a reliable measure of what coaches do after the intervention because it is self-report. In terms of coaching efficacy, this strategy does not provide information about the long-term impact of participation in large-scale coach education training programs. The other strategy consists of attending courses and collecting data with multiple data collection techniques. While this strategy is more sensitive to the context, the complexity and the time required make it less practical outside of research purposes. Lyle (2007a) recently conducted a review of the impact research on large-scale coach education training programs and concluded that no impact evaluations exist. Our review shows that there are indeed several studies that have examined the impact of large-scale coach education training programs. We believe the difference in conclusions is a result of the definition of 'impact' research. We used the term in its broadest sense to mean measurement of any variable as a result of participation in a large-scale coach education training program. Lyle, on the other hand, only considered research where the programs were evaluated against a component of coaching practice. If using this criterion then we would concur with Lyle's conclusion. The only study that has attempted to address impact, design, and delivery of a large-scale coach education training program is the Gilbert and Trudel (1999) research. However, as Lyle noted, that study was designed primarily to pilot test an evaluation protocol, not to assess program impact.

We can conclude from this overview of the literature on coach education program effectiveness that there is a scarcity of studies on this topic. In fact, Smith and Smoll's research group is the only one to have sustained a research program on coach education. Through a rigorous design and validating each step they were able to show that a well-designed workshop – even as short as 75 minutes – can have an acute impact not only on coaches but also on some of the athletes. However, as indicated earlier, the studies on CET/MAC have been limited to three sports with coaches of young adolescents (around 11 years old). With this, we are far from covering the large spectrum of coaching contexts. The few studies conducted with coaches registered in university programs demonstrates that preparing reflective coaches is very challenging and requires a considerable amount of time. Even more challenging is how to measure any changes in the coaches' reflective process. Finally, the paucity of studies on large-scale coach education training programs is surprising considering that in many countries coaches are required to be certified through these programs. One explanation for this finding could be that these programs are developed to provide training to coaches for the recreation level to the elite level and for a diversity of sports. Therefore, significant resources, and a long-term commitment would be needed to conduct a comprehensive impact study of these types of large-scale coach education training programs (Lyle 2007b).

So where do we go from here? One avenue could be to stop here and conclude that there are three main types of coach education programs with their own characteristics, purposes and ways of measuring potential impact. However, considering the limits of each program, none can claim to have found the most effective way to train coaches or how to evaluate coach education programs. Another avenue could be to look at coach education from a different approach or perspective, one that could influence researchers' and practitioners' attempts to structure and evaluate coach education programs.

Looking at coach education from a human learning approach

Generally, coach education is discussed from a curriculum design perspective, meaning that 'experts' (researchers or program designers) are in charge of selecting and delivering a specific content and, at the end of the program, participants complete some form of evaluation (Jarvis 2004). What is missing in this discussion on coach education is the learner's perspective. Three main factors lend support for the inclusion of the learner's perspective when addressing the structure and the evaluation of coach education programs. First, interviews with coaches across all types of coaching contexts clearly demonstrate that coach education programs typically play a marginal role in coach development in comparison to learning from experience. This should not be a surprise considering that most coaches accumulate many years of experience as athletes and time spent in a coach education program is minimal compared with the number of hours spent actually coaching (Gilbert et al 2006, Lynch & Mallett 2006, Werthner & Trudel 2006, Erickson et al 2007). In fact, any short coach education program could qualify as an 'episodic learning experience' (Jarvis 2006). Second, as we are now living in an information society characterised by constant technological developments along with an information explosion (Merriam et al 2007 p 17) any formal education program cannot pretend to be the sole provider of professional knowledge. For Jarvis (2004) 'Society is changing so rapidly that many of the traditional educative organizations are not able to keep abreast with the new demands and so individuals are forced to learn outside of the education system' (p 17). Third, taking into consideration the two previous factors, one has to realise that today, practitioners acquire their knowledge and develop their competencies while participating in formal education programs as well as outside of them. Therefore, it is important to find ways to recognise the learning that occurs in informal situations. In fact, there is pressure in many countries to 'identify what actions [countries] can take in designing and managing their qualifications system to promote lifelong learning' (OECD 2007 p 11). In brief, the new social context in which we live forces us to look at teaching and learning processes differently than in the past. For Merriam et al (2007) 'taking human beings rather than educational institutions as its beginning point' (p 25) can be a refreshing way of doing it. This is precisely what we want to do here by focusing on Jarvis' work. Peter Jarvis (2004, 2006, 2007) is a key author in adult education and learning who has published numerous books, including a recent trilogy on Lifelong Learning and the Learning Society.

For Jarvis, learning 'is the process of being in the world. At the heart of all learning is not merely what is learned, but what the learner is becoming (learning) as a result of doing and thinking – and feeling' (2006 p 6). This holistic and existentialist perspective suggests that 'we need to look at whole person learning in life-wide contexts. Since the whole person learns, a great deal of learning occurs in all our social living that is unrecognised, incidental, unintended and often discounted' (p 49). As we can see, Jarvis' definition of learning is far more complex than the simplistic view of what a person (coach) has acquired at the end of a few courses (coach education programs). Before we apply this human learning approach to coach education, we need to define some key terms. Differences between terms such as coach education, coach training, formal learning, non-formal learning, informal learning, lifelong education, continuing education, and lifelong learning are not always obvious. Beyond the fact that authors might have been negligent when selecting the terms, there are also historical reasons. One such example is that, in the past, education was equated with learning to prepare for a job 'which was appropriate for less technological societies, [but] is no longer relevant to contemporary society' (Jarvis 2004 p 39). Also these concepts may have different meanings in different parts of the world. As readers go through the definitions they are invited to consult Figure 9.1 to see where we have situated these concepts in relation to coach development.

Education, coach education, coach education training program

In Western societies, the term *education* is often linked with the school system and therefore 'education is regarded here as an institutionalised (and planned series of incidents) and humanistic process, it is seen as one in which the value of the human being and the quality of interaction between teachers and learner are recognized' (Jarvis 2004 p 43). Therefore, *coach education* can be seen as a

Figure 9.1 • Coach development within a lifelong learning perspective

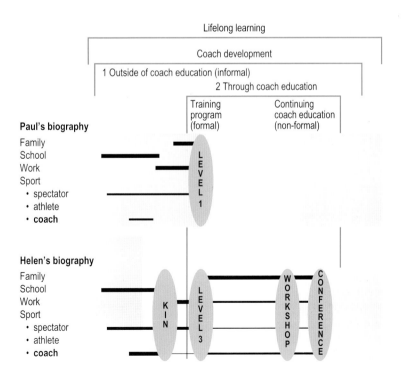

concept which regroups any planned or recognised teaching/learning activities by an institution/organisation that contributes to the development of coaches; the most popular being *coach education training programs*. Many countries have developed such programs to prepare their coaches from the recreational to the elite level. These large-scale programs generally run parallel to the post-school system.

Three main learning situations: formal, non-formal, informal

Although expressions such as formal learning, non-formal learning, and informal learning are used by many authors (Lohman 2006, Nelson et al 2006, Merriam et al 2007) we believe, as suggested by Jarvis (2006), that it is more appropriate to talk about learning in situations that are formal, non-formal or informal. A *formal situation* would refer to a situation that is supervised by an institution where the teaching is curriculum-driven and the learning recognised with grades or certifications. In the coaching field, it would be the coach education training programs that provide a certification. To complement their compulsory program for certification, coaching organisations or institutions will often organise conferences or workshops. In this case, these learning opportunities can be seen as continuing coach education and will tend to be short-term, voluntary, and have few if any prerequisites. They form the category called *non-formal situations*. Coaching organisations can encourage coaches to attend these conferences or workshops or can impose a minimum attendance at such events as a proof of their ongoing learning to maintain certification. Finally, *informal situations* refer to the learning opportunities outside of those provided under the coach education system. Thus, these opportunities can happen at any time. Within these types of learning situations, Merriam et al (2007) and Jarvis (2006) also recommend differentiating the intentional learning from the incidental learning. A coach calling a colleague or surfing on the Internet to find information is an example of intentional learning. The incidental learning is often unconscious and could include learning about the sport sub-culture. For example, only when individuals are in a coaching position will they realise that through their experience as an athlete they have unconsciously developed some coaching knowledge,

or that some of the knowledge acquired during their schooling can now be applied to their role as a coach.

Lifelong learning

Lifelong learning is an increasingly popular expression but its definition and purpose can vary widely. From an economic perspective, the Organisation for Economic Cooperation and Development (OECD 2007) proposed the following:

> Strategies for lifelong learning respond to the convergence between the economic imperative dictated by the needs of the knowledge society and the societal need to promote social cohesion by providing long-term benefits for the individual, the enterprise, the economy and the society more generally. For the individual, lifelong learning emphasises creativity, initiative and responsiveness – attributes which contribute to self-fulfilment, higher earnings and employment, and to innovation and productivity.
>
> (2007 p 10)

The limitation of using this definition in the coaching context is that the majority of coaches are volunteers and therefore we can hardly speak of long-term benefits in terms of higher earnings or employability. Arguing that human beings have a basic need to learn and therefore are lifelong learners, Jarvis (2006) proposes the following definition for lifelong learning:

> The combination of processes throughout a lifetime whereby the whole person – body (genetic, physical and biological) and mind (knowledge, skills, attitudes, values, emotions, beliefs and senses) – experiences a social situation, the perceived content of which is then transformed cognitively, emotively or practically (or through any combination) and integrated into the person's individual biography resulting in a continually changing (or more experienced) person.
>
> (2006 p 134)

Thus, lifelong learning can be viewed as an all-embracing concept that encompasses learning in many spheres of life (family, school, work, sport) and which occurs in the educational system and outside of it. While the expression 'lifelong education' suggests that 'it is the responsibility of the State and, perhaps, the employers to provide education', in lifelong learning 'the focus is upon learning, then the responsibility rests with the learners' (Jarvis 2006 p 141). Therefore, the responsibility to develop as a coach should stay in the hands of the coaches. It might include the obligation to obtain a coaching certificate delivered by a recognised institution or national coaching governing body, but it will certainly not be limited to this one way of learning.

Biography

In a human learning approach it is essential to consider the learner's past experience and for Jarvis (2006), a person's biography should include the bodily, emotive, and cognitive dimensions of previous experiences. Differences between how a group of individuals will react when participating in the same learning opportunity can be partly explained by looking at their personal biography. Werthner and Trudel (2006) using the concept of cognitive structure, which is similar to the concept of biography, have demonstrated its important role in the coaches' learning process. A person's cognitive structure/biography influences what he/she chooses to pay attention to and what he/she chooses to learn in different learning situations.

Two scenarios of coaches' development

In an attempt to be more concrete, we will use two scenarios to illustrate how a coach's personal biography influences the coach development path through formal, non-formal and informal situations. Although these scenarios are fictitious they are plausible because they are inspired by the results of many studies on coaches across coaching contexts. To the studies already cited we can add: Irwin et al 2004, Lemyre & Trudel 2004, Lemyre et al 2007, Vargas-Tonsing 2007, Wright et al 2007 and Reade et al 2008.

Scenario 1

Paul became the head coach of a youth soccer team by obligation. His daughter wanted to play soccer and he went with her to the registration meeting. The parents were told that there would be new teams only if some of them agreed to coach the teams. No coaching experience was necessary but the volunteers were required to complete a weekend coach training course if they did not already have a coaching certificate. Back home, Paul does not feel good with his decision. He has no future

plans to coach and he is doing it only because he wants his daughter to be involved in the physical activity she has chosen. His experience in sport is quite limited; he swam on his high school team but never won any races. His knowledge about soccer consists of watching some games on TV, going to the soccer stadium with friends a few times a year to cheer for the local club, and also discussing sports with friends at the bar at the end of work on Friday afternoon. If Paul is to coach, he most urgently needs examples of drills to prepare his practices and he is expecting to get this information in the training course (Level 1). The training session is held over 2 days and divided into four modules: coaching philosophy, youth development and safety, ethical behaviours, and planning a practice session. Because there are coaches from different sports, the content is not specific to soccer. However, the course conductor suggests coaches regroup by sport to complete the exercise on planning a practice session. In the last 30 minutes of the course, coaches are asked to complete a questionnaire on their satisfaction regarding the content and the delivery format. Paul found the course conductor very professional and competent but he was disappointed with the content. The information on coaching philosophy and ethical behaviours seemed obvious to him. The module on youth development and safety was useless because as a paramedic he knows more on this topic than the course conductor. The planning a practice session module was the most interesting but if you do not have a book of drills to choose from what can you plan? Fortunately, some soccer coaches at his table were kind enough to share some of the basic drills with him and at lunch time one of them suggested some books and a website where Paul could find a databank of drills. Hopefully, with this additional information, Paul should be able to complete the home assessment: development of five training sessions. As everyone was leaving, Paul had a short discussion with other coaches and he noticed that there were different opinions on the usefulness of this weekend course. For example, Louis, who had played soccer all his life although never at the elite level, found the modules on coaching philosophy and ethical behaviours very useful. He is very competitive and this module reminded him to strive for a balance between winning and having fun. The module, planning a practice session, only confirmed what he already knew and had experienced repeatedly as an athlete. The coaches also talked about their willingness to attend a workshop on soccer talent development that was announced at the end of the course. Because Paul has no intention of coaching in the future he will not attend. Louis, however, would like to coach at a more competitive level and he will have to conduct selection camps, so he is eager to attend this workshop even though it is not mandatory.

What does Paul's scenario tell us about coach education effectiveness? First, weekend courses like any other formal learning situations can hardly please every participant because of the differences in their biography – different life experiences, sport knowledge, and motives. Therefore, even if some participants are unhappy with a coach training course, it does not mean that it should be abandoned, although modifications should be made if many of the participants are unsatisfied. It is also important to recognise that, for the majority of coaches at the recreational level and for many at the developmental level, the time they have to invest to obtain their certification is very limited. Therefore, these formal learning situations have to be considered as episodic learning experiences. The possibility of learning by being involved in informal situations will always be greater although it will be very difficult to judge the quality of that learning.

Scenario 2

Helen played on the national basketball team while completing an undergraduate degree in a kinesiology program with a specialisation in coaching. She then found a job in a high school as a physical education teacher and decided to coach the elite women's team at the school. Her team was very successful for three years in a row, and she was asked to be the head coach of the provincial women's team the next year. She was pleased to see that people recognised her competencies as a coach but very surprised to learn that, as a result, she had to attend a coach education training program delivered over two weekends in order to become a certified coach at Level 3. She thought, incorrectly, that her university diploma would be recognised by the national sport governing body. They had no problem crediting her with Level 1 and 2 but not Level 3 because they felt that some of the modules contained in their coach education program were not covered in Helen's university program. When questioned about the importance of taking that specific training

programe, Helen acknowledged that the content was very pertinent but in her case it only confirmed what she already knew. She would have preferred to go into more detail on many of the topics but most of the other coaches in the courses did not have her kinesiology background and therefore struggled to understand many new concepts in a variety of disciplines (physiology, biomechanics, motor-learning, psychology, pedagogy, ethics) in such a short period of time. During the early years of her coaching career, Helen acknowledged that the most important learning opportunity was certainly the numerous discussions she had with one of her previous coaches who acted as a kind of mentor. After the birth of her first child, she was able to negotiate a part time position at the school and a part time coaching position with the provincial basketball federation. Considering the very precarious job security in coaching, this agreement seemed to be the best one for the moment (pension plan, medical care …) although a full-time coaching position would provide more opportunities to learn about coaching. A new regulation required that each certified coach must sustain a professional development record. As a result, last year Helen went to a one-day basketball workshop where a coach from a professional team talked about offensive plays. This past year she attended a 3-day national conference on coaching. She had gone through the conference program and selected the communications she thought were the most interesting, but she was disappointed in some cases because it was too theoretical, and the researchers were unable to make it relevant to the practitioners. However, other communications were very instructional, particularly one on how to use the Internet to find relevant and valid information. One of the highlights of the conference was the networking she was able to develop with coaches from different sports and from different parts of the country, as well as with a few sport scientists. However to be successful at networking she will have to be proactive; her great interpersonal skills would certainly be an asset.

What does Helen's scenario tell us about coach education effectiveness? First, as long as the sport system is not able to offer coaches a sustainable career pathway similar to other professions (teaching, health sector, and so on), the responsibility to develop as a coach should stay primarily in the hands of the individual. Helen's decision to pursue a university degree in kinesiology and then work part time in a school and in coaching impacted both her life in general (family, social) and her coaching. Regarding the recognition of her diploma by the national sport governing body this is an issue not unique to sport as countries have to create mechanisms 'to find a bridge between national qualifications systems and lifelong learning' (OECD 2007 p 3). Considering that coach education training programs are generally delivered in a short period of time, most of the coaching certificates represent the minimum of what a coach should know at a specific level. As the science of coaching expands, coaches have to find learning opportunities to stay current. National sport governing bodies can nurture that learning through workshops and conferences but they also have to be aware that these learning activities will not meet the needs of all coaches. Therefore, coaches should be actively encouraged to search out information pertinent to their particular needs. Developing skills to search on the Internet as well as developing a network of coaches seem to be essential ways to continue to learn.

Implications for measuring coach education effectiveness

By adopting Jarvis' human learning approach and his definition of lifelong learning, we have to recognise that learners (i.e., coaches) move from being individuals who are taught by experts to the owners of their development. This position contrasts starkly with the predominant view of training:

> There is an old saying that, if the learner hasn't learned, the teacher hasn't taught. This is a good philosophy for each instructor to have. It is only too easy to blame a learner for not learning…The important point is that we are measuring our own effectiveness as instructors when we evaluate the participants' learning. If we haven't succeeded, let's look at ourselves and ask where we have failed, not what is the matter with the learners. And if we discover that we have not been successful instructors, let's figure out how we can be more effective in the future. Sometimes the answer is simply better preparation. Sometimes it's the use of aids that help us to maintain interest and communicate more effectively. And sometimes the answer is to replace the instructor.
>
> (Kirkpatrick & Kirkpatrick 2006 p 49–50)

The notion of lifelong learning suggests that coaches, like any adult learner, learn how to coach through various learning situations across their lifespan. This conclusion is supported by the limited, but growing, research available on coach learning, much of which has been cited previously in this chapter. Considering that coaches learn to coach through a variety of situations (formal, non-formal, and informal), their involvement in coach education training programs will correspond generally to only a few hours of learning in their lifelong learning journey. Therefore what is the magnitude of the changes in coaches' behaviours, attitudes or reflective process that we can reasonably expect from these episodic experiences? The point we want to make here is not that coach education training programs are useless. In the literature there are many studies where coaches said they appreciated this type of learning situation (Salmela 1995, Wright et al 2007) and there is also evidence of impact on the coaches' belief in their coaching capacity (coaching efficacy) (Campbell & Sullivan 2005). The main issue is that it will always be very difficult to measure any coaches' changes outside of highly controlled research settings (Trudel et al 2000). Among the reasons is the fact that the sport milieu is based on voluntarism and therefore time and money become important factors to consider. Program designers generally try to develop training programs that require limited hours of investment from coaches and that can be accessible to a large number of coaches. This attempt to reach as many coaches as possible might increase the difficulty of measuring the impact of a coach education training program. As discussed previously, the individual coaches' biography (previous knowledge and emotions) play an important role in what coaches can and want to learn while participating in any coach education learning activities. Even if coach education training programs are usually developed for a specific group of coaches (recreational, development, elite) the chances to have participants with similar biographies are lower than in most of the education programs of other professions. For coaches, there are very few if any prerequisites required before registering in a coach education program as opposed to a specific list of credits or a diploma before starting a program in medicine, nursing, law, and so on. Also, coaches' previous athletic experience will vary extensively from one coach to the other while that type of previous experience does not exist in many professions. To have been a patient for many years is not a criterion to be a good physician. Based on the literature, and illustrated in the two scenarios, we can advance the view that in any group of coaches attending a training program there will be coaches who feel obliged to participate and therefore the impact for these coaches may be negligible. There will also be coaches who have already acquired the knowledge and developed the competencies through other learning situations and these coaches will also not show any significant changes post-program. Finally, there will be coaches who are eager to learn and the content presented corresponds to their needs. For these coaches, the training program might have an impact but it will not be easy to measure. Are we left to conclude then that the training program was not effective because some of the coaches will show no changes? If one adopts the traditional approach to evaluate training programs (i.e., Kirkpatrick & Kirkpatrick 2007), the lack of impact will mean that the instructor has failed to teach adequately the material or the program needs to be changed. However, by considering the lifelong learning perspective we are in a position to understand better the coach development process and the difficulty of measuring the effectiveness of coach education training programs.

Conclusion

We would like to conclude by providing some suggestions. First, national sport governing bodies should not expect to control the development of coaches. Considering that the majority of coaches are volunteers and the coaches that are paid generally have no job security, it is a matter of respect to let coaches be responsible for their development, which, however, will generally include the obligation to be certified. Part of the mission of national sport governing bodies should be to help coaches in their development by providing the best coach education programs they can, which will start with a well-designed and -implemented coach education training program (formal situation). The design and evaluation of any coach education training program must be sensitive to the program objectives; there is no one-size-fits-all approach. For example, if the objective of a large-scale coach education training program is to certify all coaches in a particular sport or region, then the course should be designed to be brief (few hours or one weekend), cover relevant material (as decided by the governing organisation), and be very accessible (i.e., brief, cheap, and available offline and online). In this type of situation, which is common in developed countries around the world, the measure of effectiveness will be determined by the ratio of coaches who have successfully completed the certification. One recent example of this approach is seen in the United States in the state of California, which as of 2008 requires all high school coaches to complete an introductory coach education training program. It is estimated that there are nearly 62 000 individuals who coach at this level annually (NASPE 2008). These types of coach education training programs cannot pretend to be in the business of developing coaching competencies (knowledge, behaviours, attitudes) when we see that these outcomes seldom change even in highly controlled and extended (weeks or months) research interventions (see research reviewed in section two of this chapter). If the objective of a coach education training program is to change measureable coaching outcomes (behaviours, knowledge, attitudes), or even athlete outcomes (self-esteem, anxiety, fear of failure), then the design of the program must be focused on these outcomes and the evaluation strategy must be sensitive to documenting potential changes in these outcomes. National sport governing bodies will have to be innovative in providing coaches with adequate learning opportunities. Coaching institutes are a possibility as well as the university-based coach education degrees and courses or a combination of these two.

A second suggestion is that national sport governing bodies should be innovative in planning learning activities such as conferences, workshops, and online resources (non-formal situations) to inform coaches of important developments in coaching science. They should also encourage coaches to continue intentionally to learn by developing a coaching network and to consult the tremendous diversity of information now available online (informal situations). Considering that coaching is very complex and that for most coaching issues there is rarely one proven solution, one coach education training program cannot pretend to offer 'the true way of coaching' on which coaches should be evaluated. This does not mean we should not try to measure the effectiveness of our coach education programs. It only suggests that we must be realistic about what we can measure, and more can be done if national sport governing bodies, coaches, and researchers collaborate on this important task. Such a collaborative model has recently been suggested by Lyle (2007b) in his report to sports coach UK.

References

Abraham, A., Collins, D., Martindale, R., 2006. The coaching schematic: validation through expert coach consensus. J. Sports Sci. 24 (6), 549–564.

Barnett, N.P., Smoll, F.L., Smith, R.E., 1992. Effects of enhancing coach–athlete relationships on youth sport attrition. The Sport Psychologist 6, 111–127.

Bloom, G.A., 2007. Coaching psychology. In: Crocker, P.R.E. (Ed.), Introduction to sport psychology: a Canadian perspective. Pearson, Toronto, pp. 239–265.

Boston University, 2007. Online. Available: http://www.bu.edu/online/online_programs/certificate_programs/physical_education.html.

Campbell, T., Sullivan, P., 2005. The effect of a standardized coaching education program on the efficacy of novice coaches. AVANTE 11 (1), 38–45.

Cassidy, T., Jones, R.L., Potrac, P., 2004. Understanding sports coaching: the social, cultural and pedagogical foundations of coaching practice. Routledge, London.

Cassidy, T., Potrac, P., McKenzie, A., 2006. Evaluating and reflecting upon a coach education initiative: the CoDe of rugby. The Sport Psychologist 20, 145–161.

Coaching Association of Canada, 2006. Online. Available: http://www.coach.ca/eng 9 June 2008.

Coatsworth, J.D., Conroy, D.E., 2006. Enhancing the self-esteem of youth swimmers through coach training: gender and age effects. Psychology of Sport and Exercise 7, 173–192.

Concordia University, 2006. Online. Available: http://www.cui.edu/AcademicPrograms/Graduate/Coaching/index_ektid12884.aspx.

Conroy, D.E., Coatsworth, J.D., 2004. The effects of coach training on fear of failure in youth swimmers: a latent growth curve analysis from a randomized, controlled trial. Applied Developmental Psychology 25, 193–214.

Côté, J., Gilbert, W.D., 2009. An integrative definition of coaching effectiveness and expertise. International Journal of Sports Science & Coaching 4, 307–323.

Cushion, C., 2007. Modelling the complexity of the coaching process. International Journal of Sports Science & Coaching 2 (4), 395–401.

Demers, G., Woodburn, A.J., Savard, C., 2006. The development of an undergraduate competency-based coach education program. The Sport Psychologist 20, 162–173.

Erickson, K., Côté, J., Fraser-Thomas, J., 2007. Sport experiences, milestones, and educational activities associated with high-performance coaches' development. The Sport Psychologist 21, 302–316.

Georgia Southern University, 2007. Online. Available: http://www.georgiasouthernhealthscience.com/departments/health-and-kinesiology/graduate/coaching-education-study.htm.

Gilbert, W.D., 2006. Introduction to special issue: coach education. The Sport Psychologist 20 (2), 123–125.

Gilbert, W.D., Trudel, P., 1999. An evaluation strategy for coach education programs. Journal of Sport Behavior 22 (2), 234–248.

Gilbert, W.D., Trudel, P., 2004. Analysis of coaching science published from 1970–2001. Res. Q. Exerc. Sport 75 (4), 388–399.

Gilbert, W.D., Côté, J., Mallett, C., 2006. Developmental paths and activities of successful sport coaches. International Journal of Sports Sciences & Coaching 1 (1), 69–76.

Hall, N., Jedlic, B., Muroe-Chandler, K., et al., 2007. The effects of an education program on coaches' encouragement of imagery use. International Journal of Coaching Science 1 (1), 79–86.

International Council for Coach Education, 2007. Online. Available: http://www.icce.ws 9 June 2008.

Irwin, G., Hanton, S., Kerwin, D.E., 2004. Reflective practice and the origins of elite coaching knowledge. Reflective Practice 5 (3), 425–442.

Jarvis, P., 2004. Adult education and lifelong learning: theory and practice, third ed. Routledge Falmer, London.

Jarvis, P., 2006. Towards a comprehensive theory of human learning. Routledge, London.

Jarvis, P., 2007. Globalisation, lifelong learning and the learning society: sociological perspectives. Routledge, London.

Jones, R.L., 2006. The sports coach as educator: re-conceptualising sports coaching. Routledge, London.

Jones, R.L., Turner, P., 2006. Teaching coaches to coach holistically: can problem-based learning (PBL) help? Physical Education and Sport Pedagogy 11 (2), 181–202.

Jones, R.L., Armour, K.M., Potrac, P., 2004. Sports coaching cultures: from practice to theory. Routledge, London.

Kirkpatrick, D.L., Kirkpatrick, J.D., 2006. Evaluating training programs: the four levels, third ed. Berrett-Koehler Publishers, San Francisco.

Knowles, A., Borrie, A., Telfer, H., 2005. Towards the reflective sports coach: issues of context, education and application. Ergonomics 48, 1711–1720.

Knowles, Z., Gilbourne, D., Borrie, A., et al., 2001. Developing the reflective sports coach: a study exploring the processes of reflective practice within a higher education coaching program. Reflective Practice 2 (2), 185–207.

Knowles, Z., Tyler, G., Gilbourne, D., et al., 2006. Reflecting on reflection: exploring the practice of sports coaching graduates. Reflective Practice 7 (2), 163–179.

Lee, K.S., Malete, L., Feltz, D.L., 2002. The strength of coaching efficacy between certified and non-certified Singapore coaches. International Journal of Applied Sports Sciences 14 (1), 55–67.

Lemyre, F., Trudel, P., 2004. Le parcours d'apprentissage au rôle d'entraîneur bénévole. AVANTE 10 (3), 40–55.

Lemyre, F., Trudel, P., Durand-Bush, N., 2007. How youth-sport coaches learn to coach. The Sport Psychologist 21, 191–209.

Lohman, M.C., 2006. Factors influencing teachers' engagement in informal learning activities. Journal of Workplace Learning 18 (3), 141–156.

Lyle, J., 2002. Sports coaching concepts: a framework for coaches' behaviour. Routledge, London.

Lyle, J., 2007a. A review of the research evidence for the impact of coach education. International Journal of Coaching Science 1 (1), 19–36.

Lyle, J., 2007b. UKCC impact study: definitional, conceptual and methodological review. Online. Available: http://www. sportscoachuk.org/research/ Research+Publications/UKCC+ Impact+Study+Phase+ One+Report.htm.

Lynch, M., Mallett, C., 2006. Becoming a successful high performance track and field coach. Modern Athlete & Coach 44 (2), 15–20.

Malete, L., Feltz, D.L., 2000. The effect of a coaching education program on coaching efficacy. The Sport Psychologist 14, 410–417.

McCullick, B.A., Belcher, D., Schempp, P.G., 2005. What works in coaching and sport instructor certification program? The participant's view. Physical Education and Sports Pedagogy 10 (2), 121–137.

McMillin, C.J., Reffner, C. (Eds.), 1999. Directory of college and university coaching education programs. Fitness Information Technology, Morgantown, WV.

Merriam, S.B., Caffarella, R.S., Baumgartner, L.M., 2007. Learning in adulthood: a comprehensive guide, third ed. Jossey-Bass, San Francisco, CA.

National Association for Sport and Physical Education [NASPE], 2008. NASPE National Coaching Report. Author, Reston, VA.

National Association for Sport and Physical Education [NASPE]. National Council for Accreditation of Coach Education, 2008. Online. Available: www.aahperd.org/naspe/ template.cfm?template=programs-ncace.html 9 June 2008.

Nelson, L.J., Cushion, C.J., 2006. Reflection in coach education: the case of National Governing Body Coaching Certificate. The Sport Psychologist 20, 174–183.

Nelson, L.J., Cushion, C.J., Potrac, P., 2006. Formal, nonformal and informal coach learning: a holistic conceptualisation. International Journal of Sports Sciences & Coaching 1 (3), 247–259.

Organisation for Economic Co-operation and Development, 2007. Qualifications systems: bridges to lifelong learning. OECD, Paris.

Reade, I., Rodgers, W., Hall, N., 2008. Knowledge transfer: how do high performance coaches access the knowledge of sport scientists? International Journal of Sports Sciences & Coaching 3 (3), 319–334.

Rynne, S.B., Mallett, C., Tinning, R., 2006. High performance sport coaching: institutes of sport as sites for learning. International Journal of Sport Science & Coaching 1 (3), 223–233.

Salmela, J.H., 1995. Learning from the development of expert coaches. Coaching and Sport Science Journal 2 (2), 3–13.

Smith, R.E., Smoll, F.L., 1990. Self-esteem and children's reactions to youth sport coaching behaviours: a field study of self-enhancement process. Development Psychology 26 (6), 987–993.

Smith, R.E., Smoll, F.L., Curtis, B., 1978. Coaching behaviours in Little League Baseball. In: Smoll, F.L., Smith, R.E. (Eds.), Psychological perspectives in youth sports. Hemisphere, Washington, DC, pp. 173–201.

Smith, R.E., Smoll, F.L., Curtis, B., 1979. Coach effectiveness training: a cognitive-behavioral approach to enhancing relationship skills in youth sport coaches. Journal of Sport Psychology 1, 59–75.

Smith, R.E., Zane, N.W.S., Smoll, F.L., et al., 1983. Behavioral assessment in youth sports: coaching behaviours and children's attitudes. Med. Sci. Sports Exerc. 15, 208–214.

Smith, R.E., Smoll, F.L., Barnett, N.P., 1995. Reduction of children's sport performance anxiety through social support and stress-reduction training for coaches. Journal of Applied Developmental Psychology 16, 125–142.

Smith, R.E., Smoll, F.L., Cumming, S.P., 2007. Effects of a motivational climate intervention for coaches on young athletes' sport performance anxiety. Journal of Sport and Exercise Psychology 29, 39–59.

Smoll, F.L., Smith, R.E., 2005. Coaches who never lose: making sure athletes win, no matter what the score, second ed. Warde, Palo Alto, CA.

Smoll, F.L., Smith, R.E., Barnett, N.P., et al., 1993. Enhancement of children's self-esteem through social support training for youth sport coaches. J. Appl. Psychol. 78 (4), 602–610.

Smoll, F.L., Smith, R.E., Cumming, S.P., 2007. Effects of a motivational climate intervention for coaches on changes in young athletes' achievement goal orientations. Journal of Clinical Sport Psychology 1, 23–46.

sports coach UK, 2007. Online. Available: http://www. sportscoachuk.org 9 June 2008.

Trudel, P., Gilbert, W.D., 2006. Coaching and coach education. In: Kirk, M., O'sullivan, M., McDonald, D. (Eds.), Handbook of physical education. Sage, London, pp. 516–539.

Trudel, P., Bernard, D., Boileau, R., et al., 2000. Effects of an intervention strategy on penalties, body checking and injuries in ice hockey. In: Ashare, A.B. (Ed.), Safety in hockey, 3rd volume ASTM 1341. American Society for Testing and Materials, Philadelphia, pp. 237–249.

Vargas-Tonsing, T.M., 2007. Coaches' preferences for continuing coaching education. International Journal of Sports Science & Coaching 2 (1), 25–35.

Werthner, P., Trudel, P., 2006. A new theoretical perspective for understanding how coaches learn to coach. The Sport Psychologist 20, 198–212.

Wright, T., Trudel, P., Culver, D., 2007. Learning how to coach: the different learning situations reported by youth ice hockey coaches. Physical Education and Sport Pedagogy 12 (2), 127–144.

University of Bath, 2007. Online. Available: http://www.teambath. com/?page_id=749.

University of Essex, 2007. Online. Available: http://www.essex.ac.uk/ sport/coach/index.shtm.

The learning coach…the learning approach: professional development for sports coach professionals

10

Kathleen M. Armour

Ben's story

Ben started out, like so many others before him, as a volunteer in the sport in which his children participated. Before long, Ben was persuaded to attend a couple of courses in order to gain coaching qualifications (for insurance purposes, mainly). The coaching courses were relevant and interesting, but Ben found it difficult to squeeze them in to his busy schedule and he resented having to pay for them. Nonetheless, although Ben was a busy man who had a demanding full-time job, he enjoyed his involvement in the club and was happy to donate his time to the cause. As it happens, Ben was also a good coach; caring, knowledgeable and able to connect with children. Then Ben's children lost interest in the sport and Ben moved on to other interests with them.

Jill's story

Jill started out, like so many others before her, as a volunteer in the sport in which her children participated. Before long, Jill was persuaded to attend a coaching course in order to gain a qualification (for insurance purposes, mainly). The coaching course was relevant and interesting but Jill was unemployed and although she had spare time available, she was unable to fund attendance at more than one course. Jill enjoyed her involvement in the sports club and although she was willing and able to donate her time to the cause, her personal finances were increasingly stretched. As it happens, Jill was a good coach and one of her children was showing promise as a performer. In the end, however, Jill found a job that made it impossible to ferry her children to sports activities in the evenings and at weekends. Reluctantly, both Jill and her children ended their involvement with the club and the sport.

Sam's story

Sam started out, like so many others before him, as a volunteer in a sport in which his children participated. Before long, Sam was persuaded to attend a couple of courses in order to gain coaching qualifications. The coaching courses were relevant and interesting and although Sam was supposed to fund them himself, he was delighted to find that his employers recognised and valued the skills he could gain (as documented by the Learning & Skills Council) and were happy to contribute to the cost. The coaching courses took the well-established 'learning coach' approach, and Sam found that not only was the course relevant and interesting for sports coaching, it also offered him a wide range of personal and professional development opportunities. Of particular interest to Sam was the learning support that all the coaches in the club provided for each other and access to the constantly updated on-line coaching resources, which he found to be fascinating. Indeed, as he began to learn more about children, the sport and the profession of coaching, Sam realised that the early qualifications he had taken were just the tip of a giant learning iceberg. As it happens, Sam was a very good coach. He retained his interest in coaching children long after his own children had lost interest in the sport and, last year, he resigned from his job to take up a salaried position as a Senior Coach working within a local school sports hub.

Despite the fictional nature of these coaching scenarios, this chapter is not about fantasy; it is about finding ways to make Sam's story a possibility. Its starting point is a belief that the creation of a respected profession of sports coaching is the next logical step to be taken in the development of sport in the UK. Central to that belief is the suggestion that continuing education, or continuing professional development (CPD) is the essence of a profession and the foundation upon which a new coaching profession should be built. Brunetti (1998) p 62 states, unequivocally, that 'a well developed, readily available continuing education program is the hallmark of a true profession' and in the context of the teaching profession, Falk (2001) p 137 argues that 'professional learning is *the* job of teaching'. The purpose of this chapter, therefore, is to consider some principles upon which career-long professional learning could be conceptualised, designed and organised in order to provide a secure foundation for the fledgling profession of sports coaching; thus making the 'learning coach' a reality.

Although there is, at this point in time, a relatively small body of literature specifically focused on coach professional learning, there is extensive research available in other fields and this can inform the development of coach CPD. In particular, recent research on professional development for the teaching profession is helpful, and whereas it can be argued that teaching and coaching differ in important ways, it can also be argued that they share essential common territory in their core educational functions. The rest of the chapter is, therefore, organised into five sections that reflect both the aspirations and the realities of the coaching profession:

1. The profession question
2. The learning question
3. Continuing professional development, 'what works'?
4. The learning coach...the learning approach
5. Sam's story...reprise

To be or not to be? The profession question

It seems obvious that the development of a new profession should be informed by knowledge and understanding gained from existing professions. Sports coaching needs to base the development of the 'learning coach' upon a clear vision of the features that it shares with other professions, and the unique features that set it apart. Indeed, the development of a new profession presents a tantalising opportunity both to learn from existing professions, and also to contribute to the knowledge base about professions more widely. Undoubtedly, however, the process of shared learning is complicated by

the difficulties that exist in agreeing the defining characteristics of 'a profession'.

Concepts such as 'profession' and 'professional' are contested, as even a cursory search of the literature will reveal. Analysis of phrases such as 'what makes a profession' and 'characteristics of a professional' leads directly to the heart of the controversy. There are two main ways in which discussions about professions are organised: first, the identification of specific occupational groups (e.g. law, medicine, teaching) with arguments about the relative claims each group has to the coveted status of a 'profession' (see below); and second, the development of lists of qualifying criteria to which different occupational groups can make qualifying claims. This is not the place to rehearse all those arguments, but an overview of the literature suggests the following are important considerations.

Some occupational groups appear to be very secure in their designation as a 'profession', suggesting there are few serious challenges to their status; obvious examples include medicine and law. Other professional groups seem to be less secure in their professional status; for example, in 1969, teaching was famously described by Etzioni as a 'semi-profession'. Almost 40 years later, Hargreaves et al (2007) undertook a review of the status of the teaching profession and found that 'Teachers and associated groups (teaching assistants, governors and parents) consistently perceived teaching as a less rewarded, but more controlled and regulated profession than a high status profession' (p 1).

Day (1999) concluded that professionals can be distinguished from other groups because they have, i) a specialised knowledge base – technical culture, ii) a commitment to meeting client needs – service ethic, iii) a strong collective identity – professional commitment, and iv) collegial as against bureaucratic control over practice and professional standards – professional autonomy' (p 5). In considering the development of a profession of sports coaching in these terms, it is interesting to note that:

(a) Coaching has an evolving specialised knowledge base, but it could be argued that the development, organisation, management and dissemination of coaching knowledge needs further consideration.

(b) There is a clear service ethic in coaching, but standards of provision to clients (athletes of all ages) are highly variable and disparate.

(c) Strong collective identity appears to be lacking except, perhaps, at the top levels of elite sport.

(d) There are critical issues to be addressed about professional autonomy and professional standards.

In addition to questions about 'a profession' and the characteristics of a professional, there is a further distinction to be made between being a professional and behaving as a professional. Being a professional means having the training and qualifications necessary to enter a specific profession, being bound by professional standards and a code of ethics, and having a degree of professional autonomy – all of which leads to public respect and acknowledged status in society. However, behaving as a professional is a much broader concept rooted in dedication and commitment to a job/role, and in meeting some form of agreed (or personally defined) standards when dealing with colleagues and clients. Many individuals, including coaches, could argue that they behave as professionals, even if they are not recognised as members of a profession. Thus, even in the field of teaching, which is usually acknowledged as a profession, some have argued that teachers behave as professionals but that teaching does not fulfil all the requirements for being a profession (Helsby et al 1997).

Most professions consider, from time to time, what it means to them to be a profession and what standards of professional conduct they should uphold. The case of pharmacy is both illustrative and insightful. In a paper written for pharmacy students entitled 'On being a professional', identification with and adherence to the profession's code of ethics is considered to be the cornerstone of a professional pharmacist. In their practice, it is suggested that key characteristics of a professional pharmacist are: engendering trust, exercising professional judgement and, of particular interest to this discussion, engaging in continuing education:

> If as a pharmacist you are going to perform your duties competently, then you will need to keep up to date with all aspects of professional practice. Thus, there will be a need continually to update your existing knowledge and skills, as well as acquiring new ones. Such skills and knowledge are essential if as a pharmacist you are going to be able to maintain and progress pharmaceutical standards, whatever branch of the profession you are employed in. Indeed, the Code of Ethics requires pharmacists to 'keep abreast of the progress of pharmaceutical knowledge'. So any new pharmacist, if they are to be a true professional, must embark on continuing professional education. Continuing education involves more than passively attending a few courses, it involves the pharmacist taking some responsibility for his or her own learning. Thus, as a pharmacist, you should approach continuing education in the broadest sense, using all available resources at your disposal.

> (Rees 1999 p 24–26)

This example from pharmacy makes the point eloquently: CPD is the foundation of a profession and, moreover, there is a clear expectation that pharmacy professionals will be engaged actively in the development of their situated professional learning. This would appear to suggest that a constructivist approach to learning underpins CPD thinking and the ways in which pharmacy learners are to be viewed. But how are sports coaches viewed as learners, and how is this reflected in CPD structures?

The learning question

'Learning' is a vast concept and, within it, professional learning is both complex and contested. Colley et al (2003) point out that learning looks different when viewed from different theoretical perspectives. For example, from behaviourism learning is understood as an observable, measurable change in response to a stimulus. Cognitivism focuses on individuals' cognitive structures and processes, and views learning as a change in those structures. More recently, constructivist theories of learning have become popular in a range of educational fields with their emphasis on the social character of learning, and situated learning emphasises the importance of the context and learning as part of social practice. Each of these views of learning has an impact on understanding of the most effective ways to design and conduct professional learning.

It is important to recognise that even where no specific learning theory is identified by a coach or by a professional development provider, the design of any professional learning activity will reflect an implicit learning theory. Bruner (1999) describes these implicit theories as 'folk pedagogies'; i.e. strong views about how people learn and what is 'good' for them. The problem, of course, is that even when these theories are not made explicit, they can be both limited and limiting rooted, as they are, in personal experience and strong (often unchallenged) beliefs about good, better or best ways to learn and, by default, to coach. Yet if such beliefs are not critically reviewed, it is likely that a coach may never realise the influence of personal experience, nor appreciate the ways in which powerful assumptions about what is 'best' for learners are guiding practice. In other words, the coach may have (inadvertently) developed personal coach-centred practice rather than the much-vaunted athlete-centred approach. As Wragg et al (2000) p 217 expressed it in the context of teaching: 'The way people teach is often the way they are...'.

One way to illustrate the influence of personal experiences upon beliefs about learners and learning is to conduct a critical analysis of coaches' philosophies about coaching in the context of their personal life stories. Jones et al (2004) took this approach in their study of eight top-level coaches:

> The key to analysing and understanding coaching pedagogy resides precisely in exploring the articulations ... between all the elements of the human encounter that is coaching. Coaches' lives and careers are central to their coaching philosophies that are, in turn, central to coaching pedagogy. (p 98)

Interviews with the coaches covered two main topics: their personal experiences as learners, athletes and coaches, and their coaching philosophies. Through their stories, a clear picture emerged of coaches who had built their coaching practices around their personal experiences as learners and athletes. For example, Lois Muir talked about her experiences of playing basketball; training with and being coached by men, and the 'toughening' influence this had on her practice when she became a netball coach: 'I had to work for all I got. It made me realise that you only get what you put into it' (p 86). Ian McGeechan recalled the strong influence of his teaching background: 'I'm an education man really ... I suppose I coached like I taught' (p 54).

In other words, regardless of any formal coach education in which they had engaged, these coaches developed strong personal coaching philosophies that guided their practice. Hence, it could be argued that behaviourist views of learning simply cannot capture the complexity of learning in the social practice that is coaching. On the other hand, one of the key strengths of constructivist theories of learning is the potential they offer to analyse and understand coaching as a constructive, autonomous, active, socially situated, and cooperative process of knowledge, meaning, and skill development (Imants 2002). In other words, to borrow from Wragg et al's (2000) earlier comment: 'the way people coach seems to reflect who they are'.

Constructivist theories have been employed extensively in recent education research to explain the ways in which teachers learn effectively, particularly within learning communities (Day 1999, WestEd 2000, NFER 2001, Guskey 2002, Borko 2004, Armour & Yelling 2007, Keay 2006). Linked to this body of knowledge are the widely used situated learning theories of Lave and Wenger (1991) and Wenger (1998) based on the notion of apprenticeship, and a view of learning as an ongoing process situated in social 'communities' of practice. This perspective on learning shifts understanding away from an acceptance of learning as an abstracted activity, and focuses on the combined role of social interactions *and* the environment in fostering learning. Included in this is the apprenticeship model of learning, whereby learners progress to the point where they can become full participants in a community of practice (e.g. the sports coaching community), which, in turn, they have helped to shape.

The apprenticeship view of learning highlights another important consideration in an understanding of coaches as learners: i.e. coaches are, in the main, adult learners. It has been recognised for some time that much learning theory is based on children (pedagogy), but that adults differ from children in some important ways. Tusting and Barton (2003) conducted a review of models of adult learning and concluded that adult learners:

- Have their own motivations for learning ... purposes for learning are related to their real lives
- Have a drive towards self-direction and autonomy
- Have the ability to learn about their own learning processes
- Learn by engaging in practice
- Can reflect and build upon experience
- Often learn in incidental and idiosyncratic ways, and
- Through reflection can 'see' things in different ways, leading to the potential for transformative learning (p 1–2).

This latter view of learning as 'transformative' has been developed from Mezirow's (1997, 1996, 1994, 1981) work. Mezirow's (1997) fundamental assumption is that adults progress in their learning and understanding through transforming their existing 'frames of reference' (p 5) leading to shifts in perspective.

Furthermore, Mezirow argued that individuals become autonomous thinkers by 'learning to negotiate their own values, meanings and purposes rather than uncritically acting on those of others' (1997 p 11). In the context of professional learning, therefore, it can be argued that coaches, as adult learners, need to be *engaged* in professional learning opportunities that have the capacity to *engage* them in 'transformative' learning. It is interesting to note that existing research in education, and more specifically physical education, suggests that few teachers routinely have access to such professional development experiences (e.g. Armour & Yelling 2004a, 2004b, Day & Leitch 2007).

Continuing professional development: 'what works'?

Given that engagement in CPD has been identified as the cornerstone of any profession, it might be expected that the design of CPD would be based, routinely, on a sound appreciation of how adults learn. Indeed, in the case of education-centred professions such as teaching, it is difficult to conceive of CPD being designed in any other way. Yet, research on CPD in education suggests that for many teachers, professional development signally fails to meet their needs, and evidence from the extensive CPD research literature in education can be informative because it is a field from which the fledgling coaching profession can learn. As Jones (2007) p 171 points out: 'coaching has more to do with teaching (and subsequent learning) than anything else'.

There is a growing consensus in the education literature on the key characteristics of effective professional development. In an overview of the literature, Sparks (2002) concludes that effective CPD:

- Deepens teachers' content knowledge and pedagogical skills
- Includes opportunities for practice, reflection and research
- Is embedded in the workplace and takes place in the school day
- Is sustained over time
- Is founded on a sense of collegiality and collaboration.

Research that came to similar conclusions was conducted by WestEd (2000) who reported eight school case studies in the United States that 'tell the story of students who achieve because their teachers are learners' (p 1). The study analysed low-performing schools that were 'turned-around' and where 'an exemplary professional development program' (p 1) was central to that process. In summary, the WestEd report (WestEd 2000) identified the establishment of a school-wide professional culture of learning as the key to success in these schools and defined the following six elements as central to such a culture:

- Ensure that student-centred goals underpin all professional development
- Accept an expanded definition of professional development, embracing a wide range of formal and informal learning experiences
- Recognize, value and make space for 'ongoing, job-embedded informal learning' (p 22)
- Structure a collaborative learning environment
- Ensure there is time for professional learning and collaboration
- Check (constantly) whether professional development is having an impact on pupils' learning.

Guskey (1994), however, urged caution when attempting to identify 'what works' in CPD. He argued for the importance of seeking an 'optimal mix' (p 3) of professional development activities for different teachers in different contexts. Furthermore, although there is a growing consensus in the CPD research literature about some of the characteristics of effective professional development, there is rather less agreement about the relative importance of each. Yet, as was noted earlier, growing interest in social constructivist learning theories seems to be reflected in widespread beliefs held by teachers about the value of learning with and from professional colleagues.

The development of social constructivism can be traced to the work of Dewey (1902) and latterly theories from researchers such as Vygotsky (1978). From a social constructivist perspective, Kirk and Macdonald (1998) p 377 draw upon the work of a range of authors to conclude that 'learning is an active and creative process involving an individual's interaction with their physical environment and with other learners'. It is clear, therefore, that a belief in social constructivism underpins suggestions that 'professional learning communities' (PLCs) (Wenger 1998) can be an effective mechanism for professional learning. Indeed, the desirability of establishing PLCs reverberates throughout recent professional development literature. Although a variety of different terms are given to this broad concept, such as professional community (Warren Little 2002), teacher networks (Lieberman & Wood 2001, National Foundation for Education Research 2001) and discourse communities (Putman & Borko 2000), all share a foundation in social constructivist learning theories. As Warren Little (2002) commented: 'Research spanning more that two decades points consistently to the potential educational benefit of vigorous collegial communities' (p 917). Recent research has reinforced the point further. In a study conducted as part of an extensive Teaching and Learning Research Project (TLRP) in the UK, James et al (2007) concluded:

> Classroom-based collaborative enquiry practices for teacher learning emerged as the key influence on teachers' capacity to promote learning autonomy with their pupils (p 216).

Similarly, in the USA, Lieberman and Miller (2008) conducted extensive research in the field and concluded:

> It is our belief that professional communities ... offer real alternatives to the traditional passive 'staff development' experiences that many teachers know and have come to dread ... they confirm that learning something new, whether it be new content, new forms of representation, or new ways of interacting with colleagues involves a process of unlearning and relearning and requires time and practice. Professional learning communities ... hold the promise of transforming teaching and learning for both the educators and students in our schools (p 106).

The question to be considered at this point, therefore, is to what degree are these findings applicable to coaches?

There is certainly evidence to suggest that some coaches are dissatisfied with their professional development experiences. The top-level coaches in Jones et al's research (2004) raised critical issues about their CPD; for example Steve Harrison described courses that were too narrow in scope, Graham Taylor argued that coaching is 'all down to you as a person' (p 31); Hope Powell argued that coaches need to be given the opportunity to develop their own style; and Ian McGeechan stated that, in his opinion, 'a coaching course has never produced an international coach' (p 59). Furthermore, Jones and Wallace (2005) drew upon the work of Saury and Durand (1998), Gilbert and Trudel (1999), and Cushion et al (2003) to argue that many coaches are: 'disillusioned with

professional development programmes', which they criticise as being 'fine in theory' but divorced from reality' (p 121). Moreover, Nelson and Cushion (2006) argued that coach education is characterised by individualised and ad hoc learning pathways, while Nelson et al (2006) were critical of CPD that is largely organised around traditional 'courses', delivered out of context, and without sustained follow-up support. The recent findings of Kay et al (2008) into the development of coaching as a profession largely endorsed these viewpoints. For example, Kay et al (2008) found that when interviewed, representatives from the high-performance levels of selected sports were highly critical of coach professional development:

> I think what our qualifications do is they allow people to teach gymnastics safely and confidently, but in terms of reaching the absolute pinnacle of performance then I think then we've got some way to go in terms of that route (Gymnastics)
> Qualifications aren't enough to be an international coach, they are a stepping stone (Netball)
> No real consistency or no glory in coaching part 1 or part 2 because it never meant anything ... It's kind of worthless, it feels it (Badminton)
> I don't believe courses make coaches. The glue that hangs it all together [is] the practical education, the informal learning, which is really how coaches learn (Cricket)
> (p 16)

Essentially, it would appear that many practising coaches recognise the complexity of the coaching environment and, similar to teachers, find formal professional development activities tend to lack the depth, challenge and the relevance they require. As the last quote from the cricket representative suggests, one of the solutions for coaches is to seek out informal learning with and from professional colleagues to compensate for the deficiencies of formal learning. This finding is very similar to the findings of research on PE teachers. Armour and Yelling (2003, 2007) investigated professional learning within PE departments in ten case study schools. The teachers identified activities such as going into other schools, exchanging ideas, teaching with colleagues and informal discussions with peer-delegates on PE-CPD 'courses' as productive professional learning. The researchers concluded that in the absence of effective, formal CPD, these PE teachers tended to rely on 'unofficial' CPD that is collaborative and school-based: 'They seemed to "endure" many of the courses they attended, whilst compensating for any shortcomings with their unofficial, but ultimately more valuable, CPD' (Armour & Yelling 2003 p 12).

Yet, whereas informal or unofficial CPD can demonstrably be valuable, there are also potential dangers in it: informal learning not only has the potential to enhance professional learning in positive ways; it can also lead to the reinforcement of poor practice. In both teaching and coaching, therefore, it can be argued that it is important to bring collaborative and informal learning into the formal structures of professional development in order to maximise effectiveness.

Another issue about which teachers and coaches might share similar concerns is the need for CPD to be applicable to the learning needs of both teachers/coaches and their pupils/athletes. Some PE teachers in Armour and Yelling's research (2003, 2004a) complained, not unlike coaches, that the courses they attended were not always realistic for their contexts:

> Some courses refer to PE in the ideal world, e.g. a hockey course on Astroturf, great – but back at school we've got long grass and a water-logged pitch (Armour & Yelling 2004a p 84)
>
> It's ideal so you know there's only a small number of you know kids. Everyone can have a racket and they've got space to work and you've got large groups of kids and only one court. Here that doesn't work so to me it's pointless you know...
>
> (Armour & Yelling 2003 p 8)

This issue is linked closely to another key concern for the education profession: understanding the ways in which professional developers can ensure that teachers'/coaches' professional learning leads to enhanced pupil/athlete learning (Borko 2004). Garet et al (2001) pointed out that there has been 'relatively little systematic research on the effects of professional development on improvements in teaching or on student outcomes' (p 917). Similarly, McLaughlin and Zarrow (2001) argued that many existing models of effective CPD are 'substantively and strategically incomplete' because they are missing '*data and evidence* about practice and policies at school and classroom levels' (p 99–100, italics in original). There are echoes here of comments made by Jones and Wallace (2005) who suggest that in coaching, an 'unbridgeable gap exists between the lofty and often contradictory goals inspiring coaches to act, and their capacity to attain all these goals on the ground' (p 120).

There are, however, both commonalities and differences in concerns about CPD when examined in teaching and coaching contexts. For example, if teachers or coaches are to learn effectively, and to change their practices in the best interests of their 'clients', they need to be convinced that CPD activities are relevant to their specific needs and contexts. Coburn and Russell (2008) point to the accumulating evidence that teachers who learn in effective professional learning communities are more likely to change practice, and improve student learning. In their research, effective learning communities are defined as those that include: 'shared norms and values, a focus on student learning, social trust, de-privatization of practice, collective responsibility and collaboration' (p 205). Coburn and Russell (2008) also reinforce the point made earlier about informal structures, arguing that in some cases, they are indeed more 'consequential' than formal organisational structures. Drawing on social capital theory in order to conduct a social network analysis of interactions and learning within a professional group (teachers), these authors conclude that 'social networks develop as individuals form network ties based on their perceptions of others, reaching out to those whom they see as having similar professional values...' (p 208). It would be interesting to conduct a social network analysis on coaches in order to identify, in detail, where they learn, how, with whom, from whom and why. It seems likely that such an analysis would reveal a very different pattern of networking from teachers, given the tendency for coaches to be distributed and, in many cases, professionally isolated.

It would also be interesting to relate Guskey's (2002) arguments about teacher change to the coaching context. Guskey argues that CPD providers should revise their assumptions about how and why teachers change. Rather than attempting to change teachers' attitudes and beliefs in order to persuade them to change their practices, Guskey suggests it is important to recognise that 'significant change in teachers' attitudes and beliefs occurs primarily after they gain evidence of improvements in student learning' (p 383). Klinger's (2004) research on teacher learning supports Guskey's position: 'When teachers were asked why they chose to learn one of the instructional practices and why they continued using it, their primary reason was student benefits' (p 251). Given the primacy of the focus on student learning/benefit, a characteristic that captures the essence of professionals and professions, it would seem to be crucial that further research is undertaken in coaching to determine some of the complex ways in which coach learning and athlete learning are linked; after all, this is the whole point of any CPD activity. However, a note of caution should be added here: seeking easy and direct links between specific professional development interventions and teacher/coach or pupil/athlete learning outcomes is likely to be fraught with challenges. For example, Garet et al (2008) used an experimental research design to evaluate the impact of two CPD interventions in schools and found no significant impact on measured teacher or student outcomes. What we might conclude from this is that professional learning is a more complex affair; as Desimone (2009) argues, 'the myriad of experiences that count as teacher learning pose a challenge for measuring professional development in causal studies...' (p 181).

Taken together, it can be seen that informative and critical research on teacher learning, coach learning and continuing professional development is extensive and growing. For example, Muijs and Lindsey (2008) cite research evidence that CPD is increasingly seen as 'a key part of the career development of all professionals, which is a shared responsibility with their employers because it serves the interests of both' (p 196). Given the widespread recognition of its importance, however, it is interesting to note two enduring concerns which are reflected in both teaching and coaching and which, on the surface at least, appear to be obvious and easily remedied.

The first is a concern about the ways in which CPD is evaluated. Muijs and Lindsey argue that evaluation of the impact of CPD is 'rarely undertaken in a systematic and focussed manner' (p 196). They argue that the widely used post-activity/ course 'opinionnaires' fall far short of an effective evaluation because they take no account of the way in which professional learning is subsequently applied in practice. Instead, their research suggests that Guskey's (2000) five-level approach to CPD evaluation is effective; i.e. gathering information on participant support, participant learning, organisational support, participant behaviour, and student learning outcomes (to which the authors add 'value for money'). It would be interesting to explore the ways in which Guskey's evaluation approach could be adapted to coaching. Of particular interest, given the part-time and voluntary nature of much of the coaching workforce, would be an evaluation of organisational support; i.e. which organisation would be evaluated, and how?

The second enduring concern seems to be even more obvious. Both Stein et al (1999) and Coburn and Russell (2008) point out that without effective professional development for CPD providers (i.e. coach educators) it is unlikely that providers will be able to engage teachers (or coaches) in transformative learning. Indeed, *the* key finding of an evaluation of the national PE-CPD programme in England was a clearly identified need for professional developers to be offered further support to enable them to engage teachers in effective forms of professional learning (Armour & Makopoulou 2008). There are clear lessons here for coaching. If coach professional development is to change, coach educators will need to be fully engaged in the change process.

In summary, what this section of the chapter highlights is (a) the range of knowledge available on CPD; (b) the benefits a fledgling coaching profession can gain by drawing upon that knowledge; and (c) the need for further CPD research on the unique professional context of coaching that can also contribute to the wider body of research and knowledge on professional learning.

The learning coach...the learning approach

It could be argued that if increased public funding to develop a profession of coaching in the UK becomes available, expectations about what sport and coaching can deliver will increase and, inevitably, there will be calls for greater accountability. For example, the European Commission White Paper on Sport (2007 no page number) states:

> Sport ... makes an important contribution to the EU's strategic objectives of solidarity and prosperity ... it generates important values such as team spirit, solidarity, tolerance and fair play, contributing to personal development and fulfilment ... helps to foster active citizenship ... sport has an educational dimension ... the Commission recommends strengthening the cooperation between health, education and sport sectors ...

The Commission also points out that even though it lacks direct powers to enforce its objectives for sport 'the Community must, in its actions under the various Treaty provisions, take account of the social, educational and cultural functions inherent in sport'. In such a climate, and with the approach of the London 2012 Olympics and Paralympics, it could be argued that the stage is set for a 'profession' of sports coaching to emerge, ideally comprising a workforce that has a larger salaried core than at present. Kay et al (2008) in their report to the Sportnation panel considered the difficulties to be faced in attempting to convert a largely unpaid, volunteer workforce into a profession of coaching. They argued:

> Aspirations for success in sport, from participation to performance levels, do not seem to be matched by strategies to develop a professional workforce that can deliver what is required. The proportion of volunteers within the coaching workforce should be reduced and a strong core of professional, salaried coaches developed, even if only at the youth sport level in the first instance (p 23).

Furthermore, in one of the conclusions of the report, Kay et al (2008) suggest, 'One way to address these issues would be to conceptualise coaching as a complex workforce whose constituents aspire to different levels of engagement and thus attachment to the coaching "profession"' (p 17). At the core of these suggestions are clear assumptions about what it is to be a profession or a professional (as discussed in section 2), the requirement for structures to be in place that enable professionals to learn (see section 3) and the need for sports coaching, as part of its evolution, to both draw upon and contribute to the extensive professional development research literature. There are numerous ways in which this latter aspiration might be achieved, but it has been argued in this chapter that a focus on the ways in which coaches learn, and can be supported to learn as professionals, is one way forward. Furthermore, in order to focus effectively, the complexity of coaching practice, coaching context and coaches – both as individuals and a professional group – must be acknowledged.

It could be argued that personal and professional complexity is, finally, being recognised in the teaching profession. For example, Sammons et al (2007) concluded their research on teachers' professional life phases, career journeys and professional identities as follows: 'teachers' well-being and positive professional identity are fundamental to their capacities to become and remain effective' (p 699). Similarly, Day et al (2006) suggested that teachers' identities 'are a shifting amalgam of personal biography, culture, social influence and institutional values which may change according to role and circumstance' (p 613). Fuller et al (2005) introduce the additional consideration of the 'developing biographies' of individual professionals, and the need to

remember in any profession that 'prior learning, including education, has helped construct the whole person who arrives' (p 66). Coaches as learning professionals are no less complex. A study conducted by Jones et al (2003) sought to provide an in-depth understanding of the ways in which one soccer coach constructs his expert coach knowledge. The story offers important insights for coach educators; for example, the importance of identifying structural constraints on coaches, thus helping them to become aware of 'the socialisation processes acting upon them' (p 226) and the need to understand coaches as highly adaptive, thus calling into question what the authors term the 'technical-rational' approach underpinning most coach education programmes. Indeed, echoing some of the earlier points made by Fuller et al (2005) on teachers, Saury and Durand (1998) argue that coaches have to be 'very flexible' because they need 'a "cognitive alchemy" consisting of flexible application of (social) rules, using deeply integrated past experiences' (p. 265). Yet again, therefore, there is evidence to suggest that professionals in teaching and coaching share common territory and could learn much from each other.

Darling-Hammond (2006) argued that the opportunity to engage in sustained and powerful learning is a fundamental civil right for all citizens and professionals. John Dewey's (1958) work, however, is an important reminder that the design and management of *every* professional learning opportunity needs careful consideration, because the nature and quality of current learning experiences influences how humans understand and learn in subsequent experiences. This was theorised by Dewey (1958) as the principle of *continuing of experience*. As he explained it, 'Every experience both takes up something from those which have gone before and modifies in some way the quality of those which come after' (p 27). If Dewey's view is accepted, the implication for coaches' professional learning is clear. Each professional learning activity must be designed and organised in ways that build on coaches' existing understandings but, more importantly, *extends their capacity to engage in ongoing/future learning*. Following Dewey, Claxton (2007) made a similar point with the concept of expanding learning capacity. Essentially, both authors are arguing that in order to be effective, each professional learning experience must be designed to arouse curiosity, thereby creating favourable conditions for further learning. Thus, if continuing professional learning is the cornerstone of a profession, and if coaching aspires to be a profession, it can be argued that in order to develop a learning coach:

- Coaches' professional learning should be active, situated, transformative, continuing/continuous, reflective, innovative, ever-evolving
- Professional development must recognise the complexity of coaching practice, contexts and individuals
- The core focus of professional development is the coach as learner who learns continuously in the interest of the athletes served
- Professional learning is *the* job of coaching, and each encounter with athletes is a learning opportunity
- Coaches should be encouraged to become autonomous learners within supportive coach learning communities
- Each professional learning activity should be designed to have a learning capacity-building function
- The potential of informal, collaborative learning should be harnessed in formal professional learning structures
- Coach educators need new forms of learning support to enable them to model the learning approach that will inform the development of the learning coach.

Finally, having read this chapter it is worth reading Sam's story again to consider what it would take to turn the fantasy into a possibility . . . or even a reality.

Sam's story . . . the 'learning coach' experience

Sam started out, like so many others before him, as a volunteer in a sport in which his children participated. Before long, Sam was persuaded to attend a couple of courses in order to gain coaching qualifications. The coaching courses were relevant and interesting and although Sam was supposed to fund them himself, he was delighted to find that his employers recognised and valued the skills he could gain (as documented by the Learning & Skills Council) and were happy to contribute to the cost. The coaching courses took the well-established 'learning coach' approach, and Sam found that not only was the course relevant and interesting for sports coaching, it also offered him a wide range of personal and professional development opportunities. Of particular interest to Sam, was the learning support that all the coaches in the club provided for each other and access to the constantly updated on-line coaching resources, which he found to be fascinating. Indeed, as he began to learn more about children, the sport and the profession of coaching, Sam realised that the early qualifications he had taken were just the tip of a giant learning iceberg. As it happens, Sam was a very good coach. He retained his interest in coaching children long after his own children had lost interest in the sport and, last year, he resigned from his job to take up a salaried position as a Senior Coach working within a local school sports hub.

References

Armour, K.M., Makopoulou, K., 2008. Independent evaluation of the National PE-CPD Programme – Final report. Loughborough University.

Armour, K.M., Yelling, M.R., 2003. Physical education departments as learning organisations: the foundation for effective professional development, Paper presented at the British Education Research Association Annual Conference, Edinburgh, September 2003.

Armour, K.M., Yelling, M.R., 2004a. Professional development and professional learning: bridging the gap for experienced physical education teachers. European

Physical Education Review 10 (1), 71–94.

Armour, K.M., Yelling, M.R., 2004b. Continuing professional development for experienced physical education teachers: towards effective provision. Sport, Education & Society 1, 95–114.

Armour, K.M., Yelling, M.R., 2007. Effective professional development for physical education teachers: the role of informal, collaborative learning. Journal of Teaching in Physical Education 26 (2), 177–200.

Borko, H., 2004. Professional development and teacher learning:

mapping the terrain. Educational Researcher 33 (8), 3–15.

Bruner, J., 1999. Folk pedagogies. In: Leach, B., Moon, B. (Eds.), Learners and pedagogy. The Open University, London, pp. 4–20.

Brunetti, G.J., 1998. Teacher education: a look at its future. Teacher Education Quarterly Fall 59–64.

Claxton, G., 2007. Expanding young people's capacity to learn. British Journal of Educational Studies 55 (2), 115–134.

Coburn, C.E., Russell, J.L., 2008. District policy and teachers' social networks. Educational Evaluation and Policy Analysis 30 (3), 203–235.

Colley, H., Hodkinson, P., Malcom, J., 2003. Informality and formality in learning: a report for the learning and skills research centre. Learning and Skills Research Centre, London.

Cushion, C.J., Armour, K.M., Jones, R.L., 2003. Coach education and continuing professional development: experience and learning to coach. Quest 55, 215–230.

Darling-Hammond, L., 2006. Securing the right to learn: policy and practice for powerful teaching and learning. Educational Researcher 35 (7), 13–24.

Day, C., 1999. Developing teachers: the challenges of lifelong learning. Falmer Press, London.

Day, C., Leitch, R., 2007. The continuing professional development of teachers: issues of coherence, cohesion and effectiveness. In: Townsend, T. (Ed.), International handbook of school effectiveness and improvement. Springer, Dordrecht, pp. 707–726.

Day, C., Kington, A., Stobart, G., et al., 2006. The personal and professional selves of teachers: stable and unstable identities. British Educational Research Journal 32 (4), 601–616.

Desimone, L.M., 2009. Improving impact studies of teachers' professional development: toward better conceptualisations and measures. Educational Researcher 38 (3), 181–199.

Dewey, J., 1902. The child and the curriculum. University of Chicago Press, Chicago.

Dewey, J., 1958. Experience and education. The Macmillan Company, New York.

Etzioni, A., 1969. The semi-professions and their organisation. Free Press, New York.

European Commission, 2007. White Paper on Sport, Brussels, COM (2007) 391 final. Online. Available: http://ec.europa.eu/sport/white-paper/whitepaper8_en.htm#1.

Falk, B., 2001. Professional learning through assessment. In: Lieberman, A., Miller, L. (Eds.), Teachers caught in the action: professional development that matters. Teachers College Press, New York, pp. 118–140.

Fuller, A., Hodkinson, H., Hodkinson, P., et al., 2005. Learning as peripheral participation in communities of practice; a reassessment of key concepts in workplace learning. British Educational Research Journal 31 (1), 49–68.

Garet, S.M., Porter, C.A., Desimone, L., et al., 2001. What makes professional development effective? Results from a national sample of teachers. American Educational Research Journal 38 (4), 915–945.

Gilbert, W., Trudel, P., 1999. Framing the construction of coaching knowledge in experiential learning theory. Sociology of Sport Online 2 (1) Online. Available: http://physed.otago.ac.nz/sosol/v2i1s2.htm.

Guskey, T.R., 1994. Results-oriented professional development: in search of an optimal mix of effective practices. Journal of Staff Development 15, 42–50.

Guskey, T.R., 2000. Evaluating professional development. Corwin Press, Thousand Oaks, CA.

Guskey, T.R., 2002. Professional development and teacher change. Teachers and teaching: theory and practice 8 (3–4), 381–391.

Hargreaves, L., Cunningham, M., Hansen, A.T., et al., 2007. The status of teachers and the teaching profession in England: views from inside and outside the profession. Final report of the teacher status project. DfES – Research Report RR831A.

Helsby, G., Knight, P., McCulloch, G., et al., 1997. 'Professionalism in Crisis': a report to participants on the professional cultures of teachers research project. Lancaster University, Lancaster.

Hodkinson, P., Biesta, G., James, D., 2008. Understanding learning culturally: overcoming the dualism between social and individual views of learning. Vocations and Learning 1, 27–47.

Imants, J., 2002. Restructuring schools as a context for teacher learning. International Journal of Educational Research 37, 715–732.

James, M., McCormick, R., Black, P., et al., 2007. Improving learning how to learn: classrooms, schools and networks. Routledge, London.

Jones, R.L., 2007. Coaching redefined: an everyday pedagogical encounter. Sport, Education and Society 12 (2), 159–174.

Jones, R.L., Armour, K.M., Potrac, P., 2003. Constructing expert knowledge: a case study of a top-level professional soccer coach. Sport, Education & Society 8 (2), 213–230.

Jones, R.L., Armour, K.M., Potrac, P., 2004. Sports coaching cultures: from practice to theory. Routledge, London.

Jones, R.L., Wallace, M., 2005. Another bad day at the training ground: coping with ambiguity in the coaching context. Sport, Education & Society 10 (1), 119–160.

Kay, T., Armour, K.M., Cushion, C.J., et al., 2008. Are we missing the coach for 2012? Report to the Sportnation Panel, IYS. Loughborough University.

Keay, J., 2006. Collaborative learning in physical education teachers' early-career professional development. Physical Education and Sport Pedagogy 11 (3), 285–306.

Kirk, D., Macdonald, D., 1998. Situated learning in physical education. Journal of Teaching in Physical Education 17, 376–387.

Klingner, J.K., 2004. The science of professional development. J. Learn. Disabil. 37 (3), 248–255.

Lave, J., Wenger, E., 1991. Situated learning: legitimate peripheral participation. Cambridge University Press, Cambridge.

Lieberman, A., Miller, L. (Eds.), 2008. Teachers in professional communities. Teachers College, New York.

Lieberman, L., Wood, D., 2001. When teachers write: of networks & learning. In: Lieberman, A., Miller, L. (Eds.), Teachers caught in the action: professional development that matters. Teachers College, New York, pp. 174–187.

McLaughlin, M.W., Zarrow, J., 2001. Teachers engaged in evidence-based reform: trajectories of teacher's inquiry, analysis and action. In: Lieberman, L., Miller, L. (Eds.), Teachers caught in the action: professional development that matters. Teachers College, New York, pp. 79–101.

Mezirow, J., 1981. A critical theory of adult learning and education. Adult Education Quarterly 32 (1), 3–24.

Mezirow, J., 1994. Understanding transformative theory. Adult Education Quarterly 44 (4), 222–232.

Mezirow, J., 1996. Contemporary paradigms of learning. Adult Education Quarterly 46 (3), 158–173.

Mezirow, J., 1997. Transformative learning: theory to practice. New Directions for Adult and Continuing Education 74, 5–12.

Muijs, D., Lindsay, G., 2008. Where are we at? An empirical study of levels and methods of evaluating continuing professional development. British Educational Research Journal 34 (2), 195–212.

National Foundation for Educational Research, 2001. Continuing professional development: LEA & school support for teachers. NFER, Slough.

Nelson, L.J., Cushion, C.J., 2006. Reflection in coach education: the case of the national governing body coaching certificate. The Sport Psychologist 20, 174–183.

Nelson, L.J., Cushion, C.J., Potrac, P., 2006. Formal, nonformal and informal coach learning. International Journal of Sport Science and Coaching 1 (3), 247–259.

Putnam, R., Borko, H., 2000. What do new views of knowledge and thinking have to say about research on teacher learning? Educational Researcher 29 (1), 4–15.

Rees, J.A., 1999. On being a professional. In: Mason, P. (Ed.), Tomorrow's pharmacist, 24–26. October, Online. Available: http://www.pharmj.com/students/tp1999/professional.html.

Saury, J., Durand, M., 1998. Practical knowledge in expert coaches: on site study of coaching in sailing. Res. Q. Exerc. Sport 69 (3), 254–266.

Sparks, D., 2002. Designing powerful professional development for teachers and principals. NSDC, Oxford.

Stein, M.K., Smith, M.S., Silver, E.A., 1999. The development of professional developers: learning to assist teachers in new settings in new ways. Harvard Educational Review 69 (3), 237–269.

Tusting, K., Barton, D., 2003. Models of adult learning: a literature review. NRDC for ALN, Leicester.

Vygotsky, L.S., 1978. Mind in society: the development of higher psychological processes. (M. Cole, Trans.) Harvard University Press, London.

Warren Little, J., 2002. Locating learning in teachers' communities of practice: opening up problems of analysis in records of everyday work. Teaching and Teacher Education 18, 917–946.

Wenger, E., 1998. Communities of practice: learning, meaning and identity. Cambridge University Press, Cambridge.

WestEd, 2000. Teachers who learn, kids who achieve. WestEd, San Francisco.

Wragg, E.C., Haynes, G.S., Wragg, C.M., et al., 2000. Failing teachers?. London, Routledge.

Towards a socio-pedagogy of sports coaching

David Kirk

Introduction: The centrality of learning to sports performance: the *habitus* and 'techniques of the body'

There was a time when pedagogy was not considered to be important for sports coaches or, at least, was considered to be of less importance than, say, the various sports sciences of biomechanics, physiology and psychology and the technical aspects of the sport in question. Indeed, some National Governing Body awards and degree programmes in sports coaching omit pedagogy altogether or give it a very minor role. A number of reasons for this have been suggested. First, the desire on the part of coach educators to be seen to make a clean break from school physical education teacher preparation, where pedagogy seemed to have such a central role. Second, the dominance of a bio-scientific discourse focused on performance. Finally, the relatively underdeveloped study of pedagogy in sports coaching contexts in comparison to the sports sciences to the extent that when pedagogy *was* recognised as important to coaching, writers were forced to borrow heavily from the physical education and teaching research literature (e.g. Jones 2006, Cassidy et al 2009).

With a bio-scientific performance discourse came a misguided view that the coaching of sports participants was primarily a task of enhancing performance, which involved such activities as 'training' and 'conditioning', 'drills' and 'practices'. It was rare in the language of sports coaching in the late 1970s when the author was studying for Club and Senior Coach awards in athletics to hear the word 'learning' used in relation to those who were to be coached. As we now understand, of course, learning is a fundamental aspect of enhancing sports performance, not just for beginners or junior players, but also for senior high-performance sportswomen and -men, and not just in technical sports such as gymnastics and athletics, but in all sports.

Readers need to be convinced on this basic point before we go any further because unless we have agreement that learning is fundamental to all sports performance there is nothing further to say about pedagogy and sports coaching. For those who do need to be convinced, we can draw on the ground-breaking work of French anthropologist Marcel Mauss who first set out his thesis of the 'techniques of the body' in the mid-1930s, though this work only became accessible in English in the early 1970s (Mauss 1973). Mauss' purpose was to provide a theoretical framework for thinking about the body at the intersections of the anthropological, psychological and biological, in an area of miscellany where, he argued, new discoveries can be made. He believed his framework for conceptualising the techniques of the body was indeed a new discovery.

Mauss pointed out through examples of swimming, digging, marching, walking, and running that these techniques of the body differed across nations, across gender and across time. He used the many varieties of the ways in which these techniques are practised to make two points. The first is that these are not merely biological and biomechanical phenomena. They have a clear psycho-social dimension that he captured in the concept of the *habitus* (popularised much later by Pierre Bourdieu). He explained:

I have had this notion of the social nature of the *'habitus'* for many years. Please note that I use the Latin word – it should be understood in France – *habitus*. The word translates infinitely better than *'habitude'* (habit or custom), the *'exis'*, the 'acquired ability' and 'faculty' of Aristotle (. . .) These 'habits' do not just vary with individuals and their imitations, they vary especially between societies, educations, proprieties and fashions, prestiges.

(Mauss 1973 p 73)

Mauss' use of the word *habitus* suggests these techniques are performed more or less skilfully, but habitually and routinely, apparently unconsciously. Their performance is individualised to the extent that they express something of a person's identity as it is shaped by their own unique biography of experience, nationality, social class, occupation, religion, gender, and age or generation. Furthermore, these techniques provide information about individuals both when the body is in action or repose since, as Mauss pointed out, there are different ways of relaxing and sleeping as well as moving.

While the habitual character of many of the techniques Mauss mentions such as walking, running, sleeping and so on are performed adroitly and routinely and so may appear to require no conscious effort, he makes an important second point that all of these techniques are an outcome of education.

In all of these elements of the art of using the human body, the facts of *education* were dominant. The notion of education could be superimposed on that of imitation. For there are children with very strong imitative faculties, others with weak ones, but all of them go through the same education (. . .) What takes place is a prestigious imitation. The child, the adult, imitates actions which have succeeded and which he has seen successfully performed by people in whom he has confidence or who have authority over him.

(Mauss 1973 p 73)

Some of the techniques Mauss discusses, like walking, appear to be acquired in the course of everyday life, while others like marching and swimming typically require formal instruction. But Mauss cites an example of Maori mothers in New Zealand who drilled their daughters to walk in a particular way, with a 'loose-jointed swinging of the hips' termed *onioi* and which is much admired, to make the point that all techniques of the body are learned. Closer to home, he points out that wearing shoes transforms the position of the feet when walking, something we notice immediately when we attempt to walk without them.

Mauss argued that in order to qualify as a technique of the body, an action must be both effective, that is, it must accomplish some purpose with facility, and traditional. On this latter point, he writes 'there is no technique and no transmission in the absence of tradition. This is above all what distinguishes man from the animals: the transmission of his techniques and very probably their oral transmission' (Mauss 1973 p 75). Mauss' point is that techniques of the body are meaningful actions that have a purpose and are part of a shared culture, even though there is some differentiation among social groups, nations and so on.

To illustrate these points, Mauss goes on in his paper to provide a classification of techniques of the body according to sexual division, age, efficiency, and means of transmission. He adds to this classification a biographical list of techniques that are specific to different stages of life, such as birth, infancy, adolescence and adulthood, and then elaborates his argument through a discussion of specific techniques of the body including sleep, rest, running, dancing, climbing, washing and care of the body, and sexual reproduction. Mauss' contribution allows us to appreciate the extent to which all techniques of the body are transmitted and learned, not only those which require explicit instruction. This in turn allows us to see that techniques of the body are socially constructed and reconstructed over time, that they are meaningful and value-laden, and that they are purposeful.

There are no movements in sport that do not meet Mauss' criteria for techniques of the body. All must be effective in terms of achieving some specific purpose with facility, and they must be traditional in the sense that they are part of a codified, socially approved set of practices that have developed over time within particular communities of practice. This means that all techniques of the body that construct and constitute sports performance are learned, either informally or formally, but learned nonetheless. We can see this clearly in the *habitus* of highly trained and socialised performers, in sport in the examples of gymnasts, rugby forwards, and basketball players, and in the arts in the examples of ballet dancers and opera singers; in each of these cases, the techniques of the body have been learned to a level that they seep through the individual's everyday actions as well as constituting their performances in their particular disciplines.

Since learning is central to enhancing sports performance at all levels in all sports, pedagogy is of the utmost relevance to sports coaching. Having established this point, we might now ask what it is we mean, exactly, by pedagogy, what is pedagogy's relationship to learning, and what a socio-pedagogy of sports coaching might look like? I address these questions in the next two sections, completing the first part of the chapter. In the second part, I argue that to move towards a socio-pedagogy of sport, coaches need to understand the nature of pedagogy, the pedagogical relations between different sports settings, and their moral responsibilities for cultural preservation and change in and through sport as a social practice.

Pedagogy?

While pedagogy has been defined in a number of ways, the sense in which I am using the word here refers to the interdependence and irreducibility of subject matter, learning, instruction and context (Kirk 1988, Cassidy et al 2009). Different words are sometimes substituted for each of these terms, such as teaching or coaching for instruction, knowledge and curriculum for subject matter, task for the conflation of subject matter and instruction, and environment for context. In the French tradition of *didactique*, a similar concept of the relationships among learning, instruction and knowledge features strongly while, as Amade-Escot (2007) notes, a keen object of interest in *didactique* research is to investigate the extent to which the processes of knowledge transmission and reception in contexts such as for example club sport, high-performance sport and school physical education have shared or different characteristics.

These components of pedagogy are interdependent insofar as change in one component will have an effect on each of the others. For example, if I am mainly concerned that beginner javelin throwers learn safety rules ahead of throwing techniques, I am likely to coach them in a style that is directive. In terms of context, this directive style may take a different form and indeed may be easier to implement in a school physical education lesson in comparison to a sports club. If, on the other hand, I am keen that basketball players learn to identify cues for particular actions such as when and how to shoot, pass or dribble, I would select subject matter that involved modified game play using the principles of representation (the modified game is authentic) and exaggeration (the game form encourages the learning I am looking for) (Bunker &

Thorpe 1982) and a coaching style centred on the question–answer techniques of the Socratic Method (Butler 1997). In terms of context, the age and experience of the players will determine the level of challenge I build into the modified games in terms of numbers of players, the intensity of guarding (from soft to highly intensive), size of playing area, types of target and so on (Rovegno 2006).

This clutch of components of pedagogy is irreducible in the sense that it needs to be treated collectively as a unit of analysis. This is because, as Rovegno (2006) has noted of the similar notion of the individual/task/environment triad that features in situated learning theories, it is the *relations among* these components that individuals learn rather than the components by themselves. A simple example to illustrate these notions of irreducibility and relationality is Rovegno's notion of 'throwing a catchable pass' in basketball; the thrower needs to know something about the capabilities of the catcher as well as her own capabilities, judge the speed and angle of the cut made by the catcher, where teammates and opponents are positioned, other options considered and dismissed, and so on; more of this later in the second half of the chapter.

Socio-pedagogy: sport as a social practice

The notion of socio-pedagogy returns us to Mauss and his thesis of the techniques of the body. Pedagogy is not merely the educational sub-discipline of sports coaching that sits alongside the other sub-disciplines such as biomechanics, physiology and psychology. Mauss' thesis shows very clearly that all techniques of the body are embedded in the social in the sense that they are traditional. In order to understand what Mauss means when he says that there 'can be no technique and no transmission in the absence of tradition', we might consider Alisdair MacIntyre's broader concept of a social 'practice' and the notion of intrinsic and extrinsic goods developed in his book, *After Virtue*. MacIntyre wrote

> By a 'practice' I am going to mean any coherent and complex form of socially established co-operative human activity through which goods internal to that form of activity are realised in the course of trying to achieve those standards of excellence which are appropriate to,

and partially definitive of, that form of activity, with the result that human powers to achieve excellence, and human conceptions of the ends and goods involved, are systematically extended.

(MacIntyre 1985 p 187)

MacIntyre's examples of social practices consistent with this definition include music, architecture and farming, and games such as chess and football. Providing an insight into Mauss' notion of the traditional character of techniques of the body, MacIntyre argues that standards are inherent in practices.

> To enter into a practice is to accept the authority of those standards and the inadequacy of my own performance as judged by them. It is to subject my own attitudes, choices, preferences and tastes to the standards, which currently and partially define the practice. Practices ... have a history: games, sciences and arts all have histories. Thus the standards themselves are not immune from criticism, but nonetheless we cannot be initiated into a practice without accepting the authority of the best standards realised so far. ... If, on starting to play baseball, I do not accept that others know better than I when to throw a fastball and when not, I will never learn to appreciate good pitching let alone to pitch. In the realm of practices the authority of both goods and standards operates in such a way as to rule out all subjectivist and emotivist analyses of judgement.

(MacIntyre 1985 p 190)

Applying MacIntyre's concept of a social practice to his Sport Education model, Daryl Siedentop argued that, in order to become a member of a sport practice, young people learn to accept the authority of the standards of excellence and to subject oneself to rules and traditions 'as one attempts to achieve the goods that are defined by participation in that sport and the respect and admiration of those with whom you are engaged in that sport practice' (Siedentop 2002 p 15). The coherence of this position depends on members of a community of practice having a concept of excellence, having models of excellence, and having incentives to strive for excellence. This is why Siedentop goes to some lengths to argue that heroes and heroines are necessary in sport because they stretch the limits of excellence. Without these concepts, models, and incentives, there are no authoritative standards to which one can subject oneself, and there are no 'goods' intrinsic to the practice itself.

MacIntyre argues that all practices generate both intrinsic and extrinsic goods. Intrinsic goods are unique to the practice itself, are defined by

standards of excellence, and cannot be gained in any other way than through wholehearted participation in the practice. For example, it is not possible to acquire the goods of being a tennis player, the repertoire of skills and tactics, understanding of etiquette, respect for the rules and traditions of tennis, and respect for opponents, without immersing oneself in the practice of tennis. On the other hand, someone who is an excellent tennis player can gain extrinsic goods such as money and prestige. However, these goods are not unique to tennis in the way that the skills, strategies and knowledge of traditions of the sport are.

MacIntyre accepts that it is possible that some performers may be motivated solely by goods external to a practice. But he claims the sustainability of such a person's motivation to engage in the practice may be limited. He also argues that even though such persons may exist, their achievement of external rewards from engagement in a practice is entirely dependent on the willingness of others to be motivated by internal rewards. He says that:

> External goods are therefore characteristically objects of competition in which there must be losers as well as winners. Internal goods are indeed the outcome of competition to excel, but it is characteristic of them that their achievement is a good for the whole community who participate in the practice.

(MacIntyre 1985 p 191)

MacIntyre's concept of a social practice and his useful example of baseball provides us with some content with which to expand Mauss' notion of tradition in relation to techniques of the body. All social practices including sports develop standards of excellence and generate goods both intrinsic and extrinsic to the practice. In order to become more expert in a practice, individuals must submit themselves to the discipline created by the intrinsic goods of the practice, all of which requires the exercise of the virtues of courage, justice and honesty in the face of risks and challenges. It is these goods that sustain a practice, even though extrinsic goods may also be generated. It is possible too that a practice may be corrupted if extrinsic goods overwhelm a practice to the extent that the intrinsic goods are forgotten or lost, which was a favourite claim in defence of amateurism in the face of professionalism in sport. In such a case, however, a practice could not survive, just as a sport could not survive, as Siedentop understands, without the heroes and heroines who continually set higher standards to be emulated.

A socio-pedagogy, then, recognises the deep values surrounding embodiment that find expression in social practices such as sport. Pedagogy is not merely about the transmission of tactics and techniques of games and sports, though it is centrally concerned with this process. Nor is it merely about preserving and passing on to new generations valued aspects of the physical culture of society, though it is very much about this also. A socio-pedagogy of coaching also recognises that learning the techniques of the body requires the engagement in a practice of the whole person, not merely the athlete or player. Therefore, the repetition of particular techniques of the body constructs a *habitus* expressing an individual's identity as well as competence and social worth.

Towards a socio-pedagogy of sports coaching

To embrace a socio-pedagogy of sports coaching, coaches will be required to understand at least four aspects of this concept: the relations among subject matter, learning, coaching and context; the relations among learner/s, task and environment; the relations among pedagogical settings; and, coaches' moral responsibility towards cultural reproduction and transformation.

Coaches need to understand the relations among learning, coaching, subject matter and context

A shorthand way of saying the same thing is that coaches need to understand the nature of pedagogy itself. They need to know that it comprises these four components and that the challenge is not to understand the components by themselves but rather the relations among them. This is not to say that a thorough understanding of each component is unimportant. It is instead to make the point that these components are interdependent and that coaches need to look beyond each to their relations with the others.

The least problematic component of pedagogy for sports coaches ought to be subject matter, in contrast to their colleague physical education teachers, from whom there is a salutary lesson to be learned. For physical educators, subject matter knowledge became deeply problematic with the shift in school physical education from a gymnastics-based to a sports-based subject (in Britain around the 1950s), intensified by an ongoing expansion of the curriculum ever since in terms of the number of sports that could potentially be included, and by the emergence of the sport and exercise sciences (or kinesiology) to replace physical activity in physical education teacher education courses (Kirk 2009). Not only has the range of activities in which teachers must have some expertise been stretched since the 1950s, they also have less time to master this widening range of practical knowledge since sport and exercise sciences has appropriated increasing amounts of curriculum time in degree courses. According to Siedentop, published in 2002 but writing at the end of the 1980s:

> We have arrived at a point in our history where we can now prepare teachers who are pedagogically more skilful than ever, but who, in many cases, are so unprepared in the content area that they would be described as "ignorant" if the content area were a purely cognitive knowledge field.

(Siedentop 2002 p 369)

By 'pedagogically' more skilful, Siedentop means that new teachers have high levels of knowledge of teaching and learning as processes, while they are also well-versed in kinesiology. But without detailed subject matter knowledge of specific physical activities they are unable to move beyond superficial introductory lessons, which, he claims, get taught to pupils 'again, and again and again'.

Sports coaches have traditionally tended to be specialists in one sport only, and often in one context only (such as high-performance or community-based participation). While there may be some arguments in support of coaches of beginner performers (usually children) becoming specialists in more than one sport, detailed subject matter knowledge is crucial even at this level if coaches are to design quality learning experiences for their players that make a difference to performance. Indeed, perhaps this principle of subject matter expertise is so well-established in sports coaching that it has at times been viewed as the most important and perhaps even the only component of pedagogy a coach needs to master. Indeed, such an approach has led to an overemphasis of 'what to coach' within coach education.

According to Amade-Escot (2007 p 11), knowledge lies at the heart of *didactique*. Even so, the *didactique* research shows clearly that detailed subject matter knowledge by itself is not enough to make a difference to performance. Coaches must also understand the relations among subject matter and learning, coaching and context. The recent emergence of models-based practice (MBP) in physical education (Metzler 2006) and the older Teaching Games for Understanding (TGfU) pedagogical model in particular provide an illustration of this point. The principle at the centre of MBP is that learning can be progressed most effectively when subject matter and instruction are aligned with intended learning outcomes, while taking account of context. This generic principle informs the construction of all pedagogical models, including TGfU.

TGfU came into being because Bunker and Thorpe (1982) believed that too much games teaching and coaching produced technically gifted sportsmen and -women whose performance was nevertheless limited because they rarely developed a good understanding of their game. They argued that this 'traditional' approach at its worst focused entirely on practising de-contextualised skills and drills that were rarely applied when the game was eventually played, which in itself was infrequently. They proposed that, instead, games pedagogy should be rooted in modified games, designed to exaggerate certain aspects of the tactical situations encountered in a full game while representing an authentic experience of the game. The learning outcome for the players within this TGfU approach was not to develop tactical in place of technical competence (a point regularly misunderstood by critics of the approach), but instead to produce better *players*.

In order to achieve this outcome a coach must manipulate the subject matter of the game in particular ways in order to place players in learning situations where specific, desired outcomes are likely to result. For example, in order to facilitate understanding of how to create an overlap in rugby, players may play a 3 vs 2 game on a wide playing area (e.g. 30 m x 20 m) so that they can experiment with different ways of moving defenders out of position in order to take advantage of their extra player and score a try.

The coach must also consider coaching style in this context. In the so-called traditional approach to games teaching, teachers typically and uniformly adopted a command or directive style (to use Mosston's terminology [see Mosston & Ashworth 1974]) that had its roots in the historical subject matter of physical training and more specifically

free-standing Dano-Swedish gymnastics and military drills such as marching. Applied to games teaching, this teaching style arguably made sense if the learning outcome was to improve technique but also, more likely, to maintain control of a large number of children in an outdoor space within an institution (a school) that required particular behaviours from pupils. Clearly this coaching style will not work if the learning outcome instead is to produce good players. Good players understand the game concept and tactics, and they can think independently (from the coach) and creatively while playing. They can also recognise cues that signal decisions they need to make in terms of what to do and how to do it. They are technically competent in putting decisions into practice, and can use feedback to analyse critically their own and others' performances in order to continue to improve. Barking orders and commands is likely to be counter-productive to the achievement of such a goal at the very least because this style of pedagogy denies the players' knowledge, relative independence, creativity and reflection.

Learning has already been included in this discussion of the subject matter of TGfU (modified games as a medium) and coaching styles (facilitative, using the Socratic method) through the consideration of different learning outcomes. Learning processes are also already implied in this discussion through the notion of players 'experimenting' with different ways of disorganising a defence and mention of processes such as cue perception and decision-making. The regular use of the Socratic Method of question and answer in the TGfU approach suggests that while coaches might know the answers, a more effective way to assist players to develop their understanding may be to guide them to think through issues for themselves rather than simply tell them or show them the solution. While the analogy to information processing has been a popular way of describing learning within TGfU, and while it has provided a persuasive account of the importance of cognitive processes in sports performance, it is clear that learning is much more than the processing of information. Coaches need to understand an individual's or a group of performers' readiness to learn. As we will see shortly from the vantage point provided by situated learning theory, however, cognition is distributed rather than inside individual players' heads, and there are important affective and social as well as cognitive and physical dimensions of learning.

This example of TGfU also illustrates the importance of coaches understanding the relations among subject matter/coaching/learning and context. As we will discuss below, the learning setting is one consideration in terms of context, such as the sometimes contrasting but also often similar aspects of school sport and club sport. Contextual matters that impact on the subject matter/coaching/learning relationships may also include the level of performance (participation, developmental, high performance), time of year or season, and a host of mundane, but often influential issues, such as weather, equipment, facilities, and so on.

On this account, pedagogy is a complex phenomenon, and coaches need to develop their understanding of the relations among its component parts in order to progress as a coach and to progress players' learning and performances. For example, possessing a sophisticated understanding of subject matter without understanding the relations among subject matter and learning, coaching and context will stand in the way of good coaching practice. All four components of pedagogy are vital to good coaching, not in isolation from each other but, on the contrary, in relation to each other.

Coaches need to understand the relations among learner/s, task and environment

A useful way of thinking about pedagogy at a more detailed level is provided by situated learning theory as it has been developed in physical education contexts by Rovegno (2006) and her colleagues, drawing primarily on the work of Jean Lave (1988), Barbara Rogoff (1990) and ecological research within the motor control literature (e.g. Turvey & Shaw 1995). Rovegno argues that there are three main principles identified by a situated learning perspective. The first is that the learner/s, task and environment are the primary unit of analysis. The second is that this unit is irreducible and each component is relational. The third is that cognition is distributed among or stretched across the learner/s, task and environment.

The first two principles are identical to the definition of pedagogy more broadly, with Rovego substituting 'task' for 'subject matter' but also drawing in the 'instructor', and 'environment' for 'context'. Because of the level of detail Rovegno is working at with situated learning, this difference in terminology represents a more operational and substantive version of the terms used to describe the components of pedagogy. The third principle provides a very different perspective on learning from cognitive theories such as information processing and cognitive mediation theories (see Solmon 2006). It is worth exploring here the implications of this third principle for a socio-pedagogy of coaching, while keeping in mind the other two.

The situated learning theory Rovegno has developed assumes a number of characteristics of learning that derive from constructivist perspectives, such as the notion that learning is an active process of learner engagement with a task rather than the passive receipt of information, and the idea that learners actively construct knowledge, making sense of new information in relation to their prior experiences (Rovegno & Dolly 2006). I have already introduced the example of throwing the catchable pass to illustrate the way in which learner, task and environment relate to each other. Rovegno (2006 p 119) borrows the notion of *affordances* from the work of ecological psychologists J J and E J Gibson to explain how the environment can be considered within these relations. She explains that affordances are 'opportunities for action' insofar as learners perceive what the environment 'affords (or has the capacity to provide)' in terms of an individual's or group's intentions and capabilities. A catchable pass can happen only in an environment that affords the pass to be caught, that is, a pass that is thrown in a way that is informed by the thrower's knowledge of the catcher's capabilities and intentions, and the overall configuration of the game at that moment in time.

The notion of distributed cognition can be illustrated through an example from my own coaching practice, in this case in club rugby union with relatively inexperienced youth players (i.e. under 12s). Again, throwing an effective pass is the task. Use of these so-called 'basic' skills as examples is important since they show that the techniques of the body that typically feature in sport actually are far from 'basic' in terms of their acquisition and their stable performance over time. In this case, the task was constructed in such a way as to make the process of stretching cognition across the learner/s, task and environment explicit and in so doing to offload some of the cognitive demands of the task on to the environment in order to facilitate learning.

The so-called traditional approach to coaching the lateral pass in rugby union where the ball must travel backwards and to the side, a pass typically used in back play, is to demonstrate the technique in terms of position of the hands on the ball, where to aim, the swinging action of the arms across the body, and so on, and then to have four or five players run across the pitch practising the technique of the 'pass'. This 'pass' is rarely made effectively in a game, however, no matter how well-honed technique may become through this practice. The key issue in making this pass in a game is not the technique as the first consideration (though it is important and becomes more so when the distance over which the pass needs to travel increases). The first consideration is recognising whether it is necessary to pass at all and, if the answer is yes, deciding when to make the pass.

I have used a 2 vs 1 modified game practice to coach players to throw an effective lateral pass. The game involves a player in possession of the ball who throws the pass, a second player who acts as receiver and try-scorer, and a third who defends the try-line. Within a 15 m × 15 m playing area, a 5 m × 10 m box is marked on the ground. The defender begins by standing on one 5 m line (which is also continuous with the try-line) and cannot enter the box until the player in possession of the ball enters from the other end. Any contact in the form of a tackle must take place inside the box. The player with the ball cannot make the pass until she is in the box. The receiver remains outside the box to the side and behind the player with the ball, at a distance that can be varied to suit the capabilities of the players. The defender can leave the box in pursuit of the receiving player as soon as the ball leaves the passer's hands. The challenge for the player with the ball is not to pass too early, thereby allowing the defender to escape from the box and tackle the ball-receiver, nor to pass too close to the defender, risking an interception, nor finally to wait too long and thereby be tackled before being able to make the pass.

This practice effectively offloads some of the cognitive work of the task onto the environment, particularly in relation to the passer's perception of distance from the defender and the decision when to pass. First and most obviously, the box creates a visible zone in which the action of passing must take place; the decision if and when to pass has been compressed into a specific period of time. Secondly, the requirement that the defender can only operate in the box for the first tackle effectively fixes the defender's position, again offloading this cognitive task on to the environment. The compression of the action zone is such that a decision not to make the pass – in other words, for the ball-carrier to

attempt to score on her own – will almost always result in contact of some sort being made between attacker and defender and with it the high risk to the attacker of losing possession. And thirdly, the process of cue perception is made easier because the degree of variability in the environment or, in other words, the range of affordances, is greatly reduced. As players become increasingly experienced at making effective passes, the game can be modified to increase the size of the box, add additional boxes for additional players, and then to remove the box entirely, in order to increase the range of affordances and the level of challenge for the players.

This example of distributed cognition presents some considerable challenges to coaches in terms of designing tasks or learning experiences that genuinely facilitate learning, and shows why it is of such importance for coaches to possess a profound understanding of the subject matter component of pedagogy and its relations among learning, coaching and context. These situated learning principles of unit of analysis, relationality and distributed cognition provide coaches with a powerful approach to progressing learning and performance.

Coaches need to understand the relations among pedagogical settings

It is perhaps understandable that in the early years of the development of coaching, the impulse to dis-associate coaching from physical education teaching was strong. There is some irony in this since many physical education teachers from the 1950s on (when men began to enter the workforce in larger numbers than hitherto) were also sports coaches, looking after extracurricular school sports clubs (Kirk 1992). Until the late 1980s, school was the primary site for most children to experience instruction in sport. Over the last 20 years, this situation has changed with the massive growth in club sport for increasingly younger children. It is now commonplace in Britain for young people entering secondary school at age 12 or 13 to have experienced formal instruction in a sports club setting in at least one or more sports. It is also now commonplace to find coaches running aspects of the physical education programme in many primary schools.

At this level of the upper primary and lower secondary school age range, then, within what Côté and Hay (2002) call the 'sampling years', coaches need to understand the relations among the various pedagogical settings in which young people experience sport. It is the same child who plays basketball in a physical education lesson, at the extracurricular school basketball club, and in the local basketball club. By understanding the relations between these pedagogical settings, coaches may be able to ensure a consistency and quality of experience that in all likelihood is currently unevenly distributed.

This is not a matter of suggesting that each setting ought to be the same. It is clear that schools as institutions, where attendance and participation are required, are not the same as community sports clubs, where attendance and participation are voluntary. Moreover, schools do more than teach sport, while sports clubs have a very specialised and particular focus. Accepting these fundamental differences, there is nevertheless a need for consistency of experience for young people. For example, there is a growing body of research literature that provides evidence of the benefits to young people of participation in Sport Education (e.g. Kinchin 2006). Developed by American physical educator Daryl Siedentop (1994), Sport Education seeks to produce competent, enthusiastic and literate sportspeople. It does this by recasting physical education units as seasons, requiring players to act in a number of roles in addition to player, such as referee, captain, coach, timekeeper, statistician and so on, requires a team to work together over the season as a 'persisting group', and emphasises and rewards fair play. Young people who gain a quality experience of sport in this context may be hard pressed to find an equivalent experience in club sport. And yet, the research evidence is very persuasive that even for highly talented players, Sport Education offers a valuable experience of sport (Kinchin 2006).

The question for coaches working at this level ought to be, 'how can we provide the best experience of sport for all young people, regardless of the setting?' The practice of modelling young people's experience of club sport on the adult version of a sport is in my experience widespread. Siedentop famously remarked that children would rather play on a losing team where they had their fair share of field time than sit on the bench of a winning team. If this is true then there is a considerable challenge for coaches to try to ensure that as many players as possible get to play. It would seem to make sense that every child who wants to play should be able to do so (how else are they to learn to play?), and should be able to receive a fair share of the (often) limited resource that is available in schools and clubs.

Understanding the relations between these settings is a vital first step in constructing an infrastructure for children's sport that is inclusive, fair and of high quality.

We should not limit ourselves to the sampling years and school, club and other less-formal settings. All coaches need to understand how their work at one level and in one setting relates to the work that goes on at other levels and in other settings. Again, it may be understandable that as coaching is emerging as a profession a gap has grown between so-called community coaches, most of whom are volunteers, and coaches working in high-performance youth and adult settings, increasingly as paid work. While it is unreasonable to expect volunteer coaches in particular to have an intimate knowledge of high-performance sport settings, it may be more reasonable for all coaches to have some understanding of the *pedagogical* issues among the settings.

For instance, it is often assumed that TGfU is fine for beginners but inappropriate as a means of structuring learning for professional games players. The Australian Sports Commission and some of its leading high-performance coaches such as Rick Charlesworth would disagree (ASC 1997). The intended learning outcome of TGfU is to produce better players, an outcome that would seem to be salient to all levels of sport performance. Of course, how TGfU is actually implemented will differ according to the needs and experience of the players and the expertise of the coaches. But as a pedagogical strategy, as a means of coaches facilitating the learning and performance of players, it is important that coaches appreciate how their work with the model might affect or have been affected by the use of the model in settings other than their own. For coaches in the sampling years, then, it is important that they understand the implications of their pedagogical work for players who continue into the specialising and investing years. Coaches in the specialising and investing phases likewise need to understand the basis on which they will take forward a player's learning and performance.

Coaches need to understand their moral responsibility towards cultural reproduction and transformation

If sport qualifies as a social practice in the sense set out by MacIntyre, and is a more or less formal means of developing a range of techniques of the body in the sense intended by Mauss, then coaches in all settings have inescapable moral responsibilities towards both cultural reproduction and transformation. I do not mean by this merely that all coaches should set their athletes a good example, nor that they have a duty to be of sound character, nor that they have been checked by the Criminal Records Bureau and cleared to work with young people, although each of these things is important. If Mauss is correct to argue that all techniques of the body have to be both effective and traditional and that sport consists of many such techniques, then sport is an important cultural achievement that deserves to be preserved, transmitted and reproduced. If MacIntyre is correct to argue that sport qualifies as a social practice that is constituted by standards of excellence and by both intrinsic and extrinsic goods, requiring the exercise of the virtues, then we are duty bound to ensure that only the best, sustainable aspects of this cultural achievement are preserved, transmitted and reproduced.

Consistent with these theories of Mauss and MacIntyre, the philosopher Bill Morgan has argued that

> After all, what would be the point of work or of political brinkmanship or, for that matter, of life, if there were no pursuits we humans find intrinsically satisfying that make life worth living in the first place, that is, worth all the struggle and hardship that are an inescapable part of life. And since play, games, and sports are best conceived, as the philosophical literature suggests, as just such intrinsically good things, they are among the most important and serious of human activities, and they are the very activities which things like work derive whatever seriousness they possess.

(Morgan 2006 p 102)

Morgan argues that, despite widespread misconception to the contrary in many economically advanced societies, in fact we work to live, to engage in activities we find intrinsically rewarding and fulfilling, in which we find meaning and that make life worth living. This inversion of a popular view of sport as a superficial and trivial pastime is entirely justified in light of the arguments of Mauss and MacIntyre. In making this claim, Morgan is careful to suggest that despite its high visibility, the world of professional sport, dominated as it is by external goods, is merely one form of sport and by no means a good example of the social practice of sport writ large.

If sport is indeed a major cultural achievement, an expression of our deeply held beliefs and values around embodiment and being in the world, then coaches in all sports setting have a responsibility first to understand sport's significance in society and second to seek to reproduce the very best aspects of this practice. These tasks can be undertaken and successfully accomplished in only one way, and that is through pedagogy. It is in the act of constructing quality learning experiences for sports participants appropriate to the setting and to the participants' experience and needs that coaches can fulfil this moral responsibility. There is no additional action required. If sport contains intrinsic goods, if it is constituted by standards of excellence, and if it requires the exercise of the virtues of courage, justice and honesty, then coaches have all of the material they need in sport itself.

There are, moreover, opportunities not only to preserve, transmit and reproduce the best aspects of sport as a social practice, important and difficult though this task is. There are opportunities also for cultural transformation. As MacIntyre acknowledges, the existence of standards of excellence to whose authority all sports performers must submit does not mean that the standards are above criticism and revision. To be sure, it is inappropriate for any sports performer to criticise these standards before they have engaged wholeheartedly in learning the techniques of the body specific to a sport and having understood them. But without the possibility of questioning standards of excellence sports themselves may gradually become culturally obsolete. Examples of this willingness to adapt and change sports to meet new circumstances abound, from Dick Fosbury's revolution in high jumping to whole sports embracing rule changes to engage larger numbers of spectators and participants, such as rugby union and cricket. As the arguments between traditionalists and innovators in both of these latter examples show, there are risks involved at every step of this process of critique and revision that need to be managed with great care.

The possibilities for transformation are not confined to sport forms, their rules and techniques. Sport can provide a medium and a means of wider cultural critique and transformation. A good example of this is the part sport has played in the emancipation of women. Less than 30 years ago, the longest distance women were permitted to run in athletics competition was 800 m. The first woman to run in an official marathon had to do so covertly and to be protected by friends from being physically assaulted and removed from the race by enraged male officials (McKay 1991). Now some women are running marathon times that many high-performance male athletes cannot achieve. Women's achievements in sport do not of course suggest for a moment that all women are emancipated and are treated equitably in all areas of their lives. Nor is women's participation in sport unproblematic since sport-girls and sportswomen continue to be stigmatised, their femininity and sexuality questioned, in some sports more than others (Bryson 1990). Nor can we be sure that progress made in sport can be sustained, and so there is a need to constantly refresh the struggle to maintain the gains that have been made and continue to push for even more equitable treatment. Nevertheless, with these qualifications made, we can confidently claim that sport has been both a medium and a means of cultural transformation in relation to gender and to society's quest for gender equity in particular.

In terms of this wider notion of cultural transformation in and through sport, the role of the coach in a pluralist society can never be simple and straightforward. Practices that are claimed to be cheating by one coach may be claimed by another merely to be an opportunity to take legitimate competitive advantage. Since sport will continue to offer external goods in the form of social status, wealth and other rewards, some of them fabulous in relation to the goods gained from participation in other spheres of life, there will be a constant and ongoing tension to be managed between internal and external goods, at all levels of sport. The pushy parent of folk-legend in children's sport is no less a challenge for one coach as maintaining the perspective of a millionaire teenage soccer player on life is for another. At the same time, understanding the social significance of sport as a practice is to understand the beliefs and values that underpin and find expression in sport. Interpretation will always vary as it does in all other spheres of life, including religion. This fact merely indicates the extent of the challenge to coaches to fulfil their moral obligations towards cultural reproduction and transformation.

Conclusion

The author has argued in this chapter that pedagogy is central to coaching practice, a proposition that has not always been recognised and perhaps continues to encounter some incredulity and resistance as sports coaching strives to become a fully-fledged, knowledge-based profession. The author also attempted to show through the deployment of Mauss' theory of the techniques of the body that sport is centrally concerned with learning and that coaches must, as a

consequence, understand the relations among the four components of pedagogy. Alisdair MacIntyre's work on virtue ethics was added to Mauss' theory to argue that sport is a social practice of developing meaningful and purposeful techniques of the body constituted by standards of excellence, internal and external goods, and the exercise of courage, justice and honesty. I suggested that a social practice such as sport requires a socio-pedagogy, entailing coaches' understanding of pedagogy, of relations among pedagogical settings, and of the moral responsibilities surrounding cultural reproduction and transformation.

As an emerging profession, sports coaching has much to learn from its older sibling, physical education teaching, but not for the reasons commonly supposed. While there is pedagogical research conducted in physical education settings that is of clear value to understanding pedagogy in sports coaching settings, the more profound lessons for coaches to learn are, predictably, from physical education's mistakes. In some countries such as the USA, according to their leading researchers (e.g. Siedentop 2002), physical education teacher education (PETE) has lost its way, abandoning deep understanding of its subject matter for the study of kinesiology on the one hand and content-less pedagogical processes on the other. There is evidence to suggest that a similar catastrophe has been occurring in other English-speaking countries such as Australia and Britain (Kirk 2009). There is no doubt that physical education in schools is seriously compromised by this situation in PETE.

Sports coaching must at all costs be mindful of this lesson as it moves towards the status of a knowledge-based profession, particularly as it becomes the norm for coaches to be trained, to acquire and require qualifications, and to possess undergraduate and postgraduate degrees. The knowledge that is of central importance, as the French *didactique* researchers and practitioners know, is subject matter knowledge of specific sports. At the same time, to use the technical language of philosophy, while subject matter knowledge is a necessary condition of quality coaching practice, it is not sufficient in itself. Coaches must understand the relations among subject matter, coaching, learning and context. In the preparation of coaches for all levels of sport and in all settings, this principle should be adhered to as a matter of paramount importance if sport coaching is to fulfil its full potential, which is to facilitate for as many people as possible the experience of and participation in sport as one of the major cultural achievements of modernity.

References

Amade-Escot, C., 2007. Les savoirs au coeur du didactique. In: Amade-Escot, C. (Ed.), Le Didactique. Editions Revue, Paris, pp. 11–29.

Australian Sports Commission, 1997. Game Sense: developing thinking players. ASC, Belconnen.

Bryson, L., 1990. Challenges to male hegemony in sport. In: Messner, M.A., Sabo, D.F. (Eds.), Sport, men and the gender order: critical feminist perspectives. Human Kinetics, Champaign, IL, pp. 173–184.

Bunker, D., Thorpe, R., 1982. A model for the teaching of games in the secondary school. Bulletin of Physical Education 10, 9–16.

Butler, J., 1997. How would Socrates teach games? A constructivist approach. JOPERD 68 (9), 42–47.

Cassidy, T., Jones, R., Potrac, P., 2009. Understanding sports coaching: the social, cultural and pedagogical foundations of sports practice, second ed. Routledge, London.

Côté, J., Hay, J., 2002. Children's involvement in sport: a developmental perspective. In: Silva, J.M., Stevens, D. (Eds.), Psychological foundations of sport. Allyn & Bacon, Boston.

Jones, R.L., 2006. How can educational concepts inform sports coaching? In: Jones, R.L. (Ed.), The sports coach as educator: re-conceptualising sports coaching. Routledge, London, pp. 3–13.

Kinchin, G.D., 2006. Sport education: a view of the research. In: Kirk, D., Macdonald, M., O'sullivan, M. (Eds.), The handbook of physical education. Sage, London, pp. 596–609.

Kirk, D., 1992. Defining physical education: the social construction of a school subject in post-war Britain. Falmer, London.

Kirk, D., 1988. Physical education and curriculum study: a critical introduction. Croom Helm, London.

Kirk, D., 2009. Physical education futures. Routledge, London.

Lave, J., 1988. Cognition in practice. Cambridge University Press, Cambridge.

MacIntyre, A., 1985. After virtue: a study in moral theory, second ed. Duckworth, London.

McKay, J., 1991. No pain, no gain; sport in Australian society. Prentice Hall, Sydney.

Mauss, M., 1973. Techniques of the body. Economy and Society 2, 70–87.

Metzler, M.W., 2006. Instructional models for physical education, second ed. Holcombe Hathaway, Scottsdale.

Morgan, W.J., 2006. Philosophy and physical education. In: Kirk, D., Macdonald, M., O'sullivan, M. (Eds.), The handbook of physical education. Sage, London, pp. 97–108.

Mosston, M., Ashworth, S., 1994. Teaching physical education, fourth ed. Macmillan, New York.

Rogoff, B., 1990. Apprenticeship in thinking. Oxford University Press, New York.

Rovegno, I., 2006. Teaching and learning tactical game play at the elementary school level: the role of situated cognition. In: Wallian, N., Poggi, M.P., Musard, M. (Eds.), Co-construire des savoirs: les metiers de l'intervention dans les APSP. Presses universitaries de Franche-Comte, Besançon, pp. 115–126.

Rovegno, I., Dolly, J.P., 2006. Constructivist perspectives on learning. In: Kirk, D., Macdonald, M., O'sullivan, M. (Eds.), The handbook of physical education. Sage, London, pp. 242–261.

Siedentop, D., 1994. Sport education: quality PE through positive sport experiences. Human Kinetics, Champaign, IL.

Siedentop, D., 2002. Content knowledge for physical education. Journal of Teaching in Physical Education 21, 368–377.

Solmon, M., 2006. Learner cognition. In: Kirk, D., Macdonald, D., O'sullivan, M. (Eds.), The handbook of physical education. Sage, London, pp. 226–241.

Turvey, M., Shaw, R., 1995. Toward an ecological physics and a physical psychology. In: Solso, R.L., Massaro, D.W. (Eds.), The science of the mind: 2001 and beyond. Oxford University Press, New York, pp. 144–169.

Understanding athlete learning and coaching practice: utilising 'practice theories' and 'theories of practice'

Tania Cassidy

Introduction

In the past decade scholarly interest in coaching has intensified, a situation that Lyle (2002) attributes to improved career opportunities in coaching, increased provision of coach education and access to coaching studies at tertiary institutions. A focus of some of this interest has been on the professionalisation of coaching, which Lyle credits to at least two factors: namely, the drive for the accountability of coaches, and the desire of those in the coaching community to be viewed as professionals. Increasingly, it is recognised that a characteristic of professionalism is having the ability to link theory and practice (Thompson 2003). Yet Thompson contends that theory does not have to be formal or academic theory, which he calls 'theories of practice'. Theory can also be 'practice theories', which is the informal knowledge and assumptions built up through experience and often culturally transmitted to new recruits entering specific fields. The 'theories of practice' and 'practice theories' held by coaches have implications for how they coach, or in other words how athletes are taught, and in turn have implications for how and what athletes learn or do not learn. An example of a coach's 'practice theories' is evidenced by the comments of Graham Henry (coach of the All Blacks) in Box 12.1.

In New Zealand, prior to the 2007 Rugby World Cup, the practices of the coaches and players in the All Blacks received considerable media attention. One of the policies adopted by the coaching staff was the 'rotation policy', which saw players in the squad being rotated into and out of the starting team, resulting in players having to share 'their'

position. This policy proved to be contentious for some members of the media and wider rugby community. In an interview prior to a domestic series between the All Blacks, France and Canada, John Campbell (JC), a current affairs television broadcaster, asked Graham Henry (GH) to 'look back ... to the young men he coached in the Auckland ['Blues'] team in the 1990s and compare them with the young players he is coaching now [in the All Blacks]' (For full interview see Box 12.1).

Whenever I hear Graham Henry speak I am reminded that, before he became a professional coach, he was a physical education teacher and the Principal of a large secondary school. To have succeeded in all these positions I suggest he would have built up, through experience, a body of informal knowledge and developed assumptions about how to teach and how people learn and these would in turn influence his coaching 'practice theories'.

It is often assumed (by some practitioners) that coaches only need 'practice theories'. However, I suggest coaches would benefit from having some knowledge of academic theories or 'theories of practice' because these theories can provide a conceptual framework and a vocabulary for understanding and interpreting what is observable. What is more, 'theories of practice' can focus attention on those aspects of practice that are key to finding a solution to a perceived problem (Merriam et al 2007). Anecdotally, a common problem for many coaches is that the athletes do not do what coaches tell them to do. This is illustrated in the account given by a cricket coach in Box 21.2.

Anecdotal accounts suggest that this is a common occurrence for many coaches. I suggest that coaches

Box 12.1

Postcard from the field

GH: They are different people and I think that reflects the New Zealand community, like the people today are quite different from 1996 when I coached the 'Blues'.

JC: In what way?

GH: They're less competitive, they're more supportive of each other, so there are a lot of good things that have come through society right now. Like it was 'dog eat dog' when Fitzy and Zinny used to play for the 'Blues', never give a mug a chance, like Warren Gatland sat in the stands for 44 test matches, Fitzy played 96, never got on the field Warren Gatland, now that wouldn't happen today would it? You've got Anton Oliver and Kevin Mealamu and Andrew Hore who all get an opportunity and they are supporting each other to try and make each other better and that is a reflection of society. ... for sure the player today is a different individual than the player of 10 years ago; less competitive as an individual, and I have said I think that reflects the New Zealand system, but much more supportive of each other so there are some good, very good plusses there as well.

JC: So where does this leave you as a coach? Is the net result better or worse dealing with these young men. In other words, it's not 'dog eat dog', they have a greater community sense, a community spirit in terms of their involvement.

GH: I think, I think it is a positive in many respects.

JC: Now?

GH: Yes! Yes like we would never had been able to do the rotation system without their support on that.

JC: So, 15 years ago people like Fitzy would have just totally said 'you can go and get knotted' if you had suggested that he was rotated.

GH: That is a very good expression (laughter).

JC: It was not the one I was going to use but we are on telly at 7 o'clock.

GH: Yes I agree, it wouldn't have happened 10, 15 years ago. It's happened today because it is a possibility because these guys are thinking about their fellow players and how they can improve. So there's a lot more support of each other. I am just saying that the competitiveness of the individual who enters rugby now is probably not as competitive as they were 10 years ago because of the community that they grow up in, and part of that is the evaluation system, the examination system. *Part* of that!

JC: As a rugby coach would you like us to be more cut throat? Or not? More singular? More 'dog eat dog'?

GH: Ummm, I'm fairly relaxed about that. You know you've got this support of each other. Also I think it reflects the Polynesian culture of New Zealand. I think the Polynesians have had a major effect on how we feel in the All Blacks. They look after the extended family, the whanau are important, looking out for brother and sister, grandma and grandad and so on and I think that has had a major positive effect on the All Black culture. So it's all good. (TV3 2007).

Box 12.2

Postcard from the field

'The slow (and in many cases complete absence of) progress of the players in improving their batting and bowling skills, despite my best efforts in two-hour sessions twice a week, was getting more than a little frustrating. In particular, I recall having a great deal of difficulty in getting four or five of the batsmen to correct one glaring fault.... In my view at that time, I had been doing a pretty good job with these lads – I had told them what they were doing wrong, why it was wrong and what they needed to do to put it right. Because I also understood the fear of getting hit was one potential reason why they had been getting it wrong, I took pains to explain that they had less chance of being hit if they kept their back foot still. What more did they need? Yet obviously they did need something more because, despite my coaching, they were still moving their back feet when I arrived for the next coaching session ... and the next!' (Hadfield in Kidman 2005 p 31).

often perceive the situation to be one of 'the athletes not getting it', despite the fact that they have been told over and over again what is required to improve. Coaches interpret this to be a consequence of the athletes not listening or of not being very smart. I would like to suggest that, rather than the athletes shouldering most of the blame for the lack of progress, coaches also take time to reflect on their practices and how 'theories of practice' could further assist them to interpret what they observe. One simple question upon which coaches could reflect when the athletes are 'not getting it' is, what do they know about how people learn and what does this mean for the way they work with their athletes?

The process of reflecting on the above question is highlighted in Box 12.3. In 2003 some colleagues and I were asked by a rugby provincial coaching manager to develop a coach development programme that was informed by pedagogy, sociology and psychology.

Box 12.3

Postcard from the field

Early on in the programme the coaches were asked to complete a questionnaire that introduced them to the idea that coaching was related to learning. The questionnaire was a graphic way of highlighting to the coaches that they, and their athletes, learn in different ways. The questionnaire became the vehicle for discussing ways to accommodate the learning preferences of their athletes and a catalyst for reflecting on what they already did, and could do in the future, to assist their athletes to learn.

At the completion of the CoDe programme we asked the coaches for their feedback. Six of the eight coaches said that prior to us highlighting the idea that athletes were learners they had rarely considered their athletes this way. One of the coaches said that coming to know about learning preferences had been a 'revelation' for him

and it had changed the way that he taught his players new moves. Another coach said that because he had no training as an educator it was 'nice to know' about learning preferences. Even the two coaches who were employed in educational institutions recognised the worth of having material on learning preferences included in the CoDe programme. One of them said he 'enjoyed' us highlighting how 'coaching is really about working with people and understanding how they learn'. The other admitted that while in his position as a university lecturer he would 'go to all this trouble of making sure you don't bore the shit out of them [the students] ... and I guess I hadn't really necessarily thought about applying it directly to the [players in the] rugby team' (see Cassidy et al 2006 p 151).

Consequently, we instigated a coach development initiative (which we called the CoDe programme) with representative team rugby union coaches.

I have approached the writing of this chapter from a position that assumes that if coaches wish to be viewed as professionals, or to act professionally, they should have some understanding of relevant 'theories of practice' *as well as* 'practice theories'. I do not view one form of theory to be better than the other, rather it is my position that they complement each other and that the practices of coaches should be informed by both 'practice theories' and 'theories of practice'. Coaching practice is multifaceted and as a consequence can be viewed from many different perspectives, and will be likely therefore to draw upon many 'theories of practice'. This is aptly illustrated in the *International Journal of Sport Science and Coaching* where coaching is discussed from a wide range of disciplines and perspectives. The value of having such a diverse forum is that readers can be introduced to new ideas and inter-connections. We do need to acknowledge that, while the cross-fertilisation of ideas may occur, most scholars who write about coaching do so from a particular understanding of 'how the world works' (i.e. that they have a particular ontological position). Coaches also have ontological positions, and these positions influence what questions they ask of their coaching practice and the solutions that are likely to be proposed or sought. While more often than not these ontological positions are implicit, they are nonetheless powerful. Consider how many times we do not do something

or do not agree with someone because it does not 'feel right' and how many times are we told to 'trust our gut'. These sayings implicitly recognise that individuals have ontological perspectives.

My own ontological position is that coaching involves human interaction (even if that interaction is mediated by technology) and, as a consequence of this human interaction, coaching practice can be viewed as a pedagogical process (which I describe later when discussing 'theories of practice'). I am particularly interested in gaining insight into how 'theories of practice' and 'practice theories' in relation to athlete learning are understood and enacted in coaching practice. To assist me in this endeavour I draw on 'theories of practice' associated with pedagogy. Several years ago Armour (in Jones et al 2004 p 95) made a case for examining coaching from 'the perspective of pedagogy' and suggested that pedagogy was a practical as well as analytical framework for understanding coaching practice and coach education.

The purpose of this chapter is to introduce the notion of 'practice theories' and 'theories of practice' and to discuss them in relation to: (a) coaching practices and athlete learning, and (b) pedagogical and learning theories. Linking practice and theory this way can lend support to those who wish to make a case for the professionalisation of coaching as well as highlight the gaps that may exist in the practice and theorising of athlete learning. To achieve this purpose the chapter is organised into two sections, (a) the 'practice theories' and 'theories of practice' relevant to understanding coaching as a pedagogical process, and (b) the 'practice theories' and 'theories of practice' associated with athlete learning. In each section there is a discussion of the opportunities and limitations associated with engaging with both forms of theory.

It is important to note that the literature relevant to 'theories of practice' will often be drawn from education or psychology, and not the coaching context. The reasons for this are two-fold. First, education and psychology are the disciplines from which the theoretical discussions surrounding pedagogy have emerged. Second, until relatively recently, there has been limited interest in writing or publishing material relating to pedagogical 'theories of practice' in a coaching context.

The place of pedagogy in coaching practice

In many English-speaking coaching communities, the term pedagogy has not had widespread appeal, usage, or a common understanding. Green and Lee (1995) suggest that one of the initial difficulties associated with getting some people to use the term pedagogy is that the term sounds too pretentious. I have sympathy with this position but believe it is worth persevering with the use of the term. If coaches do not engage with it, they limit their ability to engage with associated 'theories of practice', which in turn could impact on their own 'practice theories'. Despite having a lack of widespread appeal, in recent times there has been a growing recognition and acceptance that coaching is an educational or pedagogical enterprise (see Cushion et al 2003, Cassidy et al 2004, 2009, Jones et al 2004, Jones 2006a, 2006b, 2007, Penney 2006, Wikeley & Bullock 2006). What is more, there has been an increased interest in discussing and theorising learning within the coaching context (see, for example, Gilbert & Trudel 2001, 2005, Jones et al 2004, Trudel & Gilbert 2004, Cassidy & Rossi 2006, Cassidy et al 2006, 2009, Culver & Trudel 2006, Demers et al 2006, Werthner & Trudel 2006, Wright et al 2007, Culver et al in press, Rynne et al in press, and the 2006 Special Issue of the *International Journal of Sports Science and Coaching* that focused on The Sport Coach as Learner).

There is anecdotal and empirical evidence to suggest that many coaches do, at least implicitly, value 'all the elements of the human encounter' (Armour

2004 p 98) in their efforts to assist athletes to develop and learn. It would be very surprising, therefore, if coaches were not engaging with, and perhaps even being explicitly aware of, pedagogical 'practice theories'. It could even be argued that the coach's intervention or training programme must be based on 'practice theories', however, formed. On the other hand, this has not been reflected in research agendas. Very few members of the sports coaching research community have paid attention to the concept of pedagogy. In other words there has been little engagement with pedagogical 'theories of practice'. In the following subsections I highlight how the descriptions of the practices of elite coaches illustrate their pedagogical 'practice theories' and discus some of the opportunities and limitations of these accounts. This is followed by a review of work that explicitly focuses on pedagogical 'theories of practice' in the coaching context. The chapter concludes with a discussion of the opportunities and limitations of pedagogical 'theories of practice'.

Pedagogy and coaches' 'practice theories'

A common way to gain insight into coaches' 'practice theories' is through observing what coaches do and how they do it. Another way is to read a coach's (auto)biography. The appeal of this latter approach is evidenced by coaches' (auto)biographies often being ranked in lists of Top 10 best-selling sport books. As the popularity of sport-coaching courses has increased in the tertiary education sector, so too have the number of academic texts written to service the sector. Some of these texts have combined insights into what elite coaches do and how they do it with appropriate theory (to varying degrees) (see Kidman 2001, 2005, Jones et al 2004). In other words these texts have integrated discussions of coaches' 'practice theories' with formal 'theories of practice'.

In one such text, Kidman (2001) interviewed three coaches about their 'practice theories' and then discussed them in relation to an empowerment approach to coaching and what this means for coaching practice and the interaction between the coach and athlete and the coaching environment. In 2005 Kidman wrote a similar research book but this time she observed the practices and interviewed eight coaches, organising the discussion around the theme of athlete-centred coaching. This focus on what this means for coaching practice, and interactions between coach and athlete, was tempered with a discussion of some of the challenges associated with adopting an athlete-centred approach. These texts have been popular, possibly because Kidman includes large tracts of interview transcript from the coaches, which enable readers to gain detailed insights into the 'practice theories' of the coaches.

Others, such as Jones et al (2004), have also valued coaches' 'practice theories' enough to write a book about them. Jones and colleagues presented the life stories of eight coaches with the aim of providing insight into 'the coaches' lives, careers, personal philosophies on coaching and beliefs about good professional practice' (p 3). The approach adopted by these authors is that by understanding coaches' lives readers can begin to appreciate their coaching philosophies and, in turn, coaching pedagogical practices. The collection is an addition to earlier work that had a similar intent (see Cushion 2001, Poczwardowski et al 2002, Potrac et al 2002, Jones et al 2003, Light 2004).

Opportunities and limitations of focusing on coaches' 'practice theories'

There is an assumption that one of the reasons coaches enjoy reading the (auto)biographies of successful or high-profile coaches is that they learn, albeit retrospectively, about various aspects of coaching (i.e. the coaches' 'practice theories') that they may otherwise not have been privy to. Reading about the 'practice theories' of successful coaches creates a number of possibilities for 'interrogating' those practices. One of these is to visualise successful practice (in other words, to create an image of the coach in action). However, this may have only a limited value, partly because coaches may not have an appropriate vocabulary or conceptual framework with which to interpret these accounts. Although there has been an increase in the number of accounts focusing on coaches' pedagogical 'practice theories' and increasingly the term pedagogy appears both in the sports coaching literature and in coaching resources (for examples of the latter see Sport and Recreation New Zealand and the Australian Sports Commission), I believe there has not been a corresponding increase in understanding of what the term means by many practising coaches. One possible reason for this is that authors of the

literature described above and similar resources make an assumption that the readers have a common understanding of the term. As a consequence, the term pedagogy is used without any clear explanation of what it means or how it is being interpreted. Another possible reason is that many of the early discussions of pedagogy in coaching resources and literature were not robustly informed by the educational literature (see for example the Coaching Association of New Zealand *Principles of Sports Coaching: Level 2* (Hillary Commission n d and Launder 1993 respectively). Rather, these resources were based upon dictionary-type definitions of pedagogy, which viewed it as 'the science of teaching' (Oxford 1991 p 877). I suggest that the common practice in the sport coaching community of using a dictionary definition of pedagogy to inform the discussions, interpretation and subsequent use of the term has restricted the potential for many coaches and coach educators to engage generatively with a wider body of literature. This has limited the perceived value of 'practice theories' and prevented coaches from framing their practice in a pedagogical context.

Pedagogical 'theories of practice'

Any interpretation or definition of pedagogy is 'culture-bound' (Crum 1996). Therefore when entering into a discussion about the 'theories of practice' associated with pedagogy in a coaching context it is useful to recognise that there is no one consensual theory or fixed definition of pedagogy. As such it is appropriate when discussing pedagogy to be explicit about how the term is being used. One example of good practice in this regard is Armour (in Jones et al 2004) who challenged the use of a dictionary-type definition of pedagogy in sport coaching and began her discussion of coaching pedagogy with 'a theoretical analysis of the concept' (p 95). She drew on Leach and Moon's (1999) interpretation of pedagogy who viewed it as being 'about the relationships between four key elements of education: teachers, learners, learning tasks and the learning environment' (p 96). This is similar in concept to Poczwardowski et al (2002) who used a phenomenological approach to demonstrate that coaching comprises a set of reciprocal interactions between the athlete, coach and context. Reinterpreting Leach and Moon's definition to fit the culture of sports coaching, Armour defines coaching pedagogy as embracing 'the four individual but interlinked elements of teaching (and coaching), *learning*, knowledge base and *learning* environment' that also 'has an overriding focus on the unifying goal of *learning*' (in Jones et al 2004, p 94, *emphasis added*). According to Leach and Moon (1999) the interactions between the key elements occur in a 'pedagogic setting' and should be regarded as one *process*.

Like Armour, I too have challenged the use of a dictionary-type definition of pedagogy in sports coaching by suggesting that such a definition does little to add value to understanding coaches' practice. It can result in the focus being on the coaches and what they do and how they do it, rather than recognising the role that the learner, the content being taught and the context in which the coaching occurs, plays in improving practice and developing players (Cassidy 2003). Whenever discussing the term I take care to state explicitly that my interpretation is informed by the work of David Lusted (1986) (see for example Cassidy et al 2004, 2009). Lusted (1986) argues that pedagogy is the *process* of knowledge production that occurs in the interactions between the teacher, the learner and the content. To use his words – 'how one teaches [read coaches]' is 'of central interest but … it becomes inseparable from what is being taught, and, crucially, how one *learns*' (Lusted 1986, p 3 *emphasis added*). As with most attempts to improve both understanding and practice, there are limitations and opportunities from adopting 'theories of practice' such as Leach and Moon (1999) or Lusted (1986) for use in sport coaching. I will now take the opportunity to elaborate on these.

Opportunities and limitations of focusing on pedagogical 'theories of practice'

I suggest that there are at least three opportunities for coaching practice as a consequence of engaging rigorously with pedagogical 'theories of practice' and demonstrating how 'pedagogic theory' can inform coaching, which Jones (2006a) recognises is an aspect of sport coaching that needs attention. The first opportunity for coaching practice that comes about as a consequence of drawing on pedagogical 'theories of practice', such as those advocated by Leach and Moon (1999) or Lusted

(1986), is that the *complexity* of the coaching process is highlighted along with the role learning and the learner plays (see Cushion et al 2006 for a discussion about the complexity of the coaching process). Highlighting complexity can challenge the implicit hierarchies that have historically existed in the traditional interaction between coach and athlete. Rather than the emphasis being placed on the coach and instruction, which has generally resulted in an authoritarian or direct instructional approach becoming the norm, emphasis can be placed on understanding the interconnections that occur between the coach, athlete, content and the environment in which it takes place. Moreover, if coaches recognise the complexity of the coaching process they may come to recognise the importance of viewing the athlete as an integral part of the process. This may lead them to reflect upon, for example, how athletes best learn and develop, which we might argue has been a neglected aspect of coaching practice.

The second opportunity that arises as a consequence of drawing on the pedagogical 'theories of practice' of Leach and Moon (1999) and Lusted (1986) is that the interaction that occurs between the coach, the athlete and the content is considered to be a *process*. This has specific advantages for coaching practice. By viewing pedagogy as a process it allows the focus to be placed on 'pedagogy as *practice* – rather than … a disciplined body of formalized, systematized, "scientific" knowledge about pedagogy' (Lee & Green 1997 p 18 *emphasis in original*). An emphasis on pedagogy as practice may enable coaches to draw on their 'practice theories' as well as 'theories of practice'. This bodes well for those coaches who wish to be recognised as professionals since a characteristic of professionalism is having the ability to link theory and practice (Thompson 2003).

The third opportunity that can become available as a consequence of drawing on Lusted's (1986) pedagogical 'theories of practice' is that pedagogy becomes viewed as a process of *knowledge production*. Anecdotally, coaches have challenged the value of focusing on 'knowledge production' for its own sake. This may be evident in coach education, in which coaches often fail to see the relevance of distinct bodies of knowledge. This challenge may have some merit if the concept of knowledge production is understood as a process that privileges the cognitive at the expense of the embodied or practical. However, one of the opportunities of holding a Lustedian view of pedagogy is that the focus on orthodox knowledge production can be challenged in ways that could enhance coaching practice. To understand how focusing on knowledge production opens up possibilities for coaching practice in the 21st century it is first useful to discuss the concept of knowledge before turning attention to the notion of production.

Knowledge is a commonly used term, yet Gilbert (2005) argues there is no one agreed understanding of what knowledge is, how it is developed, and what is 'good' knowledge. Despite this lack of a common understanding, in recent times many Western societies have focused on developing citizens (including coaches and athletes) to work in a 'knowledge society'. Although what constitutes a 'knowledge society' is contested, one thing appears to be agreed upon and that is that for a knowledge society to operate it is necessary to a break with an 'industrial-age, assembly-line metaphor' of knowledge that has been associated with orthodox education and replace it with one that recognises the need to 'put academic and applied knowledge back together [as well as] … find ways to have rigour and inclusiveness,' (Gilbert 2005 p 153–154). Gilbert argues this is necessary because the 21st century is very different from the industrial age and as a consequence 'what people need to be able to do with knowledge (and who needs to be able to do it) is now very different' (p 154). Another characteristic of the 21st century that makes the break with industrial age metaphors necessary is the move, albeit slowly, away from viewing learning as a 'process of storing important bits of knowledge in individual minds', viewing learners as consumers of existing knowledge and viewing 'the acquisition of knowledge' as a useful 'end in itself' (Gilbert 2005 p 77). For the concept of knowledge to be useful for practice in the 21st century the focus needs to be on having knowledge *work in different ways* and *do* new things' (Gilbert 2005 p 155 *emphasis in original*). A way of doing this is to place the emphasis on *knowing* rather than knowledge because 'knowing is a process', it is a verb, a doing word, 'whereas knowledge is a thing', a noun. Knowing 'involves building relationships and connections' and as a consequence cannot be 'taken in and mastered'. Knowing 'has no end point' rather is 'always on the way to something, always in process' (Gilbert 2005 p 77).

Even if the term 'knowledge' continues to be used, Gilbert (2005) suggested that the term could be redefined to assist us to shift our understanding *and* practice out of the industrial age and to make them more relevant for the 21st century. First, she suggested redefining knowledge as being able to *do* or *produce* 'stuff' 'rather than being "stuff" that is made (usually by following certain rules) and stored away for future use' (p 154 *emphasis added*). By redefining knowledge as being able to *do* or *produce* 'new stuff' we then can have the expectation that this new 'stuff' can produce change. By viewing knowledge as a verb, recognition is given to the idea that knowledge can be developed 'through connections and relationships' and consequently when people work collaboratively together to solve problems they can 'generate new knowledge' (p 154). Redefining knowledge as 'contextual' means that the criteria being used to judge what is 'good' knowledge should recognise the 'context in which the problem is being solved' (p 155), that the criteria may 'differ from context to context' (p 154), and the importance of recognising 'the people who were involved, the brief they were given, the time and other resources they had available' (p 155). It is useful in redefining 'knowledge' to acknowledge that its eclecticism is a consequence of 'taking elements from different disciplinary areas, putting them together…and rearranging them so that they have new meanings' (Gilbert 2005 p 155).

When coaches take up the challenge to think about the production of knowledge as 'active creation' or a capacity to address contextual problems, they provide themselves with opportunities to produce new coaching knowledge and the impetus for reflecting on what they want to achieve and what they are expected to achieve. Increasingly there is an expectation by organisations such as Coaching Ireland, sport coach UK, Sport and Recreation New Zealand and the Australian Institute of Sport that athletes be recognised as active participants in the coaching process. This is a value position that permeates coach education and development. If coaches intend to involve athletes in the coaching process, they will no longer be able to rationalise practice with mantras such as 'it has always been done this way so that is why I do it ' or 'my coach did it this way and it didn't hurt me/or it worked for me, so why change?' Not only does a focus on knowledge production open up opportunities for improving coaching practice, it also has implications for administrators who should reflect on adopting practices such as appointing competent ex-players into coaching roles, a practice which is based on the assumption that because they were good players that they will have acquired the appropriate 'knowledge' to be quality coaches. Not only does a focus on knowledge production encourage coaches to be reflective, it can assist them to move away from reproducing existing practices. An over-emphasis on asking athletes simply to reproduce coach-determined activity may lead to the possibility of constraining athletes' potential to learn and develop to the best of their abilities. On the other hand, a focus on knowledge production can challenge the 'acquisition' metaphor of learning that is so prevalent in coaching communities (Trudel & Gilbert 2006). Moreover, a focus on knowledge production can provide coaches with the opportunity to experiment with their own practices. This may assist them to engage with the ideas current in various international coach education or coach development initiatives in which emphasis is increasingly being placed on athlete-centred practice.

Adopting new practices may not be particularly easy since any pedagogical innovation will have to 'compete with, replace, or otherwise modify the folk theories that already guide both teachers [coaches] and pupils [athletes]' (Armour in Jones et al 2004 p 99–100). These folk theories are often difficult to overturn because they are developed as a consequence of coaches' apprenticeship and socialisation, their skills and preferences, the content being taught, the context in which the coaching is occurring and on their 'set of beliefs' (Tinning et al 1993 p 123). There may be difficulties associated with engaging in, and experimenting with, pedagogical 'theories of practice'. However, failure to do so may will place in jeopardy coaches' aspirations to professional status.

The place of athlete learning in coaching practice

The second section of the chapter also focuses on linking 'practice theories' and 'theories of practices' but focuses on athlete learning. All coaches have views on what is the best way for athletes to learn. Nevertheless, I suggest that many coaches would have difficulty expressing these beliefs in terms of academic theories of learning or 'theories of

practice'. However, these beliefs (whether or not the coaches recognise it) do implicitly inform their 'practice theories'. For example, if a coach provides athletes with reinforcements and sanctions in an attempt to improve the latter's learning and performance, we can say that the coach's practices reflect behavioural learning theories, and that the coach is likely to be adopting instructional methods that tend to reproduce existing knowledge. If, on the other hand, a coach sets up practices that require athletes to draw from their existing knowledge, and acknowledges the social context in which the practice occurs, we can say that these practices are reflective of cognitive learning theories, and that the coach is likely to be adopting instructional methods that have the potential to produce new knowledge. In practice I would suggest that the belief systems of the coaches about how athletes learn is not 'set in concrete' rather it depends on who is being coached, what activity is being coached, and the situation in which the coaching is occurring. However, there is a danger when coaches consider 'who is being coached', that attention is given to stereotypical groupings, for example the athlete as a 'beginner', 'youth' or 'elite' rather than more detailed attention being paid to the athlete as an individual and how he or she learns best. This lends support to Galipeau and Trudel's (2006) proposal that 'understanding *who is being coached* ... could help lead to better coaching practices, better athlete–coach relationships, increased satisfaction and, ultimately, better athletic performance' (p 91 *emphasis in the original*).

At the beginning of this chapter I claimed that very few members of the sports coaching research community have paid any attention to the concept of pedagogy. As this section will show it is a similar situation in relation to the athlete as a learner. I have said elsewhere that while learning and development are integral components to the coaching process they have ambiguous status in the coaching literature (Cassidy et al 2004, 2009) and even within this body of the literature there are topics that are privileged and those that are ignored. For example, recently there has been an increased interest in, and work focusing on, learning and development in the coaching context. However, much of this work focuses on coach learning (see previous section for examples) yet only a few have focused on the athlete as a learner (see for example Miller & Kerr 2002, Cassidy et al 2006, Galipeau & Trudel 2006). The limited literature that focuses on athlete learning does make it difficult to discuss coaches' 'practice theories'.

In the following sub-sections I describe the limited literature on coaches' 'practice theories' that focus on athlete learning, before going on to discuss some of the opportunities and limitations of these accounts. This is followed by a review of work that explicitly focuses on learning 'theories of practice' used in the coaching context, which is concluded with a discussion of their opportunities and limitations.

Athlete learning and coaches' 'practice theories'

In a previous section I identified texts that had been written to service the sport coaching sector in tertiary education. These sources have adopted and adapted the genre of (auto)biography to provide insights into what elite coaches do and how they do it (see Kidman 2001, 2005, Jones et al 2004). I draw on these texts again in this section to illustrate coaches' 'practice theories' in relation to athlete learning. Not surprisingly, when reading the 'stories' from the elite coaches about their coaching practice in Jones et al (2004) the dominant focus is on coaching and the coach rather than the athlete/player. Many of the coaches in this text talk about developing supportive and caring, coaching environments, the value of having an empowering coaching philosophy, of developing players and one coach even mentioned the importance of 'establishing a "learning environment"' (p 56). In Kidman's (2001) text coaches talk about how they value their own learning and development and discuss the merits of adopting an 'empowerment' approach for increasing athlete learning, which Kidman linked to the 'Game Sense' approach. Game Sense (Thorpe 1997) is a version of Teaching Games for Understanding (Bunker & Thorpe 1982). In Kidman's text the athletes did receive some attention. In one chapter athletes gave feedback on the empowerment approach taken by the coaches and in another chapter two elite athletes discuss their perceptions of this approach. In her later text, Kidman (2005) generally focused on how elite coaches implemented an athlete-centred coaching practice and utilised strategies such as questioning. This text is a detailed description of the 'practice theories' of coaches who explicitly stated that they adopted practices that put the athlete in the centre of the coaching process.

Opportunities and limitations of focusing on coaches' 'practice theories'

The potential advantages to accrue from insights into coaches' 'practice theories' have already been outlined in a previous section. Although reading about the 'practice theories' of successful coaches can provide the reader with an opportunity to visualise successful practice, this can only occur if the practice is explicitly discussed. One limitation of the discussion by the coaches in the three texts (Kidman 2001, 2005, Jones et al 2004) is that there is little explicit mention of how the coaches view learning or how their view influences their coaching practice or 'practice theories'. For example, in Kidman (2001) one coach said that he used 'positive reinforcement' to adopt an empowerment approach, while another said he learned by 'trial and error'. There was no acknowledgement that the latter is a reflection of how learning occurs if one holds a behavioural view on learning and the former is a characteristic of operant conditioning, which is a specific behavioural learning theory. Importantly, there was no reflection by the coach or questions raised about the potential conflict or tensions of adopting the practices whilst attempting to implement an empowerment approach to coaching. Armour (in Jones et al 2004) identified a similar situation when she analysed the coaches' description of their practices. She suggested that the coaches' practices were guided by implicit assumptions about learners and what constituted 'proper' learning. This unidirectional assumption about athlete learning is reflected in Galipeau and Trudel's (2006) observation that in some situations, and 'despite coaches' attempts to be "athlete centred", athletes must still follow and execute the game plan and tactics designed by the coach'... 'even if they do not agree with coaching decisions, athletes must follow them or be faced with the possibility of not playing' (p 79).

For coaches to be guided by implicit assumptions (or at least subconscious or unchallenged assumptions) is problematic for at least two reasons. First, if coaches are not aware of the assumptions they hold about, for example, what constitutes learning, how one learns, and what learning is 'worthwhile' and 'good', there is a strong possibility that they will view their understandings as taken-for-granted and 'normal'. This situation increases the potential for conflict to occur between coaches and athletes when the assumptions they hold on these issues clash (Armour in Jones et al 2004). Second, if coaches are not explicit about, or aware of, the assumptions they hold it makes it difficult for them to reflect on their practice, particularly if reflection is considered to be the 'active, persistent and careful consideration of any belief or supposed form of knowledge in the light of the grounds that support it, and the further conclusions to which it tends' (Dewey 1910 p 6). Not being in a position to reflect on the assumptions underpinning their practice, limits coaches' capacity to change systematically their practice and improve the learning opportunities of their athletes. Once again this can have negative implications for professional status, for which being reflective and combining 'practice theories' with 'theories of practice' would be a necessary state.

The coaches in all three texts (Kidman 2001, 2005, Jones et al 2004) appeared to focus on their practice and how they understood it, whereas Armour (in Jones et al 2004) suggests that if coaches focused 'more closely on the experiences of learners' they might be 'more effective as a result' (p 102). Kidman (2001) did include the interpretations and perceptions of the athletes in the discussion on an empowerment approach to coaching. However, in both instances the focus was on the thoughts of athletes in relation to 'what' the coaches did rather that how it related to how they learned. Having reflected on the existing literature I support Armour's (in Jones et al 2004) challenge to the coaching community that it is 'imperative to place learners and learning at the heart of the coaching process, rather than coaches and coaching' (p 102). One concern I have with this challenge is how it may be interpreted. The limited explicit understanding of learning 'theories of practice' in the coaching community may lead to the challenge being interpreted to mean the adoption of practices like 'Game Sense', which is informed by a particular learning 'theory of practice'. This is not how I interpret the challenge. For me the challenge is for coaches to take responsibility for reflecting on, contextualising, and understanding the assumptions that underpin how they view learning and the learners they are working with. Becoming familiar with learning 'theories of practice' will provide them with an opportunity to experiment in an informed manner with their coaching practices in ways that provide the best possible opportunities for the athletes to learn, develop and perform.

Learning 'theories of practice'

As I argued above, there has been an increased interest in, and work on, learning and development in the coaching context. Yet the literature referenced above reflects only one aspect of the research on and about coach learning. When Trudel and Gilbert (2006) organised the coaching literature that focused on learning how to coach, they did so using Sfard's (1998) two metaphors on learning (acquisition and participation). They contended that research focusing on 'what coaches should know' and 'what coaches should do' in the process of learning how to coach could be understood as reflecting the acquisition metaphor. On the other hand, research focusing on the influence of the 'reflective process' and the 'process of becoming' in the course of learning how to coach illustrates the participation metaphor (Trudel & Gilbert 2006 p 517). The literature I draw upon in this chapter favours using the participation metaphor. When an acquisition metaphor is adopted, learning is viewed as a process of acquiring units of knowledge. I suggest that this can be loosely aligned to the behavioural 'theories of practice'. When adopting the participation metaphor, learning is viewed as occurring in context involving interaction with others and can arguably be associated with cognitive 'theories of practice'. My alignment of these 'theories of practice' with the two metaphors is contentious (see Sfrad 1998, Hodkinson et al 2008) but it is not within the scope of this chapter to debate this further and for the purpose of this chapter the debate is less important. Despite these differences I support Sfard's (1998) position that it is not desirable to favour one metaphor (or 'theory of practice') unconditionally at the expense of the other because each 'theory of practice' can assist us to explain different aspects of learning in the coaching context.

Different academic disciplines tend to support, and therefore draw upon, 'theories of practice' that reflect one metaphor on learning more than the other. Those who have an interest in understanding learning in the coaching context and align themselves with the disciplines and fields of sociology, pedagogy, and social psychology, have a tendency towards cognitive 'theories of practice', which reflect a participation metaphor. Here I broadly use the term cognitive to include those theories that can also be describe as constructivist since they all have the common assumptions that learners are 'active seekers and processors of information' (Schunk 2004 p 443) and that the seeking and processing occurs in the interaction of personal, social and environmental factors (Cassidy et al 2009). The increased interest in cognitive 'theories of practice' has occurred as academics recognise, and concede, that not everything about learning in a coaching context can be explained by focusing on what is easily observable. The work that I have referenced in this chapter draws on cognitive 'theories of practice' to understand learning in the coaching context. However, there are limitations from focusing on existing 'theories of practice' (regardless of what metaphor is used to organise them) for understanding learning in a coaching context, specifically in relation to athlete learning.

Limitations and opportunities of focusing on learning 'theories of practice'

According to Hodkinson et al (2008) key to the cognitive (and situated) perspectives on learning are 'issues of thought, knowledge and understanding of cognition' (p 30). To illustrate their position they give an example of how work that draws on Vygotsky, whose ideas are often described as relating to a situated perspective on learning, is still concerned with 'integrating the mind and its social and cultural setting' (p 30). Hodkinson et al (2008) go on to suggest that regardless of perspective on learning, the existing literature on learning has limitations. They contend that the limitation associated with the literature on individual learning is that it is often 'decontextualised' and disembodied, with little regard to the social aspect. In terms of the literature on learning theories, they suggest that the literature rarely incorporates, in detail, discussions of 'wider social and institutional structures' or the 'significance of power' (p 32). While they concede that many contemporary theories of learning do satisfy a number of these limitations, they claim that no theory 'adequately deals' with all the limitations. To rectify this, Hodkinson et al (2008) suggested that there is a 'need for a more holistic approach' (p 32), which challenges three common dualisms, namely, mind/body, agency/structure and individual/social. Drawing on the traditions of so-called 'socio-cultural' perspectives on learning they systematically unpack, develop and explain a 'cultural theory of learning'

(p 33). I suggest that this 'theory of practice' has the potential to provide sport coaching with opportunities to understand and develop practices that enable the focus to be on learners and learning rather than coaching and coaches, and as a consequence address the challenge laid down earlier by Armour (in Jones et al 2004).

The potential opportunities associated with using 'theories of practice' such as Hodkinson et al's (2008) cultural theory of learning is that it could assist members of sport coaching communities to explain 'how individuals learn through *participation* in learning cultures' (p 37 *emphasis added*). For this to occur consideration needs to be given to three issues: the place of the individual in the learning culture; recognising that learning is practical, embodied and social and that learning is about 'becoming'. While it is not within the scope of this chapter to expand on these issues (for that see Hodkinson et al 2008), I will illustrate how aspects of this 'theory of practice' are already beginning to be entertained within the sport coaching research community in an attempt to assist the 'practice theories' of coaches.

In recognising the place of the individual learner in the learning culture Hodkinson et al (2008 p 37) take the position that 'individuals influence and are part of learning cultures just as learning cultures influence and are part of individuals'. They go on to suggest that the work of Bourdieu is useful for understanding how an individual's influence on the learning culture is dependent on factors such as their 'position within' and 'dispositions towards that culture and the various types of capital (social, [physical,] cultural and economic) that they possess' (Hodkinson et al 2008 p 37). While not specifically focusing on athlete learning work has occurred in the sport coaching community that has drawn on Bourdieu to highlight the athletes' influence on the coaching culture (see Light 1999, Purdy 2005, Cushion & Jones 2006, Purdy et al in press). The challenge is to build on this body of literature by making specific links to athlete learning.

Hodkinson et al (2008) acknowledge that viewing learning as practical, embodied and social is not exclusive to a cultural theory of learning and recognise Dewey's earlier work in this area. They interpret embodiment to mean learning that involves interconnecting the physical, mental, social, emotional and practical. Hodkinson et al (2008) identified the literature that focuses on workplace learning as an example of 'theories of practice' that explicitly acknowledge learning as an embodied process since the focus is on 'learning how to do a job and become part of a workplace community' (p 31). One contributor to this body of literature is Billet (2001) whose work currently informs the work of Rynne et al (in press) in their discussions of workplace learning of high-performance sports coaches.

In a cultural theory of learning, learning is not only practical and embodied it is also social. Hodkinson et al (2008) draw on Bourdieu's work to illustrate how people are socially positioned. For Bourdieu, the 'social nature of the person with their on-going social and embodied learning' can be explained using the concept of habitus, with its associated dispositions (which are accumulated through experiences at home, school, play, work, etc.) (Hodkinson et al 2008 p 39). From this perspective, learning can be viewed as a 'process through which the dispositions that make up a person's habitus are confirmed, developed, challenged or changed' (p 39). While not specifically focusing on athlete learning, work has occurred in the sport coaching research community that has utilised Bourdieu's concept of habitus (Goodwin 2007, Cassidy et al 2009) and it is timely to make more explicit links between athlete learning and habitus. Another way to illustrate how learning is social is to reflect on the power relations that exist between athletes and coaches. While there are many different ways of viewing power it is widely accepted that discussions of social interactions cannot ignore issues of power differentials. Therefore it is an opportune time to make connections between athlete learning and the work conducted in sport coaching that has focused on power (see Johns & Johns 2000, Jones et al 2005, Denison 2007, Purdy et al 2008).

When engaging with a cultural theory of learning the third issue relates to, what is meant by 'learning as becoming'? Wenger (1998) utilised this idea of learning as becoming in his social theory of learning and linked it to identity formation. For Wenger (1998) learning is not just about an accumulation of skills and information but more about 'becoming', 'belonging', 'doing' and 'experience'. His theory is framed by two key components; theories of social practice and theories of identity, which he argues underpin learning within communities. Hodkinson et al (2008) prefer to utilise Bourdieu's concept of habitus to understand the relationship between becoming and learning. Linked this way they view learning as occurring at any time and in any situation. Yet, what is viewed as an opportunity to learn, and what is made of the opportunity, depends on a number of factors such as the 'nature of the learning culture', the habitus, social position and capital of the individuals, and how they interact with others (p 41). As a consequence of this Hodkinson et al (2008) contend that an individual is 'constantly learning through becoming, and becoming through learning' (p 41). Given that Wenger's (1998) social learning theory is a theoretical conceptualisation of communities of practice, a topic receiving increased attention by some in the sport coaching research community (see Trudel & Gilbert 2004, Cassidy & Rossi 2006, Cassidy et al 2006, Culver & Trudel, 2006, 2008, Culver et al in press) it is very likely that the coaching community will become more au fait with the idea that learning is about becoming. The challenge then becomes to understand what it means for athlete learning and coaches' practice.

Summary

In this chapter I introduced Thompson's (2003) ideas of 'practice theories' and 'theories of practice' and discussed them in relation to coaching practices and athlete learning. I suggested that this discussion may be of interest to those who wish to advocate the professionalisation of coaching since having the ability to link practice and theory is recognised as a characteristic of being a professional (Thompson 2003). The discussion may also be valuable for those interested in exploring the links between practice and theory in relation to coaching practice and athlete learning because it raised the following four issues. (1) The common practice of adopting a dictionary-type definition of pedagogy. Some may not think this is that much of an issue but increasingly the term pedagogy is being used in the coaching literature and in coaching resources. Holding a superficial dictionary-type definition, or not being explicit about how the term is used, limits the ability of coaches and coach educators to engage with broader debates about practice and ultimately improve their own practice. (2) The complexity of the coaching process. Highlighting this complexity opens up the possibility that implicit hierarchies traditionally existing between the athlete and the coach are challenged. In addition, the integral role the athlete plays in the coaching process is acknowledged. As illustrated in the chapter, to date there has been very limited recognition given to the athlete as a learner in discussions of coaching practice or the coaching literature. (3) Coaching is a process involving human interaction and as a consequence can be viewed as a pedagogical process. By viewing coaching as a pedagogical process, and adopting a particular perspective of pedagogy, coaches are provided with a conceptual framework and a vocabulary for interpreting their observations as well as directing their 'attention to those variables that are crucial in finding solutions' (Hill in Merriam et al 2007 p 277–278). Furthermore, coaches have a framework that assists them to see how (re)conceiving knowledge and knowledge production has the potential to make coaching practice more relevant to the 21st century. (4) The coaching community would benefit from drawing upon a theory of learning that recognised the social, practical, embodied and cognitive aspects of learning. In the chapter, Hodkinson et al's (2008) cultural theory of learning and Wenger's (1998) social theory of learning were described and given as examples of holistic theories that have potential to enhance further our understanding of athlete learning and coaching practice. While not specifically focusing on athlete learning, research already exists in the coaching community that could be built upon by drawing on the work of Hodkinson et al (2008) and Wenger (1998) with the aim of improving our understanding of athlete learning and coaching practice. Only time will tell if Armour's (in Jones et al 2004) challenge to the coaching community to put 'learners and learning at the heart of the coaching process' (p 102) will be heeded.

References

Billett, S., 2001. Learning throughout working life: interdependencies at work. Studies in Continuing Education 23 (1), 19–35.

Bunker, D., Thorpe, R., 1982. A model for the teaching of games in secondary schools. Bulletin of Physical Education 18 (1), 5–8.

Cassidy, T., 2004. Revisiting coach education (and coaching) in the twenty first century. Modern Athlete and Coach 42 (2), 12–16.

Cassidy, T., Rossi, T., 2006. Situating learning: (re)examining the notion of apprenticeship in coach education. International Journal of Sports Science and Coaching 1 (3), 235–246.

Cassidy, T., Jones, R., Potrac, P., 2004. Understanding sports coaching. The social, cultural and pedagogical foundations of coaching practice. Routledge, London.

Cassidy, T., Allen, J., Potrac, P., 2006. The importance of belonging: exploring the coaching process from the perspective of elite athletes. Paper presentation at the International Council for Health, Physical Education, Recreation, Sport and Dance congress, Wellington, New Zealand October.

Cassidy, T., Potrac, P., McKenzie, A., 2006. Evaluating and reflecting upon a coach education initiative: the CoDe of rugby. The Sports Psychologist 20 (2), 145–161.

Cassidy, T., Jones, R., Potrac, P., 2009. Understanding sports coaching. The social, cultural and pedagogical foundations of coaching practice, second ed. Routledge, London.

Crum, B., 1996. In search of the perspectives' paradigmatical identities: general comparison and final commentary. Unpublished manuscript, Tilburg University, Netherlands.

Culver, D., Trudel, P., 2006. Cultivating coaches' communities of practice: developing the potential for learning through interactions. In: Jones, R.L. (Ed.), The sports coach as educator: re-conceptualising sports coaching. Routledge, London, pp. 97–112.

Culver, D., Trudel, P., 2008. Clarifying the concept of communities of practice in sport. International Journal of Sports Science and Coaching 3, 1–10.

Culver, D., Trudel, P., Werthner, P., 2009. A sport leader's attempt to foster a coaches' community of practice. International Journal of Sport Science and Coaching.

Cushion, C., 2001. The coaching process in professional youth football: an ethnography of practice. Brunel University, UK Unpublished doctoral thesis.

Cushion, C., Jones, R.L., 2006. Power, discourse and symbolic violence in professional youth soccer: the case of Albion F.C. Sociology of Sport Journal 23 (2), 142–161.

Cushion, C., Armour, K.M., Jones, R.L., 2003. Coach education and continuing professional development: experience and learning to coach. Quest 55, 215–230.

Cushion, C., Armour, K.M., Jones, R.L., 2006. Locating the coaching process in practice: models 'for' and 'of' coaching. Physical Education and Sport Pedagogy 11 (1), 81–97.

Demers, G., Woodburn, A., Savard, C., 2006. The development of an undergraduate competency-based coach education program. The Sport Psychologist 20 (2), 162–173.

Denison, J., 2007. Social theory for coaches: a Foucauldian reading of one athlete's poor performance. International Journal of Sport Science and Coaching 2 (4), 369–383.

Dewey, J., 1910. How we think. Heath, Boston.

Galipeau, J., Trudel, P., 2006. Athlete learning in a community of practice: is there a role for the coach? In: Jones, R.L. (Ed.), The sports coach as educator: re-conceptualising sports coaching. Routledge, London, pp. 77–94.

Gilbert, J., 2005. Catching the knowledge wave? The knowledge society and future of education. NCER Press, Wellington.

Gilbert, W., Trudel, P., 2001. Learning to coach through experience: reflection in model youth sport coaches. Journal of Teaching in Physical Education 21 (1), 16–34.

Gilbert, W., Trudel, P., 2005. Learning to coach through experience: conditions that influence reflection. Physical Educator 62 (1), 32–43.

Goodwin, C., 2007. The weight-loss crusade: the life of an elite female distance runner. Unpublished honours dissertation, University of Otago, Dunedin, New Zealand.

Green, B., Lee, A., 1995. Theorising postgraduate pedagogy. The Australian Universities Review 38, 40–45.

Hillary Commission, n.d. Principles of Sports Coaching: Level 2. Coaching Association of New Zealand, Wellington.

Hodkinson, P., Biesta, G., James, D., 2008. Understanding learning culturally: overcoming the dualism between social and individual views. Vocations and Learning 1, 27–47.

Johns, D.P., Johns, J., 2000. Surveillance, subjectivism and technologies of power: an analysis of the discursive practice of high-performance sport. International Review for the Sociology of Sport 35, 219–234.

Jones, R.L., 2006a. How can educational concepts inform sports coaching? In: Jones, R.L. (Ed.), The sports coach as educator: re-conceptualising sports coaching. Routledge, London, pp. 3–13.

Jones, R.L., 2006b. The sports coach as educator: re-conceptualising sports coaching. Routledge, London.

Jones, R.L., 2007. Coaching redefined: an everyday pedagogical endeavour. Sport, Education and Society 12 (2), 159–173.

Jones, R.L., Armour, K., Potrac, P., 2003. Constructing expert knowledge: a case study of a top level professional soccer coach. Sport, Education and Society 8 (2), 213–229.

Jones, R.L., Armour, K.A., Potrac, P., 2004. Sports coaching cultures: from practice to theory. Routledge, London.

Jones, R.L., Glintmeyer, N., McKenzie, A., 2005. Slim bodies, eating disorders and the coach–athlete relationship: a tale of identity creation and disruption. International Review for the Sociology of Sport 40 (3), 377–391.

Kidman, L., 2001. Developing decision makers: an empowerment approach to coaching. Innovative Press, Christchurch, NZ.

Kidman, L., 2005. Athlete-centred coaching: developing inspired and inspiring people. Innovative Print Communications, Christchurch, NZ.

Launder, A., 1993. Coach education for the twenty first century. Sports Coach 2 January–March.

Leach, J., Moon, B., 1999. Recreating pedagogy. In: Leach, J., Moon, B. (Eds.), Learners and pedagogy. Paul Chapman, London, pp. 265–276.

Lee, A., Green, B., 1997. Pedagogy and disciplinarity in the 'new university. UTS Review 3, 1–25.

Light, R., 1999. Social dimensions of rugby in Japanese and Australian schools. Unpublished doctoral dissertation, University of Queensland, Australia.

Light, R., 2004. Coaches' experience of Game Sense: opportunities and challenges. Physical Education and Sport Pedagogy 9 (2), 115–132.

Lusted, D., 1986. Why pedagogy? Screen 27 (5), 2–14.

Lyle, J., 2002. Sports coaching concepts: a framework for coaches' behaviour. Routledge, London.

Merriam, S., Caffarella, R., Baumgartner, L., 2007. Learning in adulthood: a comprehensive guide, third ed. John Wiley, San Francisco.

Miller, P., Kerr, G., 2002. The athletic, academic, and social experiences of intercollegiate student-athletes. Journal of Sport Behavior 25, 346–367.

Oxford, 1991. Concise Oxford Dictionary, eighth ed. Oxford University Press, London.

Penney, D., 2006. Coaching as teaching: new acknowledgements in practice. In: Jones, R.L. (Ed.), The sports coach as educator: re-conceptualising sports coaching. Routledge, London, pp. 25–36.

Poczwardowski, A., Barott, J., Henschen, K., 2002. The athlete and coach: their relationships and its meaning, results of an interpretive study. International Journal of Sport Psychology 33 (1), 116–140.

Potrac, P., Jones, R.L., Armour, K., 2002. It's about getting respect: the coaching behaviours of a top-level English football coach. Sport, Education and Society 7 (2), 183–202.

Purdy, L., 2005. Coaching in the current: the climate of an elite men's rowing training programme. Unpublished doctoral dissertation, University of Otago, Dunedin, New Zealand.

Purdy, L., Potrac, P., Jones, R., 2008. Power, consent and resistance: an autoethnography of competitive rowing. Sport, Education and Society 13 (3), 319–336.

Purdy, L., Jones, R.L., Cassidy, T., 2009. Negotiation and capital: athletes' use of power in an elite men's rowing programme. Sport, Education and Society 14 (3), 321–338.

Rynne, S., Mallett, C., Tinning, R., in press. Workplace learning of high performance sports coaches. Sport, Education and Society.

Schunk, D., 2004. Learning theories. An educational perspective, fourth ed. Pearson, New Jersey.

Sfard, A., 1998. On two metaphors for learning and the danger of choosing just one. Educational Researcher 27, 4–13.

Thompson, N., 2003. Theory and practice in human services. Open University Press, Maidenhead.

Thorpe, R., 1997. Game Sense: developing thinking players (video recording). Australian Sports Commission, Belconnen ACT.

Tinning, R., Kirk, D., Evans, J., 1993. Learning to teach physical education. Prentice Hall, London.

Trudel, P., Gilbert, W., 2004. Communities of practice as an approach to foster ice hockey coach development. In: Pearsal, D.J., Ashare, A.B. (Eds.), Safety in ice hockey, vol. 4. ASTM International, West Conshohoken PA.

Trudel, P., Gilbert, W., 2006. Coaching and coach education. In: Kirk, D., Macdonald, M., O'Sullivan, M. (Eds.), The handbook of physical education. Sage, London, pp. 516–539.

TV3, 2007. Interview with Graham Henry, 16 April (video recording).

Wenger, E., 1998. Communities of practice: learning, meaning and identity. Cambridge University Press, Cambridge.

Werthner, P., Trudel, P., 2006. A new theoretical perspective for understanding how coaches learn to coach. The Sport Psychologist 20, 198–212.

Wikeley, F., Bullock, K., 2006. Coaching as an educational relationship. In: Jones, R.L. (Ed.), The sports coach as educator: re-conceptualising sports coaching. Routledge, London, pp. 14–24.

Wright, T., Trudel, P., Culver, D., 2007. Learning how to coach: the different learning situations reported by youth ice hockey coaches. Physical Education and Sport Pedagogy 12 (2), 127–144.

Coaching workforce development

13

Alan Lynn and John Lyle

Introduction

This chapter will set out a series of problems and choices that currently face the development of the coaching workforce in the UK. While not currently a traditional 'academic' area for coaching, workforce development is a relevant topic that demonstrates practical consequences for issues such as coaching, coaching domains, coach education, and professionalisation. We aim to define what workforce development means and to describe the challenges of developing the coaching workforce, and to do so with a 'critical edge'. It is clear that an examination of a system-wide management and development of the existing workforce in the UK has central to it issues such as a surveillance culture within the 'voluntary sector' in sport, 'system' development versus individual development, and contested assumptions about what 'development' means. We have attempted to open up this area as one that will become fertile ground for researchers and writers. In this chapter we have resisted the temptation to flood the text with references to existing work related to 'development issues' – we believe that this has been done by other authors (see Chapters 8 and 9; also Green & Houlihan 2005, Lyle 2007, Bolton & Smith 2008, Kay et al 2008, Lyle 2008). Rather, we report our 'active research' from having been significantly involved in the promulgation and implementation of this development planning, and we hope to have drawn attention to an aspect of sports coaching provision and practice that will merit much more detailed study. Our intention to be polemical takes the form of asking questions, and, in aggregation, creating a research agenda.

In this chapter we take workforce development planning to mean a managed approach to the supply and demand for sport coaches, the perceived quality of that workforce, its employment and deployment, and arrangements for appropriate education and training. There have been a number of recent 'drivers' towards workforce development planning for the deployment of coaches in the UK. The government agency SkillsActive has produced a *Sector Skills Agreement* (SkillsActive 2006) for the sector of the economy that includes sport. This document emphasises the role of coaching and coaches, but acknowledges that workforce planning is underdeveloped, and much of the workforce needs to be upskilled (as the term implies, this refers to improvement in a set of recognised coaching skills, knowledge and practical competences). Sports coaching is thus drawn into more general employment and training policy; although recognising that the concern is largely with entry-level qualifications, and acknowledging that the voluntarism in the coaching workforce creates particular issues. Upskilling generally refers to a skills deficit; that is, recognising that the implicit quality or competence of the workforce could or should be better. The issue of the employment profile of the workforce (proportion of full-time jobs, career opportunities, and so on) is a separate concern within the overall professionalisation debate.

The United Kingdom Coaching Framework (UKCF), launched in April 2008 (sportscoach UK 2008), also emphasises the need for evidence-based policy making and identifies five 'Strategic Action Areas' and 12 'Specific Actions' over a 3–7–11 year timeframe, many of which assume a systematic, audited approach to coaching workforce planning. This implies databases of active coaches, licensing of coaches, and a more regulated matching of coaches (and coach education) to athletes' needs.

In addition, the United Kingdom Coaching Certificate (UKCC 2003) has been introduced (sports coach UK n d). The UKCC is an endorsement of National Governing Body of sport (NGB) coach education certification against a set of standardised UK-wide criteria for sports-specific coach education programmes. Learning programmes, coach educator training, mentoring and other coach education support structures are judged against these standards. The guidance criteria are based on National Occupational Standards (NOS). Government-recognised Occupational Standards identify the skills, knowledge and understanding required to carry out a job to nationally recognised levels of competence (see www.ukstandards.org). This is further alignment of sports coaching within the more general employment framework.

Sports that choose to have their coaching qualifications UKCC-endorsed are charged with producing an implementation delivery plan, and this has turned attention to the existing arrangements for awarding bodies, qualification structures, coach educators, mentors, and assessors. Arrangements for governance, quality assurance, data gathering, funding, monitoring, growth and development are also increasingly required to be evidence-based. Thus, strategic and development planning of the coaching workforce asks fundamental questions about the existing scale (and perceived quality) of coaching provision, and the relationships between this and growth projections within the sport. As we will discuss later, a more all-embracing management of the workforce makes assumptions about the coaches' motives, sense of community, comparability of roles, and the very 'boundary markers' of coaching itself. The responsibility placed on the NGBs is reflective of a greater accountability for governance and government policy-related outcomes – an accountability that may be questionable in terms of the NGB's traditional coach education and training role and the disparate nature of the coaching workforce.

The recent strategy document in Scotland: *Reaching Higher: Building on the Success of Sport 21* (Scottish Executive 2007) makes considerable reference to the importance of coaching in achieving a wide range of policy objectives for sport, as does *Grow, Sustain, Excel*, the 2008–2011 Sport England strategy (Sport England 2008). Whilst we may argue that these claims are aspirational, and are based on a set of practice-based, but ultimately untested, assumptions about the contribution of the coach to the development of sport, there seems to be little doubt that the more evident emphasis on the coaching workforce has enhanced the role of coaching and consequent resource allocation. Nevertheless, there is a recurring theme in both documents of increasing the quantity and quality (a contested term, to which we will return) of coaches with attention to an upskilling agenda. Each strategy states that having the 'right coaches in the right place at the right time' is a valuable policy marker, even if a little simplistic. However, there will also be sport-specific issues that drive workforce planning in each sport. Examples of these might include the balance of volunteer/paid employment, perceived under-qualification leading to safety issues, the traditional role of the coach, geographical distribution, gender balance, the reward environment, and so on. A more specific position report is provided by the document *Coaching Scotland* (Vaga Associates 2006), which emphasises the need for increased attention to the coaching workforce. There is a general exhortation to improve coaching provision and quality, although it is not entirely clear at this stage whether this constitutes a skills shortage, skills deficit, growth-leading or growth-dependent shortfall.

The documents identified so far are generally predicated on the assumption that the existing knowledge about the coaching workforce in each sport is unsatisfactory; that is, the extent, characteristics, and qualifications of the workforce are not known in detail. In addition, it seems likely that the proportion of unqualified coaches is higher than would be wished and there is an under-representation of women, disabled persons and black and ethnic minorities (Townend & North 2007). A number of the *Coaching Scotland* report's recommendations refer directly to workforce planning: (a) coaching audits and workforce development plans to be carried out, supported by better data management systems, (b) more flexible coach education delivery, (c) increased attention to volunteer recruitment and management, (d) increased funding for and marketing of the UKCC in Scotland, and (e) a recruitment and retention drive (Vaga Associates 2006).

In the context of these policy drivers the opportunity to generate coaching audits and workforce development plans for a range of Scottish Governing Bodies of sport (SGBs) was both significant and highly relevant. The authors were employed to carry out this work, and the research required to devise these audits and plans provided an opportunity to gain insights about the particular circumstances of workforce development planning for coaches in the (predominantly) voluntary sector. Thus the overall process has resulted in a form of 'research in action', from which we have drawn attention to some critical questions about the workforce itself and how it is represented. This chapter examines the concept of workforce planning, describes the process of workforce development planning with 19 SGBs, and provides a critical interpretation of the process that establishes links to conceptual issues about sports coaching.

Workforce development planning

According to the Employers Organisation document *Workforce Development Planning: Guidance Document* (2004), workforce development is directly related to organisational performance and the achievement of corporate goals. This is particularly important in service or people-directed occupational sectors:

> Effective people management and development is fundamental to achieving service improvement. Unless (an organisation) can attract, retain, develop, manage and motivate skilled people it will find it difficult to keep pace with the increasing demands for high performance, improvement, modernisation and efficiency. All (organisations) need to carry out workforce planning and use this as a basis for their Workforce Development Plan. This Plan should identify their strategies for building the relevant skills and capacity needed for organisational success. Workforce planning is the process of getting the right people, with the right skills, in the right jobs at the right time. (2004 p 3)

The document stresses the need to clarify the 'key service priorities' in the short, medium and longer term. Assessing 'demand' in this way is necessary in order to identify the consequent jobs or roles and their characteristics, and whether the people who can satisfy this demand are currently available or can be recruited. In other words, it is necessary to be clear about what the organisation intends to achieve, in order to identify its workforce requirements. Therefore, workforce development plans should be based on workforce planning analysis, which involves (a) identifying the current and future skills and number of employees needed to deliver new and improved services, (b) comparing the present workforce and the desired future workforce to highlight shortages, surpluses and competency gaps, and (c) comparing the (organisation's) diversity profile with that of the population more generally.

A literature review carried out for the Employers' Organisation for Local Government (2003b) identifies a number of key features of workforce planning: (a) workforce planning can be driven by competition, building capacity, skills shortages, demands of modernisation, and/or demographic changes; (b) the process is beneficial for focusing on 'key' aspects of the organisation; (c) the danger is that the Workforce Development Plan is perceived as a predictor of the future. It is more about setting an agenda and acting as a decision-making filter for the organisation. It should be flexible, on-going and responsible to a changing environment; (d) it must not be perceived as solely a 'numbers game' – the qualitative aspect is important; (e) all strategic plans within the organisation need to be reconciled; (f) the Workforce Development Plan is acknowledged to have benefits beyond the plan itself. The organisation benefits from thinking ahead, coordination, and integration within the organisation; and (g) models of workforce planning can be complex, including the use of software. However, the target is a simple, focused and effective workforce plan. The underlying assumptions about a cohesive workforce and asset of consensual objectives may not apply to a coaching workforce that is more disparate and with multi-agency deployment. Nevertheless, recognition that there are benefits simply from paying attention to the nature of the workforce, and being ready to embrace change, should commend the process to coach developers.

It is also important to focus on how workforce planning should be conducted. The Scottish Integrated Workforce Planning Group (SIWPG 2002a) was established to consider and advise on the principles and key issues for workforce planning in the National Health Service in Scotland. The SIWPG provides a useful template around which to structure workforce planning. The principles of workforce planning identified by the Group (amended from SIWPG 2002b p 4) are shown in Table 13.1 along with some implications for sport and coaching.

The SIWPG template identifies nine elements to be clarified in setting the context: timescale,

Table 13.1 Workforce planning principles

Principles	Implications for sport/coaching
Workforce planning is a continuous process that includes monitoring and evaluation and it should be sufficiently flexible to accommodate both incremental and quantum change	Recognition of its ubiquitousness and capacity to respond to a changing sport policy environment; implications for data management, for targets/capacity building, and for education and training
Workforce planning cycle iterations should be linked to planning for other purposes	This has implications for corporate planning, and implies that complementary 'development' strategies are available. In particular coaching workforce plans should be integrated fully with planning for education and training, player/athlete development, performance development and club/infrastructural development
Workforce planning should improve the balance of supply and demand of skills in the context of continual change	As a 'supplier' of personnel there are implications here for governing bodies of sport. As a training provider rather than a significant employer, such an agency has to ensure that it manages the balance of supply and demand through regulation, data availability, promotion, encouragement, and support
Services are normally delivered by groups of employees (for example, of coaches or teachers) and workforce planning should aim to achieve the appropriate mix of skills within the team	There are implications here for workforce planning at individual organisational level. Workforces (for example, in a sports club) need a balance of qualifications and experience. However, we should acknowledge that many coaches operate alone
Workforce planning should recognise and influence mechanisms that affect supply and demand	Insofar as adequate recruitment to coaching is always an issue, there is a need to introduce evidence-based practice to calculations of supply and demand. The message is that it is the contributory factors that are important, rather than the setting of targets
Workforce planning information and mechanisms must be linked across all delivery levels, all time horizons, and all sectors	Given multi-sector, multi-agency delivery, with very distinctive employment/deployment practices, this is a challenge for national sports organisations whose influence may be limited

geographical situation, type of service, nature of demand, scale of service change, organisational scale, planning focus, client group, and employment categories. Thereafter, the plan should move to a consideration of demand, supply, imbalances (gaps), risk assessments/business case, resource implications, and recommended actions. The importance of these nine elements cannot be overstressed, and they provide a data-gathering agenda for workforce developers. They set the parameters or assumptions on which planning should be based. At this stage, it becomes clear that coaching workforce development on a national scale, and encompassing all agencies, is likely to present significant challenges. It is useful to note that the nature of demand is further divided into 'initiated' (promotion/development by a lead agency, such as a Governing Body of sport), 'managed flow' (balance within existing provision), and

'reactive' (unforeseen demand) (SIWPG 2002a). In the same document, the scale of the service change is divided into 'quantum change' (significant scale in short period of time), 'incremental' (moderate growth over longer period), and 'maintenance' (maintain existing service levels). Incremental and/or maintenance change was thought most likely for SGBs because of their reliance on a limited infrastructure, and in the context of modest growth, and this assumption was very strongly borne out by our experience.

The document *Guide to Workforce Planning in Local Authorities: Getting the Right People with the Right Skills in the Right Place at the Right Time* (Employers' Organisation for Local Authorities 2003a) is also helpful for providing a generic template for workforce planning. The document stresses that information needs should be gathered from a mixture of quantitative and qualitative sources, and dealt with in a simple cyclical planning process: preparation, data collection, assessment of current position, future needs (and scenario planning), gap analysis, strategies and action plans, evaluation against initial plans, and process evaluation. Interestingly this (incontestable) process makes assumptions about existing planning processes being in place. Furthermore, there is a proposal for the minimum data required for effective workforce planning. This comprises details of employee roles, personal characteristics, vacancies, sources of recruitment, turnover and wastage, and qualifications and skills data. It is interesting that the Guide assumes, perhaps not unreasonably, that the (coaching) workforce is a known entity.

However, experience would suggest that this is not the case with the coaching workforce of many sports organisations, and for that reason a coaching audit is a necessary first stage in a workforce planning project. Before embarking on the planning projects undertaken by the authors, it became evident from sports agency representatives that data on the coaching workforce was 'patchy' at best, with a mix of membership lists, databases, local government employment records, coaching association records, and general lack of 'collation' of all sources. Table 13.2 illustrates the questions that arose from the guidance documents to which reference has already been made. In initiating the WDP process, these questions were the ones that needed to be addressed by sports, and acted as a framework for the procedures to be adopted. However, it becomes apparent from examining these questions that there are implications for professionalisation, coaching practice, the boundaries of the role, sports coaching policy, and how we conceive of 'provision'.

In addition to these, often quite specific, questions about the nature of the existing workforce, there are a number of 'political' considerations. Recognition within the sport of the contribution of coaches and coaching, and the level of support for change from the traditional pattern of provision may be facilitating or constraining. Having established the scope of coaching workforce development, we now examine some of the particular challenges that are presented when operating in the context of governing bodies of sport. Once again we emphasise that these insights have been gained from first-hand experience of working with a considerable number of these agencies.

Coaching workforce characteristics of national sports organisations

There are a number of features of workforce planning and management that will help to explain the relevance of some of the barriers to be overcome when national sports organisations attempt to develop their coaching workforce. First, workforce planning is normally carried out by or on behalf of an employer or an organisation (reflecting demand) but not always with an accompanying responsibility for workforce education and training (i.e. supply), if this is not carried on in-house. Second, workforce planning may also be sector-wide (and we will return to an example of this). However, this implies a close relationship between supply (for example, from further or higher education) and employment. This is perhaps most appropriate in publicly funded education and training, and in controlled employment environments (public sector job markets).

In this instance, Scottish governing bodies of sport employ directly a relatively small number of persons; ranging from a small sport such as Shinty with six full-time employees to a much larger organisation such as Scottish Swimming that has five times this number. The principal employers and deployers for the coaching workforce are the sports clubs and local government authorities. However, as previously stated, SGBs tend to be 'authority regulators' of matters relating to education and training, quality assurance, and working practices (for example, coach–athlete ratios or safety standards). For these reasons, many workforce plans implicitly acknowledge this limited influence and have a 'supply planning' focus, in that they emphasise recruitment, education and training requirements (in the context of a 'deficit demand').

Not surprisingly, coaching workforce planning cannot be seen in isolation from other personnel and organisational planning issues. Five priority areas are likely to impact on workforce planning; namely, leadership capacity, organisational development, the resources available, effective arrangements for developing skills and capacities, and pay and rewards. Each national sports organisation context is a complex one and will differ with respect to these factors. However, there is some commonality in that pay and rewards are a mix of almost completely intrinsically driven voluntary activity within sports clubs, and

Table 13.2 Questions to guide data collection

Baseline	Future thinking
What are the key priorities for the organisation?	What are the indications for growth (in participation, membership)? Are these aspirational, policy-driven, or based on extant demand? How will strategic changes impact on coaching; are they dependent on them?
What are the key environmental issues?	What external factors will impact on the organisation in the future? For example, would the UK Coaching Framework provide a change agenda?
What are perceived to be the current skills shortages? Is any part of the 'business' held back by skills shortages?	Which of the policy aspirations/growth targets for the sport are dependent on the quantity or quality of coaching?
Does the organisation have effective leadership?	Is there adequate leadership for those elements of organisational activity related to coaches and coaching? What is the relative status of coaching within the sport?
What are the financial implications of education and training?	Who pays for coach education and training? How much subsidy might be expected for 'public service'? Would the quality of the 'service' justify provision through further and higher education?
What are the current levels of turnover and retention of coaches?	What is the qualifications profile of the workforce? Are there barriers to progression? How might coaches' motives for coaching be better satisfied?
What are the 'regulations'/ recommendations for staffing levels (coach–athlete ratios)?	Is it anticipated that these might change? Is there any monitoring of these regulations? Would licensing of coaches make a difference?
Who is responsible for the recruitment of coaches into the sport, and what is the balance of volunteer and paid deployment?	Is there any expectation that changes in the 'reward environment' (particularly payment), increasing professionalisation, or licensing will impact on the coaches' motives and demand for certification?
What is the balance of provision, and the characteristics of deployment across the public, voluntary and commercial sectors?	Is change anticipated or planned in the balance of these provision sectors?
Which of the sport's different 'populations' do coaches serve? Are different roles recognised within the sport?	How much of provision is 'coach-dependent'? Does the sport recognise different roles for sports teachers, instructors and coaches?
Are there characteristics of coaching practice that renders it less susceptible to management?	The majority of coaches are part-time volunteers. It is clear that the coach's effectiveness can be evaluated with any confidence? Individual coach's motives may differ from those of the participants or the organisation. These are generalisations but they suggest limitations to the management of the workforce

(usually to a lesser extent) paid employment (both full- and part-time) within local government authorities, national agencies, and the commercial sector. It is important to note that workforce planning attends to the capacity of the sector to deliver not only current and perceived future demand with appropriate quality standards but also 'builds in' a capacity and flexibility to react to changes in the environment. For example, this may be achieved by affording opportunities for coaches to 'move through' a structured qualifications system that offers both progression and specialisation. This 'horizontal and vertical' dimension is an ambition that is a feature of the recently instituted UKCC endorsement framework.

Workforce planning acknowledges the distinction between skills shortages (lack of coaches with the appropriate skills, evident in vacancies and recruitment difficulties) and skills gaps or deficits (lack of appropriate skills of persons in post). The former is an issue largely of recruitment, and the latter one of retraining and upskilling. The skills gaps may also be of two kinds; (a) the coaching population is perceived to be too lowly qualified (sport-specific qualifications), and/or (b) the coaches/employees are perceived to have a deficit in more generic competences (communication, client handling and person-related skills). In general, the SGBs in this series of projects reported somewhere between 14–20% of their total coaching workforce as 'unqualified'. A common assumption is that these individuals are operating at the lower levels of sports participation, but whilst this is true in the majority of cases, interviews conducted with many of the sports revealed that there were appointments to 'performance coaching' positions for which coaches were either unqualified, or had 'lower-level' awards.

Therefore, a key feature of workforce planning is skills analysis. The 'skills framework' approach breaks the workforce into sub-groups of similar functions, and considers whether existing capacity is sufficient or growth/change is required. This is the approach adopted with coaching workforce planning, although the boundaries of the workforce are not uncontested. Coaches may be defined by being in coaching roles within clubs, by their qualifications, or in large-scale surveys, by self-report (Townend & North 2007). The principal occupational group is sports coaches (normally with an 'inclusive' approach to definition), but these are characterised by their level of award, coaching domains, and discipline specialisms. There is an assumption within each sport that coaches with these different levels of expertise are discharging a distinctive function (that is, coaching athletes with particular needs and aspirations within a particular organisational context). This may suggest a 'neatness' that does not accurately reflect practice. For example, the sport of Gymnastics was concerned that highly qualified coaches, in this case those expected to work with higher-level performers, were being too commonly deployed at the recreational and participation levels. It is also worth noting, as a number of chapters in this book will attest, that an unproblematic approach to 'skills' is unwarranted when coaches' expertise is not well understood. 'Skills' in this planning sense are equated with qualifications, and the education and training assumed by that award.

In addition, the coaching context has a number of specific characteristics. First, there was a widespread concern within the sports with which we worked that coaches might be discharging a function 'above' that for which they are qualified. This is a skills gap. Second, the skills analysis is at a fairly general and superficial level, since the detailed skills and competences are already subsumed within the awards/certification system. Third, the remedies to a skills gap resulting from a training needs analysis might be influenced (even limited) by the nature of workforce management within national sports organisations. These governing bodies of sport do not draw from a ready pool of labour. Also, coaches generally need to begin at entry level, and there is a very limited movement of coaches between clubs. The implication is that recruitment is generally a more significant issue than simply matching skills to needs within a responsive, mobile and dynamic workforce.

There are a number of issues that are specific to those organisations with a largely voluntary workforce. The general pattern is that Governing Body services to their members (within the voluntary sector) are delivered within a voluntary coaching commitment. This means that there is no coaching 'career' in a progressive employment sense, and this must impact on the coaching workforce development plan in terms of incentives and motives for recruitment and training/education. Progression may be measured by status and level of athlete coached. In some sports, there are a significant number of coaches in local government authority employment who are employed on a full-time basis, or nearly so (swimming is a good example), but there is currently no evidence that this, along with the voluntary sector, forms part of a structured career framework. Clearly this impacts on the expectations that coaching might have for being recognised as a profession.

National sports organisations receive a significant proportion of their funding from government, and this brings with it a climate of target setting and developmental ambitions ('enforced' by quangos such as Sport England) that not surprisingly coincide with the policy perceptions of government. These are driven mainly by policy areas such as health, social equity, and sporting success. One of the characteristics of coach education/workforce development planning is to base demand on developmental aspirations, without a realistic assessment of their likely successful outcome. In the authors' experience, the aspirational nature of strategic and development planning is characteristic of much of sports planning, and we comment later on this in recent coaching documentation (North 2009). Although it is understandable that strategic documentation should have a 'political' dimension and demonstrate ambitions that assume that existing constraints can be overcome, this approach is less helpful in the context of service-provision planning, wherein realistic assumptions of growth are important for setting targets (and committing resources). This is particularly important since the availability of coaches and the developmental outcomes are often perceived to be mutually dependent.

In the Scottish context, from which we are deriving this analysis, there are many SGBs that are relatively small, employ few full-time members of staff, and rely on volunteers to carry out many of their services. Workforce development planning for coaches is a challenging process in largely 'amateur' organisations such as these. For example, to date there has been limited planning for, or attempted management of, the coaching workforce, either in the sector or in individual sports. The expressed intention has been to attract as many coaches as possible to attend coach education courses, and to join clubs, but without a specific workforce strategy. There is an overwhelming (and, based on our data gathering, for the most part, accurate) assumption that coaches are 'generated' from within the sport. In our experience, such agencies have tended not to have sophisticated databases of coaches, and this clearly impacts on the setting and monitoring of targets. Without a licensing system (not simply certification), it is difficult to estimate 'churn' (the level of replacement necessitated by coaches leaving the sport each year) in the workplace. This is exacerbated by coaches in some sports operating without having membership of their Governing Body. These factors result in some real challenges for these bodies: intrinsic incentives, absence of recruitment strategies, limited demand analysis, and limited supply monitoring.

The recruitment of coaches to the workforce is a major element on workforce planning. However, there are a number of factors that militate against the straightforward setting of recruitment targets:

(a) In general, sports do not operate with a pool of trained labour (coaches) available for immediate employment/deployment. This is exacerbated by coaches (at least from the evidence generated in Scotland) not generally being recruited from extended further- or higher-education courses. National sports organisations may therefore have difficulty in providing 'training against future growth' because there is no incentive for individuals to engage in training without immediate deployment. This may be a little different for upskilling-related training provision, where 'better service' objectives can be more clearly established. Coaching workforce development planning has therefore tended to be reactive in this sector. The separation of proactive recruitment and training from extant demand may depend on future career incentives. Current consideration of the role of higher education and the setting of 'threshold' coaching standards in the development of coaching may be pointers to future developments.

(b) Workforce development planning in coaching (at least in the voluntary sector) has an additional issue in that, in general, employers (clubs) can only attract at the new-entrant level. There is limited movement of coaches between clubs. Unlike other employment sectors, coaches do not 'switch' sports in mid-training, and individuals do not (directly) qualify at middle levels. As a result, there is a time lag in increasing provision across levels.

(c) The environment is always fluid (although this is no different to business or local government sectors). However, because of a reliance on government funding for many national organisations, the sector is constantly subject to development initiatives, partly because of government policies and because sports participation is never sufficient to match policy objectives. The outcome is an often uneven and discontinuous demand for coaches, usually through public-sector-led initiatives.

(d) In sport, the service/product (athlete participation) can be amended to match the provision (coaching) available. This is different to a fixed service level agreement or a task analysis-led production quota. The tendency, therefore, is to 'work with what you've got', and, by implication, to cloud the relationship between growth or provision and coach numbers. Coaching provision is therefore considered to be 'elastic'. Additional demand may be dealt with by absorption into existing provision or the coach may provide additional

Table 13.3 Illustration of strategic options analysis

Workforce element	Coach education infrastructure	Upskilling agenda	Recruitment	Deployment	Career development
Status	Working well	Significant requirement	No process in place; Expectation of certification low	Some quality control; Part-time volunteers	Volunteer club sport; Payment opportunities
Mediation	Period of transition to UKCC qualifications	Demand uncertain; Role clutter (instructor, coach, leader)	Proficiency requirement Recruitment from within the sport	SGB staff largely in performance focus; Recreation emphasis in clubs	Commercial sector Outdoor activity/ education paid sector
Issues	Absence of control of recruitment by SGB; Potential resistance to change	Competition orientation demand from SGB	Attention required to coaching motives	Club autonomy; Coach buy-in;	Changing expectations to UKCC framework; Rewarding volunteers
SGB Influence	High	Moderate/limited	Moderate	Moderate/limited	Limited
Action	Prioritise	Prioritise	Prioritise	Advise/regulate	Advise

sessions. It is also the case that new initiatives or growth are often staffed initially by the existing workforce, until the growth in demand becomes more stable. The result is a dynamic, often untidy, calculation of skills shortages.

(e) Continuing professional development (CPD) provision is also part of workforce development. The voluntary nature of much of coaching may again be an issue in the extent to which coaches can be attracted to take part in CPD activity, despite its obvious role in maintaining the currency of skills and knowledge, and relevance to licensing of coaches. Traditionally governing bodies have limited influence in this because of the restricted reward environment, the absence of a career pathway, and modest, if any, performance monitoring.

Part of the initial stage of workforce planning is to construct a strategic analysis of the factors that will influence strategic objectives. Not surprisingly, such an analysis will reflect many of the characteristics of workforce deployment in national sporting organisations, as we have described above. It is important to note that when we say NSO or SGB, we imply the full range of organisations and agencies in that sport. The extent to which governing bodies

of sport can exert influence or control over workplace planning in the sport as a whole is problematic. Table 13.3 illustrates the strategic options for one SGB with which we worked. The evidence for these judgements is not provided, we merely wish to illustrate the limited impact that the Governing Body of sport may have: nevertheless, the analysis provides a useful example of a workforce profile.

Coaching in the wider employment context

Although the Governing Body of sport context is quite particular in its implications for coaching workforce planning, it is important to be able to site these workforce developments within the broader context of trends within the sport and leisure sector. The documents available to support such an analysis (e.g. Experian Business Strategies 2005) are somewhat limited in their utility by being focused on paid employment, which does not characterise the greater part of the 'coaching sector'. The most recent and comprehensive is the *Sector Skills Agreement* (2006) produced by SkillsActive, which is the Sector Skills Council for Active Leisure and Learning in the UK. Sector Skills Councils are the government-recognised agencies with responsibility for the strategic direction of the recruitment, training and education needs of each employment sector. The Councils are led by employers, with representation from national agencies, partner organisations and training providers. SkillsActive has recently published a *Sector Skills Agreement for Scotland*, which identifies the skills needs of the workforce in Scotland and how these will be addressed.

The *Sector Skills Agreement* is a valuable document for identifying skills gaps, although not all of the evidence was gathered from the voluntary sector with its particular employment/deployment working practices and motives. Nevertheless, there are some clear messages for the coaching workforce. A number of factors (including the establishment of the UK Coaching Framework and Active Schools [http://www.sportscotland.org.uk/activeschools/]) have created a dynamic but potentially rewarding employment sector. There is recognition that this is a people industry in which communication and other 'people skills' are crucial to the quality of service provided. The place of employers is recognised to be central, but similarly the volunteer status of many workers is acknowledged. In relation to sports coaching and SGBs, local government authorities, and commercial sector providers, there is acknowledged to be some lack of clarity in roles and responsibilities for training. Table 13.4 is a selective review of the objectives outlined in the *Sector Skills Agreement*, accompanied by a commentary related to sports coaching, in order to illustrate the particularities of the coaching workforce.

It is clear that organisations dealing with volunteer workforces may have some difficulty implementing many of the recommendations in the *Sector Skills Agreement*, no matter how appropriate they appear to be. Many of the developmental aspects of professionalisation of coaching and the development of education and training are embraced by the policy document, *UK Coaching Framework* (sports coach UK 2008), which complements the SkillsActive recommendations. The sports coaching workforce is characterised by distinctive roles and levels of qualification (and a fairly catholic approach to defining a coach). Moving between levels is a way of upskilling, although this may not lead to a different role. Experience suggests that national sports organisations and local government authorities can identify skills gaps and shortages However, the limited role for coach education in the development of coaches' expertise (see elsewhere in this

book) may be part of the reason for some reluctance by coaches to undertake 'higher' coaching qualifications. One of the questions we pose is whether coach education certification is more a mark of status than a training award. Part of the problem may be that it is not clear that this perceived lower quality of service (the skills gap) can be redressed through coach education, or that it impacts on the level of demand.

National projections versus sport-specific projections

The *Coaching Workforce 2009–2016* document (North 2009) was prepared by sportscoach UK for the Coaching Summit 2009 in Glasgow. Its relevance is that it highlights a mechanism for calculating workforce needs that might be described as 'top-down'. This is in contrast to the sport-specific 'bottom-up' approach undertaken by the authors. The 'top-down' approach requires an audit or baseline position from which to project the demand for coaching by using national participation targets to calculate the additional number of coaching hours required to meet these targets. This can be done in each of the coaching domains. For example, national survey data can be employed to estimate the number of coaches (and coaching hours) in children's, participation, talent or performance development, and high-performance coaching domains. Clearly this is a 'broad-brush' approach.

A workforce audit provides the information from which to shape 'strategic and operational decision making and planning for the coaching workforce' (North 2009 p 15). The *Coaching Workforce 2009–2016* document identifies the number of existing 'guided sport and sport coaching hours per week', that is, the current supply of coaching (note that there is some differentiation between coaching and other sport leadership roles). When interpreted in the light of information about coaching group size, coaches per group, and participation–coach ratios, it is possible to provide an estimate of the current 'supply' of coaches and coaching. The current participation rates are compared to national target participation rates and the demand for coaching hours can be calculated. The difference between this 'demand' and the existing supply is intended to inform policy makers and to influence resource requirements, particularly coach recruitment. However, it is particularly noteworthy that

Table 13.4 Sector skills agreement related to sports coaching

	Scotland sector skills agreement objectives	Commentary on sports coaching
1	Improve the quality and range of services	It would be difficult to disagree, but measurement of 'quality' remains problematic
2	Engage employers in addressing the skills and training needs of the sector	The role and influence of governing bodies and clubs in relation to volunteers needs to be taken into account
3	Align training and qualifications in the sector to the drive to meet government agendas and customer expectations	There needs to be a clearer identification of the rationale for training. Aspirational demand assumptions may be problematic
4	Disseminate good practice to employers and training providers across the sector	There is limited tradition in sharing best practice across governing bodies of sport
5	Improve recruitment and retention / Match training supply to employer demand	The good advice in this category needs to account for the fact that training is not characterised by being pre-service or based in further or higher education
6	Improve interaction between the sector and training providers	National sports organisations are the training providers, but 'employers' are very diverse
7	Improve the relevance and responsiveness of further and higher education provision	Need clearer research on coaching career pathways. Higher education shows interest in 'higher' qualifications for which students may be less appropriate
8	Embed sector qualifications in further and higher education	This is a current ambition, particularly at the higher levels of certification
9	Improve standardisation and transferability of skills and qualifications	The sports specificity of technical skills limits transferability. However, the multi-skills, multi-sports agenda for 'community coaches' may impact positively on this
10	Professionalise and upskill the existing workforce	Clearly a current preoccupation in coaching policy (c.f. UK Coaching Framework)
11	Address the skills and training needs of the existing workforce (paid and volunteer)	As the chapters in this book will testify, there is limited agreement on the coach's expertise and how it is best developed
12	Improve the take-up of vocational qualifications by volunteers	Most coaches are volunteers, and certification is an expectation in most circumstances
13	Make qualifications more accessible to people seeking to develop their skills	Previous experience suggests that there are barriers to provision. There is general agreement that a form of public subsidy for training would improve uptake, particularly in the context of increased costs for UKCC-endorsed courses
13	Address the personal training and qualification needs of employees	Coach education has tended to be provided at the 'system' level, although the UKCC-endorsement framework has inspired more targeted provision, and the rhetoric of coach development is 'needs-related'
14	Increase sector investment	There has been significant investment in sport in the UK, partly as a result of hosting the 2012 London Olympics
15	Make volunteering experience count towards career development	Although identified in policy statements, there is no clear evidence of a transition pathway from volunteering to paid employment

Continued

Table 13.4 Continued

	Scotland sector skills agreement objectives	Commentary on sports coaching
16	Encourage employers to embed training in their business plans	This may be common with local government authority employment/provision, but voluntary sector clubs may have limited resources
17	Attract funding to address employers' workforce development needs	Some public funding has been made available to meet part of the costs of coach education
18	Re-direct funding from public sources to meet the skills needs of sector employers	
19	Reduce barriers to accessing training – more local, flexible work-based training provision	This is an accepted principle but, although coach education is increasingly experiential, the voluntary sector may not be well placed to support this. Feedback from coaches in the project identifies the availability, geography and cost of coach education as barriers

this document identifies the opportunity to address the demand for increased coaching hours by changing the profile of the coaching workforce (the proportion of full-time and part-time paid coaches) rather than by simply recruiting increased numbers of coaches.

Clearly there are advantages and disadvantages to this 'national approach'. The positives are the use of national survey data, and the opportunity to adopt a sector-wide perspective. This broad perspective is most appropriate for national policy and resource considerations. On the other hand, the national approach loses the context and specific circumstances of individual sports, and the projections have limited value for individual-sport planning. A more obvious limitation is that projections are based on aspirational (government) participation targets, and may encourage an overestimation of coaching needs. Although the details of the document's recommendations are not discussed here, the three-fold increase in coaching hours that are identified in the document may bear out the aspirational nature of the demand projections.

Discussion

Coaching workforce development is a practical exemplar for many of the conceptual issues that have arisen throughout this book and are current within academic writing. Coaching workforce planning is a microcosm of the challenges to professionalisation and illustrates the fragile nature of the voluntary sector in coaching in the UK. A number of critical questions can be asked about this process. Is there such a thing as a 'coaching workforce'? Can coaching be conceived of as a 'service', as a commodity? Is the concept of 'upskilling' too mechanistic an approach for what we know to be a complex set of competences, knowledge and experience that goes beyond coach education certification? We briefly address each of these questions.

Inevitably our discussions will often focus on a distinction between practical interpretation and conceptual nicety. There is no doubt that we can describe a coaching workforce for each sport with which we have worked. It is possible to identify those individuals who 'coach' in the club, school, local authority, and commercial sectors (and including development officer teams and high-performance institutes and centres). These individuals can be captured in national surveys (Townend & North 2007) and in our 'bottom-up' surveys. However, this does not mean that there are no issues about the workforce. There is no doubt that it is a disparate group. The range of deployments, from the one-hour introduction to primary school children to full-time Olympic preparation, and with very different experience and levels of certification, tests the notion of a cohesive group. It may be more appropriate to conceive of the workforce in its domains (for example, children's development/participation/performance sport), rather than as a sport-specific aggregation.

While carrying out our development work with SGBs we had several lengthy debates about the scope of the workforce: should instructors be included, were PE teachers included, were youth leaders included? Was there a threshold of involvement to be considered part of the workforce? These were often debates about the scope of the 'development reach' of the Governing Body, but the implications for professionalisation of coaching are clear. The workforce existed but it was largely unregulated, had qualified and unqualified coaches, and was largely volunteer. This is an important point because it suggests that the unifying factor is the sport, and not a validated threshold level of expertise or a commonality of occupational practice and expectations. This absence of cohesion and the lack of clear 'markers' of what being a coach means are limitations that the professionalisation process has yet to overcome.

A number of themes will have emerged in this collection of chapters: the concept of coaching as a negotiated interpersonal relationship that is sensitive to the socio-cultural context in which it is practised is certainly one of them. The notion of coaching as a 'service' provided by a Governing Body and commodified by the calculation of the supply and demand for coached hours may seem very much at odds with this concept. However, this does appear to be one of those occasions when the perspective adopted provides the lens through which our perceptions are evaluated. Governing Bodies of sport, local authorities, schools and other agencies have a responsibility to oversee and provide opportunities for participation in their sport. This creates an environment (sometimes with more and sometimes with less control) that all of the coaches in our researches have to operate within. There are participation and performance targets that are held to be in the public interest, and therefore worthy of receiving public funds. Accepting that one of these responsibilities is to ensure that a sufficiency of well-educated (usually meaning certificated) coaches is both available and operating in appropriate ways (related to the needs of the participants), it is difficult to imagine how this could be achieved other than at the 'system' level. Does this smack of a 'techno-rational' approach, and does it seem to ignore the 'attachment' of the individual practitioner? Yes, of course, that is what the 'system' approach means, and is no different to the other caring professions in which workforce planning is necessary, but the quality of the individual attachment is valued.

It is important to appreciate, however, that this system-wide approach need not prevent academics and others from striving to disseminate understandings and insights about coaching practice in ways that influence coach education and training, deployment practices, and career transitions. Our experience has shown that coach development pathways are not well understood (Gilbert et al 2006, Erikson et al 2007) and certainly not yet evident in development policy. It does seem a very mechanistic approach to reduce the need for a more skilled workforce to an incremental improvement in the profile of certification within the sport. However, this is what we mean by the microcosm of practice and concept. Academics have views on the development of expertise, what it means to have 'better coaching', how to measure coaching effectiveness, and the influence of distinctive domains and participants' needs. The practitioner might ask whether this body of knowledge is sufficiently well-organised to provide an alternative approach. Perhaps a simple beginning would be to maintain the notion of improved certification levels, but to ensure that this validation of expertise was based on a coach education and training process that better reflected the research available.

Workforce development remains a practical challenge for the Governing Bodies of sport and a potential area of research interest for academics in coaching. The subtleties of how individual coaches can best be 'developed', how coaching practice can be improved, how quality can be evaluated, and theories of how coaching outcomes can best be achieved have to sit alongside a responsibility to deliver on a national scale, and to be held accountable for both practice and outcome. Projecting growth, and subsequently demand for coaching, is a challenging exercise for governing bodies of sport. They have traditionally wrestled with the issue of 'needing coaches in order to stimulate growth' although it is not clear that there is evidence to substantiate this development principle. It is also possible that an increased number of coaches would simply result in a better service to existing numbers of participants (that is, better player–coach ratios) rather than increased capacity.

Another way of describing this development conundrum is the relationship between supply and demand. Should supply reflect existing demand? Of course – this is a basic principle otherwise skills shortages will result, but existing demand seems to be elastic in sport in general in that the throughput of players/athletes may not be directly dependent on the supply of coaches. However, absorbing potential or aspirational demand may also be dependent on the supply of coaches. Should supply reflect potential demand (measured by waiting lists or other indicators of demand)? It seems incontrovertible that potential demand should be taken into account, but 'top-down' estimates may create recruitment targets that seem unattainable.

There is also a degree of flexibility in the relationship between the 'role' and the 'service' provided. Although there are factors such as productivity increases and overtime working (to borrow from other occupations), there is normally an assumed relationship between the job and the contribution to the service (even in a voluntary context). However, there is a potential in coaching for (a) variable group/squad/class sizes, (b) part-time/casual working providing flexibility (e.g. local government part-time workers may increase capacity by 'taking on' more hours. This increases capacity but does not require a greater number of coaches, and was one of the options provided in the *Coaching Workforce 2009–2016* document), (c) scheduling being varied to accommodate coaches' availability, or (d) demand being displaced to another provider with some supply capacity.

For many sports that we worked with the number of coaches recruited into the sport is not unmanageable. At the entry level within the voluntary club workforce, the motivations are those most common in voluntary activity – former participants, parental commitment, and a desire to help. It does seem that the majority of persons who join the 'workforce' have a connection with a club or a participant, and certainly the sport, before certification. To date, our experience suggests that it would appear that supply is a local reaction to a demand issue; there has been no strategic management of the workforce. However, it would seem that, in developmental terms, capacity building is not able to precede growth or development. Supply is regulated to some extent by the reward environment created within the sport. The obvious complications here are the distinctive motives of individuals based on volunteering within the club sector, and remunerated activity within the public and commercial sectors.

Coaching workforce planning is a welcome and necessary element in the development of coaching. It has the potential to bridge the gap between individualised and systemic development. As this chapter has demonstrated, the ambition of national sports organisations to manage recruitment, supply and demand in their sports in a planned fashion is a challenging exercise, and raises issues that are practical manifestations of those that researchers attempt to confront. Coaches and coach developers operate in a policy context in which planning and accountability form part of the landscape and are inevitable. Although we raised issues about the boundaries of the coaching workforce, the concept of coaching as a commodified service, and the system versus individual concept of coaching, the implications are most challenging for the professionalisation agenda. Coaching workforce development is, in part, driven by this agenda, but its operationalisation demonstrates that many of the building blocks towards professionalisation have yet to be realised.

References

Bolton, N., Smith, B., 2008. Sport development for coaches. In: Jones, R.L., Hughes, M., Kingston, K. (Eds.), An introduction to sports coaching. Routledge, London, pp. 73–84.

Employers' Organisation for Local Government, 2003a. Guide to workforce planning in local authorities: getting the right people with the right skills in the right place at the right time. Online. Available: http://www.idea-knowledge.gov.uk/idk/aio/5689268 12 Feb 2007.

Employers' Organisation for Local Government, 2003b. Workforce planning: the wider context. Institute for Employment Studies. Online. Available:http://www.idea-knowledge.gov.uk/idk/aio/5549965 12 Feb 2007.

Employers' Organisation, 2004. Workforce development planning: guidance document. Institute for Employment Studies. Online. Available:http://www.idea-knowledge.gov.uk/idk/aio/4465769 26 Feb 2007.

Erikson, K., Cote, J., Fraser-Thomas, J., 2007. Sport experiences, milestones, and educational activities associated with high-performance coaches' development. The Sport Psychologist 21, 302–316.

Experian Business Strategies, 2005. The future of active leisure and learning. SkillsActive, Scotland.

Gilbert, W.D., Côté, J., Mallett, C., 2006. Developmental paths and activities of successful sports coaches. International Journal of Sport Sciences and Coaching 1, 69–76.

Green, M., Houlihan, B., 2005. Elite sport development: policy learning and political priorities. Routledge, London.

Kay, T., Armour, K., Cushion, C., et al., 2008. Are we missing the coach for 2012. University of Loughborough/Sportnation. 9 June 2009 www.thelssa.co.uk/lssa/Sportnation/SportnationDiscussion.pdf 9 June 2009.

Lyle, J., 2007. UKCC impact study: definitional, conceptual and methodological review. Online. Available: http://www.sportscoachuk.org/research/Research+Publications/UKCC+Impact+Study+Phase+One+Report.htm 9 June 2009.

Lyle, J., 2008. Sports development and sports coaching. In: Hylton, K., Bramham, P. (Eds.), Sports development. Routledge, London, pp. 214–235.

North, J., 2009. The coaching workforce 2009–2016. National Coaching Foundation, Leeds.

Scottish Executive, 2002a. Planning together: final report of the Scottish Integrated Workforce Planning Group. Online. Available:http://www.scotland.gov.uk/library3/health/.

Scottish Executive, 2002b. SIWPG stage 1 report, April 2000. Online. Available:http://scotland.gov.uk/library2/doc15/siwpg-02.asp 13 April 2009.

Scottish Executive, 2007. Reaching higher: building on the success of Sport 21. Online. Available:http://www.scotland.gov.uk/Publications/2007 13 April 2009.

Skills Active, 2006. Sector skills agreement Scotland. Online. Available: http://www.skillsactive.com/resources/research 13 April 2009.

Sport England, 2008. Grow sustain excel: Sport England strategy 2008–2011. Online. Available:http://www.sportengland.org/sport_england_strategy/ 13 April 2009.

sports coach UK, 2008. The UK coaching framework executive summary. Coachwise, Leeds.

sports coach, no date. UK coaching certificate. Online. Available: http://www.sportscoachUK.org/investing+in+coaching/UK+Coaching+Certificate/13 April 2009.

Townend, R., North, J., 2007. Sports coaching in the UK II. sports coach UK, Leeds.

Vaga Associates, 2006. Coaching Scotland, Research Report No 133. sportscotland, Edinburgh.

Coaching practice and practice ethics

14

Hamish Telfer

Introduction

When the word ethics is mentioned, often the first reaction is to assume that what follows is a 'right' and a 'wrong' way of doing things. This is not necessarily the case. The determination of what is 'right' and 'wrong' is more complex, relying on situational factors that are often unique. Sports coaching is characterised by such situationally unique factors with environmental and performer variables contributing to performance outcomes and processes that are often unpredictable. The role and function of the coach is to bring to bear upon these factors a degree of judgement about correct or 'right' actions. These judgements contribute to a nuanced practice environment within which coaches are increasingly judged on performers' successes and failures (and especially so against a backdrop of funding for sport that is primarily based on medal success). Coaches may have to make decisions about and within their practice against the backdrop of sets of conditions that may challenge their values and their decision making. Moral or ethical decision making has the potential to isolate coaches when they are presented with practice dilemmas that question the basis of their attitudes, values and beliefs, especially when confronted with others whose views may be different. These dilemmas challenge not just *what* the coach decides is appropriate, but also *how* they go about coaching their performers, particularly in terms of interpersonal relationships.

However, as our understanding of coaching practice has evolved, key principles underpinning the practice of coaching and the behaviour of coaches have evolved in parallel. As coaching in the United Kingdom moves towards a more 'professionalised' approach, more widespread and more accountable educational structures and systems have also emerged. Improved guidance, resources, and principles of good practice have also evolved to support coaching practice. Ethics of practice, however, appear to become relatively taken-for-granted; something that coaches are assumed to understand and grasp intuitively. In the event of a dilemma or the need for guidance, codes of ethics, conduct and practice are relied upon with the questionable assumption that the implementation of these codes will create morally sound coaches. The essence of applying ethics to practice goes beyond codes, and coach education courses are now placing increasing emphasis on coaches becoming aware of and understanding the implications of their 'duty of care' and the nature of the trust and power relationship between the performer and the coach. The advent of screening and checking the suitability of coaches to work with children and young people in the UK and elsewhere has acted as a catalyst for thinking about the personal qualities deemed desirable in those coaching sports performers. However, we might reasonably expect that this debate will go beyond dealing with young performers to encompass all coaching domains and the broader moral compass that this implies. In this respect performer welfare is one area of growing interest and awareness within coaching (see Brackenridge et al 2007).

It is a reasonable expectation that the occupation of coaching should be underpinned with an understanding of an ethical base for practice. This is at least in part to gain a foothold on what is seen as an integral part of any profession, namely, a set of ethical or guiding principles. Formalised in various forms of codes, it is through these codes that professions are seen to be accountable for the practice of those who claim to belong to such a profession. Accountability is also the means through which professions gain a form of acceptability as a profession (McNamee 1998). For example, being able to justify player selections, being able to articulate an understanding of the need to realign practice with the needs of coaching children or performers with a disability, or indeed being able to justify the way coaches speak and interact with others as good self-reflective practitioners are examples of relevant ethical contexts. Each of these contributes to a client or participant focus that ought to be embraced by coaches, and codes play a part in aligning practice so that the performer is at the centre (or heart) of this process; in essence, emphasising the principle of 'performer-centred – coach-led'.

Codes therefore have a role to play in establishing good practice and usually encompass broad guiding principles enshrined within Professional Codes of Practice (sometimes also variously known as Codes of Conduct or Codes of Ethics depending on their use and function). These codes are supported by National Occupational Standards for Coaching, Teaching and Instruction (NOS for CTI). Additionally, the law often determines how our practice must fit within broader societal expectations. Examples of this are the recent changes to the law in the UK regarding working with children and young people (see The Children Act 2004 and the Safeguarding Vulnerable Persons Act 2006). Similar legal minimum standards and expectations in relation to equity are also defined for those working with individuals who have a disability as well as in relation to race and ethnicity, gender and sexual orientation.

These measures however are poor substitutes for individual probity and the objective of this chapter is to outline basic and current principles of practice ethics, as well as exploring areas where coaching is still less than robust in its acceptance and application of ethical practice. This is evident in the power position of the coach in relation to their duty of care and trust, responsibility, working with performers at the 'stage of imminent achievement' and being able to support and evidence practice. Evidence-based practice is a key element of 'practice ethics' and allows coaches to identify, apply and

demonstrate good practice. The principles outlined throughout the chapter reflect current thinking in relation to good coaching practice and should inform and underpin the day-to-day work of coaches.

The chapter concludes with an exploration of the function and expectations inherent within 'codes', adopting the position that they should be interpreted as sets of guidance rather than 'rules'. It will be argued that coaches ought to have a robust sense of the ethical underpinning of the process and outcomes of their coaching in order to be able to interpret the guidance offered and to function autonomously as ethical practitioners. This will also enable them to audit and be accountable for their own behaviour and practice (see McNamee 1998).

Setting the scene: ethics, sport and coaching

There is no doubting the interplay of ethics, sport and coaching. Lyle (1999) in his review of the coaching process makes a strong claim for a humanistic approach to coaching. In his later work he illustrated the ways in which ethics impacts across a range of sporting contexts and can challenge such a humanistic approach (Lyle 2002). Coaches often work across the performance spectrum being responsible for beginners as well as more established performers. This demands a level of sophistication in the coach's capacity to apply good practice principles across what is an increasingly demanding range of performance levels and stages. What may be deemed acceptable as a way of conducting practice at one level may not be as appropriate at another. Identifying appropriate ethical decisions and behaviours at each stage of the performance spectrum can be problematic, both for the individual practitioner and also for the coaching profession. The implication is that coaching practice, in relation to ethical judgement, is complex, situationally dependent, and offers a dynamic set of practice catalysts. In such a context, it is reasonable to question whether common principles can be identified and applied effectively.

Nevertheless, what underpins ethical behaviour, and our sense of what it is, are links to moral values. Russell (2007) argues that the distinctiveness of the moral values of sport is not easily distinguishable from those of society at large. He argues that while sport may be able to contribute uniquely to the promotion of these values, it still has a commitment to human dignity and needs to be rooted in integrity. Moral values are of course notoriously slippery concepts to articulate with any degree of certainty. The way in which moral values (or ideals) form the basis of our ethical framework in practice is constantly subjected to moral evaluations often variously applied depending on the varying situations in which we find ourselves. Societal norms impact upon our personal attitudes, beliefs and values (and these are not always interchangeable) and shape our views, behaviours and practice as coaches. In a sense, it is inescapable that our values and attitudes are shaped and influenced by the expectations of our wider society. This of course may not always be for the good of sport, our performers or ourselves as coaches, as it assumes that those from outside the community of sport understand and subscribe to what sport means to those involved in it. This is not intentionally to mythologise sport but merely to highlight that there may be competing or uninformed values at play.

Sport generally benefits from being considered 'a good thing'. It might therefore follow that the process and outcomes of sport involvement are generally beneficial for those involved. To be a sports performer, coach or volunteer may be seen as possessing some virtuous quality, or at least benefiting from the moral qualities that sport is assumed to possess. Rules are formulated to enable those involved in sport to share an understanding of engagement as well as to protect this mythical quality of the 'good' of sport. McFee's (2004) work expands further on this relationship between the values of sport and the necessity and nature of rules.

The assumptions inherent in the view that sport is 'a good thing' and that it therefore follows that those involved in sport are 'good' is contested ground. Dealing with performers who are on the whole young and impressionable and led by coaches whose education and training may be limited to a mere handful of hours over a few weekends demonstrates a clear need for greater investment in the way in which sport seeks to develop expertise in their coaches. Expertise takes time to develop and there is certainly an argument that novice coaches should be made more aware of the limitations of coaching individuals or teams armed only with the most basic coaching level award. Although governing bodies of sport generally try to emphasise that an early coaching role should be that of supporting more qualified coaches, this is poorly regulated.

Ethical debate in and around sport has tended to focus on crisis events and rule violations such as the use of ergogenic aids, violence and various forms of deception. There has been little attention to the more all-embracing practice of coaching. Since coaching practice is 'contoured', fluid and dynamic and rarely completely predictable, this presents the coach with ever-changing circumstances and problems, thus contributing to the notion of the 'craft' of coaching (Knowles et al 2006). This notion of coaching as having 'craft' qualities is only now beginning to receive attention and builds on the work of, for example, Abrahams and Collins (1998). Practice ethics, as an essential part of the skill set of sports coaches, is still however, a generally neglected area in the development of this 'craft'. This perhaps indicates a relatively underdeveloped awareness, or understanding, of duties associated with professional practice. One explanation is that coaches already possess a well-rehearsed sense of ethical behaviour, and this need not therefore warrant significant attention in coach education. This is a mistake, as coaches should not operate to a default setting of only being able to articulate a sense of their practice as ethical when things go wrong. It is essential for professional development that coaches are able to articulate a sense of what constitutes ethical practice and what it means for their own coaching principles and practice. It is important to note here that words such as *duty* and *obligations* are central to an understanding of ethical practice. These are too often relegated to a brief consideration within Codes of Conduct.

In setting the scene, perhaps nothing more acutely focuses the attention of coaches than the balance between the need to achieve outcomes (e.g. winning), and the means by which coaches work with performers to achieve this. The dilemmas inherent in this simple equation bring into sharp relief the nature of coaching practice across the performance spectrum. The outcome orientation of performance sport, felt most intensely at international or professional levels, contrasts with the use of sport for various social agendas, for example, combating obesity and engaging young people in developing physically active lifestyles. For many coaches the reality of their coaching experience embraces this continuum.

The demands and expectations at the various stages of performer development present coaches with practice dilemmas, not only in terms of the appropriateness of progression strategies, skill selection and the choice of appropriate methodologies of practice and team selection, but also in relation to consideration of the nature of any authority exercised, the nature of the power relationship and the boundaries that are consistent with the exercise of such power and the position of trust. This is seldom addressed in depth within coach education programmes but is exemplified in how coaches are recognised as good practitioners. The balance between rewarding process as opposed to outcomes could usefully be given more considered attention by the coaching community.

What are ethics and what are they not?

At this point it is relevant to consider what we mean by ethics. Ethics should not be interpreted as a *restriction*. Rather they should be viewed as the manner in which coaches, as practitioners, exercise their own morality. To act ethically is to be considerate of the interests of others. Ethics are also about the interests or the rights of others and indeed, are at the heart of questions relating to practice dilemmas and decision alternatives that invite coaches to ask, 'what should I do?' In essence they constitute our set of personal laws, especially in relation to context-specific behaviours. These are not necessarily independent of what is rightfully expected of a practitioner since there should be consonance between what sport and society expects of us and our personal actions. However, they do allow for practitioners to be reactive to particular situations.

Our ethical behaviour is determined by what we as practitioners do rather than what others may do or indeed impose upon us. Ethics therefore are a set of duties we impose upon ourselves as practitioners while taking account of what sport and society expects of us. This might conjure up the notion that there are a variety of appropriate responses to ethical dilemmas. While this might be the case, ethical decisions are nevertheless subject to some universal understanding and agreement. For example, sport has defined appropriate conduct by coaches as requiring them to be subject to a principle that demands that they do not covertly or overtly administer banned substances to their performers, or that they do not use physical chastisement as a means of coercion within their practice. This is based upon what individuals within sport and indeed society expect of sport. Therefore, ethical practice is about making moral decisions based upon a majority consensus on universal principles.

A key consideration within this exercise of moral judgement is the notion that those that we coach, instruct or lead are often considered by the nature of the coaching environment to be 'situationally vulnerable'. This means that the coach is in a position of trust and that trust can, if developed without check, create an unwitting power imbalance. This can lead to a negative coaching environment, potential dependency and indeed in extreme cases, an abusive relationship (see Brackenridge 2001). This trust extends beyond the mere ability to ensure that coaches select the appropriate number of sets, repetitions and intensities, but also to the way in which they are able to interact with their performers and use their power position for the good of the performer. This notion of client service or good will be discussed later.

In performance sport, coaches are most often evaluated by the performance outcomes of their athletes. For some this offers a number of opportunities to 'take short cuts'. These actions create moral dilemmas and inevitably, in such circumstances, we generate self-justificatory arguments to defend our behaviour. An understanding of, and reflection on, professional ethics allows us to consider this rationale for behaviour in the context of key principles and processes, although this may not reflect 'firm ground'. Jones and McNamee (2003, p 42) recognise that 'sport is a complex cultural practice that is neither entirely synonymous with the rest of society nor separate from it.' It is within this contested ground that coaches operate. Thus the ability to differentiate between options as moral agents is important in being able to act as client-centred professionals. What is required of practitioners is judgement. The knowledge of what moral rules are and the principles on which they are founded help practitioners make better judgements.

At this point it will be useful to consider the nature of ethical decision-making that guides practice ethics in most professions. Although there is no one particular process for arriving at a morally 'right' position or decision, there are key theories that help us formulate our arguments. Most of these will be familiar, with the key tenet of 'do unto others as you would have them do unto you' the most obvious. This tendentious and often elusive ambition is frequently a tipping point between good and poor practice. However, it forms only part of our moral reasoning. These moral guides or markers are important in arriving at a shared understanding of what our practice should look like both to ourselves and to those that we coach. Shields and Bredemeier (1995) suggest that for the purposes of making a decision about moral actions there is a staged process:

1. Interpreting of moral cues – what is the significance of this event?
2. Exercising judgement – this might depend on the moral maturity of the individual involved (and supports the case that ethics and ethical behaviour need to be given increased emphasis in the education and training of coaches).
3. Selecting a course of action (value choice) – based on what is perceived to be the most appropriate course of action, depending on the context of the moral judgement and individual choice.
4. Implementing action – to act in a manner that underpins the judgement made.

However, the relationship between *what* coaches do and *how* they should do it as part of critical self-analysis of whether it is a 'good' action is seldom considered. It is important to be able to distinguish between 'good' (for the client) and 'good' (as in virtuous). This distinction is at the centre of how we make ethical decisions as coaches. What sometimes helps practitioners in the interpretation of these principles, and the construction of actions, are action principles. Kant's 'categorical imperatives' form part of the most widely known, accepted and understood set of underpinning rationales in ethical theory. There are three key imperatives and *simply* interpreted, they are expressed as follows.

1. Laws should be universal. That is to say, an action is good only if the principle of it can be applied in practice to everyone. Therefore to act in a moral manner is based on the understanding that everyone might act similarly.
2. You should consider yourself as subject to any act. In other words you should only do to others what you would do to yourself.
3. Never treat others as a means to an end (see Hursthouse 2001 for a good summary).

Although the key tenets of Kant's categorical imperatives are laid out somewhat simplistically above, they are nevertheless recognisable as guiding principles. The underlying premise of Kant's rules is that they provide overarching guidance based on moral principles that apply to all contexts and to all persons. From this perspective, actions are based on rules, duties and obligations as we navigate our way through the complexities of professional practice. Thus, particular actions are good or bad, and there is little leeway in this. For example, intrinsically good acts in coaching practice might be always telling the truth and always keeping promises (such as in selection) irrespective of the situation. Intrinsically bad acts might be inflicting physical or emotional harm or deliberately and wilfully breaking rules (such as the administration of banned substances).

There are other competing principles however, since this is contested ground. The notion that Kant's principles can be universally applied in all situations is somewhat simplistic. For example, Brown (2003) argues that moral considerations arise out of moral obligations, which in turn arise out of conflicts. These conflicts are the product of what we might call our personal inclinations on the one hand and our duties on the other. It is our ability to act as a moral agent in distinguishing between the two that will determine our effectiveness in dealing with situations involving those that we are entrusted to coach or lead. Indeed, as the choices inherent within coaching practice come under increasing scrutiny, sport practitioners must confront the consequences of their decisions, and be comfortable in opening their practice to such scrutiny. This scrutiny may suggest to the coach that some aspect of the situation has been ignored or not recognised, or that alternative courses of action were possible. This sort of reflection may also highlight any conflict between our personal or core values and the action that seems appropriate.

An alternative approach is utilitarian or consequentialist theory, which requires practitioners to consider the outcome or consequence of their actions. This approach emphasises the end result of our actions in determining how we should act. Inevitably, the 'rules' can be seen as somewhat flexible, with the action decision in one situation not necessarily being applied in another apparently similar situation. What is important in this approach is that it defines the moral worth of an action or decision as maximising happiness to the greatest number. Thus the right action or outcome is that which achieves this. Outcome-based decision making may not always be in the interests of the individual performer. This approach in many cases can also appear to indicate a limited set of choices for the coach since the best outcomes may appear predetermined. Achieving the outcome of maximising happiness for the majority may thus overtake the benefits to some individuals.

Cross and Wood (2005) make it clear that this approach could mean an abdication of decision making by practitioners as they need only cite the outcome and therefore this justifies the means. The practitioner therefore in this approach may exercise little individual moral judgement. If the ends and means argument is followed through then individual autonomy is compromised, an approach which sports practitioners should in general guard against since this clearly puts the practitioner at potential odds with what are regarded as sport's key principles. If the 'ends indeed do justify the means' then this may imply performers being used as a means to that end and not being treated as ends in themselves, that is, with regard to their own individual worth. The use of talent identification programmes and athlete funding become an issue within this particular argument since funding follows those who achieve the targets. Those targets are usually set in relation to achievement against a fixed criterion (usually medal prospects). Thus the performer is expected to achieve against criteria that are reflective of the demands of the sport system rather than for their own intrinsic worth. This however is generally seen as a 'fair' way of distributing scarce resources since within a national agenda it will increase the sum of happiness, and, of course, the criteria are relatively transparent. Performance outcomes are of course transitory in the case of sport, and practitioners need to guard against expediency in exercising this consequentialist approach.

An ethical pluralist approach is often used to address the issue of conflicting principles. Ethical pluralists weigh multiple possibilities and attempt to balance both of the previous approaches. This demands a degree of moral character based on reasoning and has the advantage of generating as many options or propositions as possible in order to arrive at a correct decision. In sport the time for (relatively) rational consideration of alternatives in order to weigh up possibilities is not always available, since decision making in training and competition environments is often rapid and intuitive. Linked to this approach is the notion of 'virtue ethics'. These invite us to consider not only what we do but also the nature of who we are. In other words as Sim (1997) suggests, morality is about agent-centred as well as act-centred

considerations. Virtue ethics is concerned with character traits that should be displayed as practitioners. There is a danger that coaches might assume that they have the right virtues and are always able to produce the right actions or decisions. This is clearly not the case and indeed Kohlberg (1981) suggests that the notion of virtue is a highly subjective one with little consensus on what virtues are. Notwithstanding Kohlberg's arguments, it is important that coaches should understand that moral virtue is required of them and not just their actions. This is an important distinction. Very often the inherent character of sport and its association with 'being a good thing' gives the practitioner, by association, a perceived position of moral authority based on some sort of moral virtue. This may not always be the case. It is therefore necessary to consider what these key moral virtues or principles might be in relation to practice ethics for coaches.

Key ethical principles

There is a conceptual basis for ethical decision making, which forms the starting point for ethical analysis. Sim (1997) argues that an ethical principle is one that should be based on a fundamental belief or value that justifies an action or decision. Practitioners should weigh their decisions and actions against these principles. He then goes on to suggest a set of primary principles. These are easily and very relevantly applied to coaching practice.

The principle of *beneficence* (doing good) and *non-maleficence* (not doing harm) is fundamental to good coaching practice. In any profession or indeed in any power relationship, there should be the tacit assumption by those under the guidance and control of others that those to whom they give their trust, will exercise that power in a way that will promote their interests and well-being, and indeed will remove potential harm. Beneficence therefore is a positive requirement of us while non-maleficence requires us to refrain from acts that render the performer worse off. Non-maleficence within coaching practice, however, is a difficult area to negotiate since within training and performance there may be situations where there is a requirement to push the human body to its physical and emotional limits. The line between harm and appropriate endeavour is sometimes a fine one and certainly this is an enduring debate in relation to coaching the child or young performer.

The consequence of neglecting our duty to ensure the performer does not suffer harm is potentially more problematic and may lead to coaching practice becoming more conservative.

Autonomy and the right to determine for oneself a course of action is often thought of as the ultimate goal of the good coach–performer relationship. As relationships mature and develop decision making by coaches on behalf of the performer often changes towards a more autonomous self-determined role for the performer. Coaches should protect the self-determination of those they coach and promote greater autonomy. The principle of autonomy is enshrined within individual liberty and as such is considered a human right. Coaches can often undermine this autonomy by restricting choices, freedom of action or by distorting or restricting information. This unbalanced power relationship in coaching is often evident in the early stages with the coach controlling much of the decision making and the performer accepting the power position of the coach. It is within this stage of the relationship especially that coaches must exercise care in order to develop within the performer a capacity to be able to identify and exercise choice later in their careers.

However, within this concept of autonomy there is also the principle of 'professional autonomy'. This is characteristic of professions in their quest to regulate and control their activities independently (often of government). Coaching (in the UK) currently does not have an autonomous, independent body and thus any tension between performer and professional autonomy cannot be resolved by the profession. Practice therefore is 'regulated' by an amalgam of sports governing bodies that assume the role of arbitrator in coaching practice and other national agencies such as UK Sport and the British Olympic Association who may be asked to give a view of specific situations. In extremis, recourse to law may be sought.

Aligned to autonomy, the principle of respect for persons requires coaches to be able to demonstrate that they value the inherent worth of each and every performer. In a target-driven sport environment, there is always a danger that the individuals (both the coach and the performer) are subsumed into a wider 'good', thus depersonalising and anonymising the coaching experience. When viewed in this way, the individual is part of a process that contributes towards achieving (often national) targets. In doing so, individuals may lose their individuality. This can be taken to extremes with target-driven agendas, and the policy, funding and selection decisions that

are a consequence. This principle of respect for persons is enshrined within Kant's imperative of never using others as a means to an end (especially one's own ends). This principle is closely and fundamentally aligned to the notion of individual dignity. Not only is this a key principle in coach–performer relations but it is also a necessary principle within coach-to-coach relationships. Coaches should recognise the values and merits of colleagues, and indeed codes of practice in sport are now addressing the increasing problem of coaching behaviour that does not give due accord to the opinions, skills, achievements and aspirations of colleagues.

The principle of justice is based on fairness. This is also linked to individual merit. This causes some difficulty since sport, at least competitive sport, is clearly designed to distinguish one set of sporting abilities from another. Rewards tend to go to the winners but it is essential that opportunities are not denied to any group of performers. Treating everyone in the same way may solve one part of this dilemma. However, there are individual differences between athletes that may militate against this, and justify different treatment; the merits and needs of individuals need to be balanced. The particular type of justice most appropriate to coaching practice is that of 'distributive justice', that is to say the weighing of benefits and costs of certain actions or decisions. This is evident in deciding the length of time spent with some performers as opposed to others, the selective seeking of additional assistance for some but not others in their team, or making decisions about inclusion or exclusion from teams or squads.

Justifying and analysing ethical practice

Being able to justify one's actions as a practitioner is an essential part of the claim of being a professional; practitioners should have a rational basis for justifying their actions and decisions. Competing views and the validity of these views often make it difficult to arrive at a consensual justification since much of what seems personally rational can be collectively subjective. In the quest for impartial objectivity in practice, what is important is that personal bias can be accounted for as well as predilections. It is important to recognise the significance of arriving at the correct decision by the right means as well as achieving the desired end result. Getting the process right ensures that coaches can identify when their individual preferences are in danger of intruding into a process. It is implied that coaches ought to act in such a way as to keep the performer's needs sharply in focus rather than their own.

The staged approach of Shields and Breidemeier (1995) can be applied to rationalising ethical decision making, and Johnstone (2004) suggests a looped approach to evaluating and understanding ethical decision making. By actively assessing situations, identifying the moral dilemmas, setting goals and actions, and then implementing action plans to achieve the desired outcomes we can more consciously evaluate our coaching practice from an ethical perspective.

However this assumes that practitioners have developed to a point at which they are sensitive to the moral demands of practice and that they are capable of producing morally appropriate actions. The need for ethical training within coach education courses is clear. The ability to assess, identify, action plan, implement and evaluate practice based on little or no training in the basic principles or understanding of practice ethics will only ever at best result in sports practitioners relying on their own, perhaps ill-considered, judgement of what a right action might be. This optimistic perspective relies on the notion that sport succeeds in attracting practitioners who have morally acceptable character traits. For this reason, it might be necessary to argue that sport itself needs to articulate what its moral boundaries are in relation to sports practice. Loland's (2002) work in defining a moral norm system in sport goes some way to being able to ground our thinking. He comments, importantly for the sports practitioner, that 'norms are shared when two or more parties are aware that they are consenting to an interpretation of the basic rules. That is to say, there exists a consensual perception . . . .' (p 7). In other words, sport tends to 'work' only when all parties share a common view as to what is 'right' and what is 'wrong'. He goes on to state the case for fairness and fair play as inherent characteristics of a moral norm system within sport, thus at least setting some sets of boundaries for the context within which practitioners might test the moral outcomes of practice.

Ethics in practice

Clark (2000) reminds us that the promotion of a multiplicity of values may lead only to confusion and inertia. However, there must be a set of core values, which professional ethics embrace. He states

that, 'Values . . . must be few. Professional ethics however, may helpfully be laid out in different formulations to suit a range of different practical problems and situations' (Clark 2000 p 26). Therefore, sport should have a clear set of core values and sensibilities that oblige us to act in a certain manner and which are capable of being applied across a range of coaching situations. This sense of the prescriptive and the critical are necessary parts of the same continuum. On the one hand there is the need to work within carefully defined parameters in order that practitioners maintain a degree of uniformity in the way in which they go about the business of coaching. On the other hand it is important that sports practitioners are able to function at a critical level in working out for each situation the relevant response within the prescriptive. Prescription in this sense is only a set of fundamental parameters within which practitioners then need to be able to act independently. Clark (2000) suggests a set of rules for good practice in respect of the qualities demanded of practitioners.

The practitioner has to assess, plan, implement, manage and evaluate not merely the outcome of practice but the implementation of it, and its impact on the performer. This requires of the practitioner a degree of sensitivity and reflection. Being able to reflect about and upon practice engages the practitioner with both the outcome effect on the performer and also the range and nature of their own behaviours and effectiveness as coaches. Hawley (2007) goes further in suggesting that practice that actively accounts for its ethical dimension is quality practice. Without taking account of our actions therefore we cannot claim to be offering or engaging in quality practice. Knowles et al (2005) advocate the use of reflective techniques as one means of engaging with evidence-based practice, which is the primary means through which practitioners validate their actions and decisions.

Quality practice based on sound ethical principles needs to be transparent, safe, culturally sensitive, respect autonomy and conform to the accepted technical and methodological practice of the sport. In this sense much of our accepted approaches and belief systems about what is ethically correct come from socialisation within our respective sports. We learn the dominant values from peers and from colleagues in education and training who transmit something of the culture and nature of sport (although recognising the limited influence of coach education in comparison to other socialising mechanisms). We learn as practitioners to be able to deal with 'what is' as well as 'what ought to be' (Banks 1999). These lessons are transmitted from coaches to athletes, as the performers become 'occupationally socialised' into sets of attitudes, values and beliefs from the way coaches go about their practice. This socialisation can, and should be, highly contested since values are seldom static. The 'received wisdom' transmitted during education and training should always be open to question and re-appraisal.

Ethics in practice therefore is about clarity of engagement. Sports practitioners should ensure that the voice of those they coach is heard. Parrot (2006) highlights four key values associated with service professionals: the ability to listen; engaging empathetically; being clear about what practitioners can and cannot do, and being able to provide basic and effective support at a range of levels including socio-emotional support. Despite these apparently compelling principles, sports practitioners face a number of unique dilemmas as practitioners. Sport is a contested activity in the very sense of the word. It is essentially about winning or being able to exact the very best in performance from the human body. The coach's role in this therefore is to be able to work with performers in a way that maximises abilities of the performer while minimising or redressing their limitations. In determining training loads, delivering interventions, defining tactics and in preparing for competition, coaches themselves can be said to compete. Therefore, coaching is in itself a contested activity as one coach seeks advantage over another through the efforts of their respective performers. Since performance coaches tend to be evaluated on whether their performers win, there is an incentive to select and train those who are most likely to achieve these goals.

As pressures grow in challenging the limits of human performance so ethical pressures also grow. Critical ethical issues in sport tend to focus on the concept of fair play and how this concept is grounded in sport. Hurka (2007) and Simon (2007) discuss what it is to be a 'good sport' as well as a cheat and offers some guidance in navigating our way through the arguments. Additionally and importantly they encourage the argument that the notion of fairness is embodied in a form of implicit contract or agreement between participating parties. The notion of 'sportsmanship' therefore is one that the coach, as a key 'moral agent', should be central in transmitting, demonstrating and inculcating. Indeed, the notion

of the coach as a form of custodian and transmitter of sports values is one that deserves further attention.

Ethics in practice should be about the demonstration of the moral authority of practitioners in their service to their clients. The moral authority of coaches is grounded in their ability to underwrite the trust placed in them as they guide performers to achieve their goals. McNamee (1998) in his seminal work on the conduct of coaches based his arguments on Koehn's seven conditions for the moral authority of a professional. It is worthwhile reprising these here.

1. The professional must aim at the client's good (whose desires do not simply define that good).
2. The professional must exhibit a willingness to work towards this aim.
3. Such willingness to act thus must continue for as long as is necessary to reach a determination.
4. The professional must be competent (in the appropriate knowledge and skills).
5. The professional must be able to demand from the client (specific appropriate knowledge and performances).
6. The professional must be free to serve the client with discretion (which, as with (1) above, need not be consistent with their desires).
7. The professional must have a highly internalised sense of responsibility (adapted from McNamee 1998 p 149).

Inherent in these conditions is the notion of the trust relationship at the heart of professional practice, and the promotion of good. McNamee (1998) goes on to situate the debate within the requirement of a profession to codify its practice in sets of rules laid out as codes of professional conduct. While putting forward the notion that codes are attempts to arrive at some sort of moral certainty, he suggests that codes define and delimit the actions of professionals. Codes of ethical and professional practice are seen as a form of professional pledge as well as serving to eliminate what McNamee calls 'caprice or arbitrariness' (p 151). However, as McNamee states 'the rule book will not do the work for us' (McNamee 1998 p 160).

Codes of professional conduct and ethical practice

Banks (2004) outlines the purposes of codes from her examination of codes across a range of professions. The common characteristics include statements about the core purposes of the profession, the characteristics or attributes of the professional, ethical rules and principles, principles governing practice, and rules governing practice. These codes seek to claim a level of accountability over the practitioner since with such accountability comes the ability to regulate better the profession, enhance professional identity and enhance status. It also, according to Parrott (2006), makes the practitioner justify actions and counters external criticism.

Codes also assist in determining the extent to which legal redress can be sought. The law often seeks advice from professions as to how they regulate practice and determine standards. However the law, it should be remembered, only operates to a threshold of interest (known as *de minimis non curat lex* – 'the law does not concern itself with trivial matters'). Therefore there is an overlapping relationship between ethics, law and prudence in defining the relevant actions and decisions of sports practitioners. Furthermore, the attempt to arrive at some common consensus of professional standards also has to keep in focus sets of competing rights; the performer, the practitioner and sport more generally. It is these sets of nuanced relationships that can make codes important in the determination of ethical boundaries. They have the potential to identify standards, evaluation criteria, help resolve conflicts and of course set out the boundaries, which, if transgressed, allow organisations to exclude individuals from practice. In addition to setting out what practitioners can do, they also often disallow actions. We also have to acknowledge that a key criticism levelled at codes is that they perhaps encourage a blame culture and a 'compensation mentality' by removing the responsibility for perceived failure from the client to the practitioner.

Banks (2004) is also critical of codes for encouraging a rule-based approach to ethical practice rather than laying out key principles and encouraging the practitioner to engage in reflective thinking about their practice. This is a view McNamee (1998) supports in his criticism that rules seldom take account of differing roles and contexts as well as the difficulties and ambiguities in applying them. Indeed Banks (2004) argues that codes of ethics are a contradiction in terms since ethics are open-ended and are formed as result of a critical deliberation that runs counter to sets of rules that are intended to apply uniformly. The scope, application and interpretation of rules are also problematic. Would sport wish its practitioners merely to follow 'the rules'? This would be a morally impoverished view

of professional practice and remove a key element of the 'professional', which is the capacity to exercise judgement within practice. The scope of codes often includes the extension of their 'reach' into the personal life of the practitioner. The practitioner is expected to uphold the standing of sport both within practice as well as in the varying roles they fulfil within society. This is particularly problematic given that the majority of coaches are not full time and serve on a voluntary basis.

Nevertheless, codes of professional conduct may serve as guidance as well as regulation. The United Kingdom has developed and refined a code governing the activities of those in coaching positions. This is intended to apply to all individuals in a coaching role irrespective of payment or time engaged. The code has developed from a Code of Ethics and Conduct through to its present form of a Code of Practice for Sports Coaches. The Code has four key sections of Rights, Relationships, Personal Responsibilities and Professional Responsibilities (sports coach UK n d).

There remain critical issues relating to the identification of the role and function of the sports practitioner at the heart of developing such codes. First, sport in the UK is in transition, with significantly increased funding for elite sport. This has witnessed the growth of new stratum of sports professionals and practitioners. The extensive range of engagement from volunteers in the community, often possessing high levels of expertise, to full-time employment at national level, demands a code that takes account of these deployments. McNamee (1998) makes a particular point about the capacity and scope of such rules in being able to account correctly and appropriately for the range of such deployments. Second, the interpretation of the coaching role places increasing emphasis and importance on the coach–performer relationship. Thus coaches, in addition to their technical skills, are also expected to be able to engage with performers in a way that encourages them to be advocates. Third, there exists a new relationship into which coaches increasingly have to adjust, namely that of sport support professionals such as sports scientists, physiotherapists, sport psychologists, specialist sports medicine professionals, and so on. The challenges are obvious: promoting legitimacy across such a range of roles and purposes will be problematic for both the individual and the coaching community. Achieving this without a professional body is perhaps reflective of the current stage of professionalisation.

To what extent do codes legitimise the power of professionals? Furthermore, to what extent do codes defend the rights of the practitioners? Clark (2000 p 104) states that 'Professions function in a social and political context that legitimates their operations and organisations.' In sport therefore any code must reflect this legitimacy by emphasising and promoting the craft or expertise of coaches in its social context. It must also operate within the law since any exercise of professional power can only be taken within the legal context within which it resides. Thus legitimacy of practice is reflected by codes that on the one hand regulate to ensure safeguards and militate against abuses of power, and, on the other hand, advocate and promote the authority, competency and expertise of the practitioner. As suggested above there must be some uncertainty about the professional status of sports coaching, and we might ponder whether the code or the appropriate occupational status should come first.

Summary

Parry (1998) suggests that the development of ethical practice in sport has been characterised by a piecemeal approach. Certainly the development of a robust ethical critique of sports practice (if such a thing can be defined) is generally lacking in sport. The notion of what the sports coach is, what coaches stand for, and the nature of the process of coaching from a moral and ethical standpoint demands constant examination. Practice ethics in sport are of importance, not least because of the changing nature and utility of sport but also as sport 'professionalises'. With this professionalisation comes an increasing regulation, scrutiny and accountability for practice that questions the autonomy of the coaching community.

If coaching practice is characterised by the making of ethical decisions, often in relation to and on behalf of others, then coaches need to be able to understand the process of how these decisions should be made. Decisions need to be underpinned by a clear ethical understanding and there is a need to impress upon sports practitioners the danger of purely emotional responses. Ethical frameworks for coaching also give a shared understanding for practitioners. However, it is also essential that coaches examine their own beliefs and values rather than adopt codes of professional conduct unquestioningly. Improved awareness of practice ethics also allows practitioners to explain and justify their action decisions and judgements.

The role and status of sport within society is constantly changing. Outcome orientation in performance sport is important but must be balanced against the process by which we gain such success. This helps balance the ends versus means dilemma that is often evident in elite sport. Being able to exercise judgement as a coaching practitioner demands of the coach an awareness of the issues and a determination of moral actions on the basis of moral values. An understanding of how ethics are constructed, their 'laws' and principles, and how they might be exercised, helps coaches to develop their practice so that it is robust, inclusive and acceptable. As new 'professionals', being able to justify practice is one key hallmark of professional practice and allows us to become more accountable and legitimate. In turn, and as reflective practitioners, coaches can develop ethics-related abilities that validate their practice.

In this respect codes can help but cannot, nor should they ever, replace the exercise of moral judgement in practice. Codes are one way of establishing rules. It is the implementation of these rules that relies on human agency. The capacity of the coaching community to regulate and police itself is important. Without this, it is much more likely that the law will intervene. On the other hand, if the coaching community understands and accepts the importance of ethics, the coaching community will find itself accorded the status and reputation that follows from being able to demonstrate that it works in a morally and ethically sound way.

References

Abraham, A., Collins, D., 1998. Examining and extending research in coach development. Quest 50, 59–79.

Banks, S., 1999. Ethical issues in youth work. Routledge, London.

Banks, S., 2004. Ethics, accountability and the social professions. Palgrave MacMillan, Basingstoke.

Brackenridge, C., 2001. Spoilsports: understanding and preventing sexual exploitation in sport. Routledge, London.

Brackenridge, C., Pitchford, A., Russell, K., et al., 2007. Child welfare in football. Routledge, London.

Brown, W.M., 2003. Personal best. In: Boxill, J. (Ed.), Sports ethics: an anthology. Blackwell, Oxford, pp. 144–152.

Childrens Act, 2004. OPSI. HM Government, London.

Clark, C., 2000. Social work ethics: politics, principles and practice. Palgrave, Basingstoke.

Cross, M., Wood, J., 2005. The personal in ethical decision-making: living with our choices. In: Tribe, R., Morrissey, J. (Eds.), Handbook of professional and ethical practice. Brunner-Routledge, London, pp. 47–59.

Cross, N., Lyle, J., 1999. The coaching process: principles and practice for sport. Butterworth-Heinemann, Oxford.

Hawley, G., 2007. Making decisions that are ethical. In: Hawley, G. (Ed.), Ethics in clinical practice: an interprofessional approach. Pearson, London, pp. 214–241.

Hurka, T., 2007. Games and the good. In: Morgan, W., Meier, K., Schneider, A. (Eds.), Ethics and sport. E&FN Spon, London, pp. 21–34.

Hursthouse, R., 2001. On virtue ethics. OUP, Oxford.

Johnstone, M., 2004. Bioethics: a nursing perspective, third ed. Harcourt Saunders, Sydney.

Jones, C., McNamee, M., 2003. Moral development and sport: character and cognitive developmentalism contrasted. In: Boxill, J. (Ed.), Sports

ethics: an anthology. Blackwell, Oxford, pp. 40–52.

Knowles, Z., Borrie, A., Telfer, H., 2005. Towards the reflective sports coach: issues of context, education and application. Ergonomics 48, 11–14.

Knowles, Z., Tyler, G., Gilbourne, D., et al., 2006. Reflecting on reflection: exploring the practice of sports coaching graduates. Reflective Practice 7, 163–179.

Kohlberg, L., 1981. Essays on moral development, Vol 1. The philosophy of moral development. Jones, C., McNamee, M., 2003. Moral development and sport: Character and cognitive developmentalism contrasted. In: Boxill, J. (Ed.), Sports ethics: an anthology. Blackwell, Oxford, pp. 40–52.

Loland, S., 2002. Fair play in sport: a moral norm system. Routledge, London.

Lyle, J., 1999. Coaching philosophy and coaching behaviour. In: Cross, N., Lyle, J. (Eds.), The coaching process: principles and practice for sport. Butterworth-Heinemann, Oxford, pp. 25–46.

Lyle, J., 2002. Sports coaching concepts: a framework for coaches behaviour. Routledge, Abingdon.

McFee, G., 2004. Sport, rules and values: philosophical investigation into the nature of sport. Routledge, London.

McNamee, M., 1998. Celebrating trust: virtues and rules in the ethical

conduct of sports coaches. In: McNamee, J., Parry, J. (Eds.), Ethics and sport. E&FN Spon, London, pp. 148–168.

National Occupational Standards, 2004. Skills Active, London. Online. Available: http://www.skillsactive. com 21 Aug 2008.

Parrott, L., 2006. Values and ethics in social work practice. Learning Matters, Exeter.

Parry, S.J., 1998. Introduction. In: McNamee, J., Parry, J. (Eds.), Ethics and sport. E&FN Spon, London, pp. xi–xv.

Russell, J., 2007. Broad internalism and the moral foundations of sport. In: Morgan, J. (Ed.), Ethics in sport. second ed. Human Kinetics, Champaign, IL, pp. 51–66.

Safeguarding Vulnerable Persons Act, 2006. OPSI. HM Government, London.

Shields, D., Bredemeier, B., 1995. Character development and physical activity. Human Kinetics, Champaign, IL.

Sim, J., 1997. Ethical decision making in therapy practice. Butterworth-Heinemann, Oxford.

sports coach UK, no date. Code of Practice. sports coach UK, Leeds.

Simon, R.L., 2007. Internalism and internal values in sport. In: Morgan, K., Meier, K., Schneider, A. (Eds.), Ethics and sport. E&FN Spon, London, pp. 35–50.

Coaches' expertise

Paul G. Schempp and Bryan McCullick

'Leaders are made, they are not born. They are made by hard effort,
which is the price which all of us must pay to achieve any goal that is worthwhile'

Vince Lombardi, American Football Coach

Introduction

To even the most casual spectator, the superior athlete is readily distinguishable from their less-accomplished counterparts. Superior athletes simply go about the task of sport performance at a higher level of proficiency and with consistently greater results. Superior athletes, in the main, are faster, stronger, better skilled and demonstrate remarkable judgement. But turn your eye to the coaches on either side of the pitch or court, and it is far more challenging to detect the subtleties that characterise coaches who consistently outperform their coaching peers.

It is important to understand the differences between those who find ways to guide their athletes to success time after time, and those who do not. In recent years, a growing body of research has contributed greatly to identifying the characteristics, skill, and knowledge that distinguish the great from the good in coaching. Research has, for example, revealed that expert coaches see things differently from the less expert (Woorons 2001); but *what* exactly do they see? Research also reveals that expert coaches can, for the most part, say the right thing to the right player at the right time (Webster 2006), but *how* do they know *what* to say and *when*

to say it? The results achieved by expert coaches over time suggest that, in the main, they know when and how to make the decisions that lead an athlete or a team to success, but do we understand *how* expert coaches make decisions? In this chapter, we will explore the traits of expert coaches identified by systematic, scholarly inquiry (Gilbert et al 2006, Schempp et al 2006b). From this work, three elements consistently emerge as contributing to the expertise of a coach: (a) experience, (b) knowledge, and (c) skills. These three elements will, therefore, comprise the main structure of this chapter.

Expert coaches' experience

There is no substitute for experience when it comes to developing expertise. Simply put, no one achieves expertise in coaching without substantial experience. There is no empirical evidence to support the notion that an inexperienced coach can consistently outperform a coach with extensive experience. To the contrary, research has repeatedly revealed that it takes extensive experience – a minimum of 10 years in most fields – to reach the level of expert (e.g. Ericsson 1998). While it takes more than just experience, clearly one cannot become expert without substantial experience in one's craft. It is in these experiences, and as a result of these experiences, that skills and knowledge unite to define the coach's level of competence and performance. To be considered an expert coach, one must prove it in the practical experience of coaching. Put another way, one's record of success and failure is forged in the experiences one has as a coach, and, by definition, the best coaches have established the best records by consistently outperforming their peers over time (Tan 1997).

However, experience provides something more than a means by which to exercise skill and knowledge. Experience offers an unparalleled opportunity to learn. All too often, however, coaches ignore the lessons offered by their experiences and simply repeat, again and again, the same ineffective patterns of performance. Coaches who consistently reach the pinnacle of successful do so, in large part, because they have mastered the skill of learning from their experiences – and from the experiences of others (Vickers 2008). This process means that by thoughtfully analysing the events of their experiences outstanding coaches identify what they did well and what could be improved (Schempp et al 2007). Put another way, outstanding coaches continually evaluate and critique the quality of their performance to search for what might be improved in their coaching practice. Knowing what was good (or rather, effective) and what could be done better are equally important, for both suggest insights that can lead to improved performances. Perhaps as a reflection of their limited practical experience, novices find 'real world' experience to be their most important source of information for increasing expertise (Schempp 2003). Like novices, expert coaches embrace the lessons they learn from experience, but unlike novices, they realise that there are other sources that are equally valuable for increasing skill, knowledge and performance. We will return to this in the next two sections of the chapter.

A greater diversity of coaching experiences (e.g. different people, situations, purposes) offers even more benefits (Schempp 2003). Different experiences represent opportunities to apply skills and knowledge in unique and untested ways. When a coach modifies and adapts her or his skills to meet the changing environmental demands, those coaching skills become stronger and more robust. Likewise, when a coach works through the challenges of different athletes, opponents, competitive demands and the like, the deeper their knowledge base grows. In essence, there is a clear relationship between experience and knowledge; indeed, from experience comes knowledge.

Experience alone, however, will neither increase expertise nor improve a coach's record of success. This point is made clear by Dr. Anders Ericsson (Ericsson et al 2006), arguably the world's leading scholar on developing expertise, when he writes:

Improvement in performance of aspiring experts does not happen automatically or casually as a function of further experience. Improvements are caused by changes in cognitive mechanisms mediating how the brain and nervous system control performance and in the degree of adaptation of physiological systems of the body. The principal challenge to attaining expert level performance is to induce stable specific changes that allow the performance to be incrementally improved.
(2006 p 698)

In other words, it is deliberate, systematic and continual change that brings about the improvements leading to expert performance. Experience is a critical, but clearly not a singular key to developing expertise (Ericsson et al 2006). In addition to extensive experience, great coaches share two other characteristics: extensive knowledge and highly developed coaching skills. In the next section, we will explore the knowledge of an expert coach.

Expert coaches' knowledge

While it perhaps seems obvious that an expert coach has an extensive knowledge base, the importance of this characteristic to their success demands that it be scrutinised thoroughly. There are many lessons for developing coaches in knowing what an expert knows – and how they came to know it. Experts make a significant investment in learning all they can about their subject, their athletes and their coaching (Schempp et al 1998a, 1999). Attend coaching workshops, clinics or conferences, and you will be likely to see expert coaches there. Many of the experts will be the presenters, but experts also attend as learners. This may seem counterintuitive but we know from our study of these extraordinary coaches that while it appears experts are the least likely to benefit from attending a workshop, they become expert because they seldom pass up opportunities to learn – from anyone, at any time, and anywhere. This point was pressed upon us in a study with the highly successful American football coach Bobby Bowden. After listening to another coach for a lengthy period of time, coach Bowden was asked why he listened so intently to someone who was not nearly as accomplished as himself. His reply was 'You never know where the next great idea is going to come from' (Vickers 2008).

In contrast, those who fail to achieve the experts' level of competence are the ones who stop reading, going to workshops or talking with colleagues because they believe they 'pretty much know every-thing there is to know.' Further buttressing this notion of 'continual improvement' is the research suggesting that expert coaches monitor their prog-ress consistently and vigilantly by setting goals for their performance and concocting strategies to achieve those goals (Schempp et al 2006, 2007).

Sources of knowledge

Experts enjoy talking almost endlessly about their subject, gather others' views on pertinent topics, and have compiled extensive libraries devoted to their subject (Ericsson & Charness 1994). This enables them to assemble a large store of knowl-edge. Experience and other coaches have been most often identified as important sources of knowledge; but books, workshops, certification programmes, journals and magazines, athletic experiences and even athletes have been identified as important sources for coaches' knowledge (Fincher & Schempp 1994, Schempp et al 1999). Walk into a coach's office and look at her or his library. If there are no, or few, books to be found, it isn't likely that the person who works there is an expert. They may be good at what they do, but they are not at the top of their profession.

What may be surprising about some of the books on expert coaches' shelves is that they are likely to have come from other areas that, on the surface, appear to be less relevant to coaching. However, having learned the lessons of experience, proficient coaches look to sources outside their own coaching for fresh information. Other coaches and resources like conferences, books, videotapes and the like are important sources of information for these coaches (Schempp 2006). Experts are sponges when it comes to absorbing new knowledge. Less-expert coaches are satisfied with what they know. To stop learning is to stop getting better. Experts know that.

Types of knowledge

In his research with teachers, Shulman (1987) found that teachers have specific categories or types of knowledge. Shulman's typology of teachers' knowledge identified seven forms of knowledge needed for teaching. These included knowledge of their subject, learners, learning environment, pur-poses, curriculum, pedagogy, and a special form of knowledge uniquely the province of a teacher:

pedagogical content knowledge. Like teachers, coaches appear to have specific types of knowledge necessary for guiding their decisions and actions. In our research on expert coaches, we found that they possess extensive knowledge of their sport, their players, and coaching (Schempp et al 1998, Schempp 2006). It is these three types of knowledge that allow them to convey their sport knowledge to their players efficiently and effectively in order to achieve maximum performance from their athletes (DeMarco & McCullick 1997).

Skilled coaches are able to synthesise their knowledge about a skill or sport into meaningful information for athletes to comprehend and apply (Siedentop & Eldar 1989). By having an extensive knowledge base, coaches have at their disposal an array of options when presenting information intended to promote athletes' skill, knowledge and performance (Bian 2003). Due to their extensive knowledge base, it is the expert coach that recog-nises when a player misunderstands an initial expla-nation and can then offer alternative explanations, demonstrations, training aid, or other communica-tion strategies. Coaches with less expertise, and consequently, less knowledge, often find themselves restricted to far fewer options for conveying infor-mation (Woorons 2001, Bian 2003).

The superior knowledge of expert coaches allows them to use their coaching environment (i.e. equip-ment, facilities, and resources) to greater effect than can the less-expert coach. For example, they demonstrate greater flexibility in using equipment to facilitate athletes' learning (Housner & Griffey 1985). They know different ways of using the same equipment for multiple purposes. A broom handle might, for example, be used by an expert coach for a fitness activity, a target, training aid, or some other creative purpose. The novice would likely see the broom handle as simply a broom handle. Perhaps the famous words of Robert Kennedy assist us in expressing this notion better: 'There are those who look at things the way they are, and ask why . . . I dream of things that never were, and ask why not?' Knowing that he was 'ahead of his time', we can only surmise that Senator Kennedy was referring to his expertise when he said this.

Despite knowing more about their sport, their athletes or coaching than virtually anyone, experts do not see themselves as knowing everything. Rather, they recognise that there is still a great deal to learn and new knowledge is continually available. When expert coaches come across information with which they are unfamiliar, they take measures to gain an understanding of the area and seek ways in which it may benefit them or their athletes (Schempp et al 1998b). In fact, they take pains to talk with people who are experts on topics outside their own coaching expertise, read pertinent material and even work on developing new coaching skills. Experts know the importance of information that can be brought to bear on their success.

Developing strategic knowledge

Strategic knowledge allows expert coaches to distinguish the important from the unimportant when observing an athlete's performance (Chi et al 1988, Ericsson et al 2006). In strategic knowledge, the ultimate goal or 'bigger picture' is placed before short-term goals and everyday rules. This knowledge permits the expert coach to use tactics such as ignoring or flexing standard rules and traditions as the situation dictates. A coach may, for example, overlook a player missing practice due to a family emergency and thus break the 'no missing practice' rule, if the emergency and circumstance warrants the pardon. A coach with less experience or expertise would be likely to enforce the rule 'because it is a rule' and thereby damage both team morale and player loyalty.

Beginning coaches are schooled to keep feedback positive in order to create a 'positive' atmosphere and bolster an athlete's self-esteem (Martens 2004). Following this principle, new coaches may be heard uttering 'good job', 'nice try' and other well meaning but instructionally worthless responses to player efforts. Because a 'positive' atmosphere or an athlete's self-esteem may not necessarily represent the ultimate prize to the expert coach who strives for performance over emotion, feedback may take a different form and matter. The expert coach knows that praise in certain circumstances may actually communicate low expectations and there are times when constructive criticism serves as more effective feedback in prompting a superior athletic performance (Berliner 1994). Again, strategic knowledge provides the expert coach with the wisdom to know what to say and when to say it.

To acquire strategic coaching knowledge requires a combination of coaching experience and knowledge of athletes, sport, and coaching (Schempp et al 1999, Schempp 2003). It is in the trial and error of coaching experience and the constant pursuit of new information to improve oneself as a coach that strategic knowledge is incubated and grown. Beginners who do these three things will develop strategic knowledge: (a) gain experience, (b) use reflective practices about their coaching to learn all they can from their experiences, and (c) experiment with different decisions to see their results while accepting that some will produce failure or, at least, little success (Schempp et al 2006b). An examination of expert coaches' careers usually reveals that success was not immediate and some relative failure typically preceded success. It is by experimenting with coaching practices and seeking information to spur coaching improvement that a coach becomes skilled in knowing what to do and when to do it – strategic knowledge.

Expert coaches' skills

While knowledge provides the foundation for the expert coach's decisions, a second factor that sets them apart from those with less expertise is the skill set they employ in their coaching practices (DeMarco & McCullick 1997, Schempp et al 2006b). In other words, it is both what they know and what they do that defines the expert coach. Expert coaching is thus comprised of large quantities of experience, knowledge and skill (Dodds 1994, DeMarco & McCullick 1997, Martens 2004). In this section, we focus on the skills of the expert coach, but before doing so we offer one note of caution – do not confuse skills with characteristics. Many tend to believe that what a coach *does* is the same as the type of person a coach *is*. This should be of some comfort to those aspiring to increase their expertise, as skills can be learned whereas personality traits are much more difficult to change.

Planning

Expert coaches recognise that being fully prepared to perform at peak levels requires thoughtful and extensive planning. Success in sport happens by design, not by accident. Even with extensive years of experience, experts are aware of the need to devise detailed practice plans in order to meet their target goals. American football coach, Bobby Bowden, plans each practice thoroughly, places an outline of that practice on one side of an index card, which he places in his back pocket. As practice progresses, he pulls the card out for reference, and turns it over to make notes to discuss various parts of the practice with his coaches when practice concludes. Bowden considers his planning skills a prerequisite to coaching success (Smith 2004).

A beginning coach or, for that matter, any coach who believes he or she can coach well without planning is much like the person who enters an unfamiliar city without a map and sees no need to ask directions to his or her destination. At best, they waste a great deal of time in reaching their destination and at worse, they never get where they intended to go. While planning may seem like a tedious and unnecessary task to a coach who has conducted similar practices many times throughout his or her career, it is reassuring to be reminded that planning becomes less tedious as experience grows (Schempp 2003).

Predict outcomes

At times, the predictive skills of expert coaches make it appear that they have a crystal ball to forecast the future. Research has found that experts do have predictive skills, but it is not because they have a crystal ball or magical powers. Rather, these coaches are extraordinarily skilled at recognising similarities across situations, and because they have seen similar situations time and again, they can predict potential outcomes of unfolding events with a high degree of accuracy and precision (McCullick et al 2006). This was demonstrated in a study of expert teachers who were asked to view a series of slides of classroom events and comment about what they were thinking (Carter et al 1988). The teachers provided rich commentaries about their observations, and drew upon their own experiences to make judgements about what they viewed. The teachers 'made many assumptions about what they saw, appeared to be looking for the meaning of events portrayed in slides in this task, inferred relationships between actions and situations in the slides' (Carter et al 1988 p 28). Expert coaches, like expert teachers, possess predictive skills as was found in research on coaches in tennis (Woorons 2001), swimming (Leas & Chi 1993) and volleyball (Bian 2003).

A skill that provides the expert with an advantage over other coaches is the ability to analyse a situation with the thought 'if I do this, then this will likely happen, but if I do that then this will likely happen.' This ability to have contingency plans ready to go if needed is a step in decision making that coaches with less expertise never take (Fincher 1996). The less-skilled coach normally acts on the strategy or solution that first popped into their head, or that they have used before – even if previously the results were mediocre. The ability to predict potential outcomes proves to be useful for the expert coach in selecting activities because only those practice activities and game strategies with the greatest chance of success are selected (Leas & Chi 1993).

How does a coach develop the skill of predicting likely outcomes? First, it takes years of coaching experience. Having seen situations and events occur time and again and having analysed the outcomes of their decisions over years gives the expert coach insight into which decisions and actions stand the greatest chance of success and why they are likely to be successful. As with experts in any field, constant experimentation, reflecting on past decisions and actions, networking with other coaches and a passion for always trying to find a better solution to coaching challenges leads to a coach developing predictive skills (Ericsson et al 2006). As one grows more familiar with the situations continually encountered in the coaching environment, the more often one is able to test the veracity of solutions and strategies used in meeting the demands found in that environment.

Intuitive decision making

As coaches increase their proficiency, instructional routines become so familiar that coaches respond instinctively to a situation rather than having to give the situation careful and rational analysis before coming to a decision (Smith 2004). At this point intuition is developing and is gaining prominence in the coaches' decision-making. The coach no longer has to consciously consider every action they take, and therefore their coaching activities take on a natural fluidity and timing. Intuitive decision making stands as a major divide between the expert and less expert (Berliner 1994, Ericsson et al 2006). Experts use an intuition polished by years of experience and founded upon extensive knowledge to make many of their decisions. They get 'gut feelings' and have the confidence to go with those feelings – even if those feelings run counter to accepted logic or convention (Smith 2004). This would be a dangerous practice for beginning, or perhaps even competent, coaches but it is a standard operating procedure for the expert.

Through the continual analysis of the flow of events in a practice or game expert coaches can select from a large repertoire of possible actions that will have the largest impact on player performance (Woorons 2001). Because coaches are intimately familiar with their environment and can call on a large knowledge store (McCullick et al 2006), they identify critical cues as situations develop. These critical cues trigger the intuitive responses and actions. It is much like driving a car. After a significant number of hours behind the wheel of a car, one does not consciously have to consider which foot to use to depress the brake pedal or even give thought to the location of the brake pedal. The response is instinctive and when certain environmental cues arise, like a pedestrian stepping into the path of the car, the braking process begins instinctively. Similarly, expert coaches are skilled in reading pertinent cues, anticipating likely events and responding to shifting conditions in player performances (Woorons 2001, Bian 2003).

Communication

A recent study highlights important differences between expert and novice teachers from a communication perspective (Webster 2006). Perhaps in concert with their extensive knowledge of their athletes, experts approached coaching communication with the intent to individualise instruction (Jones 2006). In contrast, novice coaches focused mostly on using behaviours that, while proven to be effective, were not necessarily player-centred but were reflective of their self-concern for clarity rather than student understanding. Further, expert coaches expressed more concern for the effectiveness of their communication than did novices. The substantially higher number of expert concerns suggested that the experts placed a higher priority on communication effectiveness than did novice coaches. The central theme of the novices' communication concerns indicated a strong focus on finding ways to help the student understand the lesson content from the coach's perspective. Conversely, the experts' concerns centred on seeking to understand ways to communicate more effectively based on

their understanding of the player's perspective. The communication challenge, as the expert coaches saw it, was to develop the level of empathy that allowed them to find ways into players' shoes and select communication strategies or techniques on the players' terms (Webster 2006).

Automatic coaching behaviour

The intuitive decision making and well-honed communication skills of expert coaches give their actions a fast, fluid, and natural appearance (Berliner 1994, Smith 2004). Extensive experience and constant practice to improve coaching skills such as communication are important prerequisites in developing coaching behaviour that is automatic. Most often, it is the daily routines of an expert's coaching practice that become automatic – performed regularly with little or no conscious thought (Baker et al 1998). These routines are the repetitive activities that seemingly occur with little planning, practice or forethought. The automatic behaviour of an expert is attributable to their ability to identify information early and respond quickly (Siedentop & Eldar 1989). The analysis of expert coaches' working memory has revealed that when shown a picture that is of a familiar situation, he or she responds not only with a high volume of recall but that the recall includes what appears to be the most relevant information from the picture (McCullick et al 2006).

As previously mentioned, it is in the routine tasks of coaching that automatic behaviour is most quickly identified (or developed for aspiring coaches). Perfunctory duties such as practice openings, closings, demonstrations, explanations, practice activities, player movement, equipment distribution and even interactions with athletes are often performed with what seems like little effort, but achieve remarkable results. Coaches seeking to raise their level of expertise should look to the routines they currently use, or consider developing routines that allow for more coaching time and less administrating or organising time during practice or a game.

The atypical gets attention

When observing an expert coach in action, whether it is in practice or during competition, it is often to watch a person who appears to be casually observing the scene. In reality, the coach is comfortable if the observed events unfold as s/he would anticipate (recall the previously mentioned skill, 'predicting outcomes'). What moves the expert to respond is when s/he detects an anomaly; something atypical has happened and the coach seizes the opportunity for action. On the radar screens of expert coaches, it is the atypical that causes blips to occur, and action to follow. For example, a tennis coach may spot something a bit different in a player's stroke. Upon closer inspection and analysis, the coach connects the anomaly with other differences in the swing and immediately begins a plan of action or actions to correct the defect (Woorons 2001).

Similarly, Carter and colleagues (1988) found that expert teachers assess events as either typical or atypical, and that the assessment of typicality affected the way experts processed information. When the situation was assessed as 'typical', experts passively let the event unfold. When the situation appeared 'atypical', experts worked to make sense of the anomalies and then take appropriate action. While observing a basketball practice, for example, an elbow out of line with the body when shooting free throws may strike the coach as not typical for that particular player. Once the 'atypical' action is spotted, the expert coach then seeks to discover its cause and take appropriate action. In this particular case, the coach might suggest to the player that s/he keep the elbow in front of them during their shot to gain greater accuracy and consistency. What did not happen was the coach assessing every aspect of the player's shooting technique in the search for improvements. Rather, a casual observation led to detecting the atypical and a response followed.

It is when the atypical event is recognised by the expert that they take action – normally a corrective action. A study of expert coaches revealed that they often perceive themselves to be 'repair people' (McCullick et al 1999). That is, they find a fault and fix it. More specifically, a swim coach may be monitoring athletes swimming their required warm-up laps. For a while, nothing seems out of the ordinary. Then the coach recognises that one particular swimmer is lifting her arm out of the water at a different angle than is normal for that swimmer. After seeing this pattern repeated once or twice, the coach steps to the swimmer to ask about the arm. Perhaps it is an injury, or the athlete's attempt to improve form, or they may be completely unaware of the action. The coach can then respond to the new information and 'repair' the problem. It

is the intimate and substantial familiarity with their environment and their athletes that permits the expert to know what is typical and what is atypical.

When tending to the atypical, experts draw upon their extensive and highly organized knowledge to efficiently and economically sift the information to determine their next set of actions (Woorons 2001, Bian 2003). When things are working in a normal pattern, however, they tend not to reflect on what is occurring, but rather simply monitor the process until something seems out of the ordinary. The skill of attending to the atypical permits the coach to reserve both energy and time, but still allows them to identify and respond to the critical aspects of performance – and often with a great deal more accuracy than less-expert coaches.

Solving problems

Every coach faces many challenges, on many levels, with many issues. However, the quality of the solutions derived is noticeably different between the expert coach and the less expert. Research has uncovered, at least in part, the problem-solving skills of experts that lead them to superior solutions (Ericsson et al 2006). First, experts invest more time identifying, defining, and analysing a problem before searching for a solution than do people with less expertise. They realise if they don't get the problem right, there is no hope of getting the solution right.

While experts may, at times, be slower than novices in the early stages of problem solving (i.e. time spent on analysing the problem is longer for experts), it seems time well spent as experts may still ultimately solve problems faster than novices and they solve them with greater accuracy and permanency (Chi et al 1981). In other words, when experts solve problems (or 'repair' a fault), those problems tend to stay solved. In contrast, less-expert coaches often guess a solution, try it, declare 'It doesn't work!' and move on to another ill-founded solution. To them, time is of the essence, whereas experts believe that accuracy is what matters most. When it comes to winning a gold medal at the Olympic Games, which do you think matters most, how quickly a coach offers a solution or how appropriate and accurate the solution is? You can answer that one, and see it manifested in elite sport each day.

One way in which the expert takes greater care in solving problems is by spending more time gathering all the facts before making decisions or attempting solutions (Chi et al 1981, Bell 1997). It always seems that quick decisive action is a trait (or skill) that many see as a mark of a good leader. However, 'haste makes waste' and experts know this. When it comes to coaching athletes, whether elite or youth, waste is not a word with which anyone would like to be associated. Consider this example; expert coaches will spend significant time analysing the problem, attempting to identify all facets and components of the situation in an effort to link specific occurrences in coaching to the purpose or goals of the player or team. In solving routine problems, expert problem-solvers tend to work 'forward' from known facts to the unknown solution. Interestingly, people with lower levels of expertise tend to work 'backwards' in their reasoning. That is, they see a problem and a solution comes to mind almost immediately. They then tend to work backward from the solution using the facts to justify their initial solution. Those facts that don't fit the solution are often discarded as irrelevant (Patel & Groen 1991).

In contrast, the expert has learned that assembling all facts first, and linking them into a logical order will allow them to understand the full nature of the problem, and then derive a solution. In other words, they collect and examine each fact pertaining to the problem and think 'forward' to a solution. For example, an expert basketball coach may notice that one of their players appears to be putting little effort into the game. He or she then begins to recall the player during the previous practices, takes note of any unusual actions by the player (e.g. limping or harsh words with teammates), or any other 'atypical' action on the part of the player. The coach may then pull the player from the game, give them a brief rest, and then question them a bit in search of information that might explain their lack of hustle in the game. Once all the information possible has been collected, the coach plans a solution to the problem of the player's lack of effort. A novice coach, upon noticing the lack of effort by the player, immediately decides to pull the player from the game for not hustling. The solution is then justified by recalling examples of a lack of effort during practice and warm ups. The player is then pulled from the game and banished to the bench with a few harsh words with the real reasons for the lack of effort never really known to the coach.

Self-monitoring

Becoming an expert is the result of learning and exerting conscious effort toward applying what is learned to improve coaching performance (Cassidy et al 2009). And when one becomes expert, it does not mean the learning stops. If it does, the expert today will become a 'has-been' tomorrow and replaced by those who continue the pursuit of knowledge and skills. In our research with expert coaches, we've often heard the self-critique 'Just because I know more than most people about coaching this sport, doesn't mean I know everything there is to know' (e.g. Smith 2004). There is an interesting phenomenon in coaching; less-expert coaches often have a great deal more confidence in their knowledge and actions than do the experts. It seems experts are far better at recognising the limits of their knowledge and skills, are more analytical and critical of the quality of their coaching, and have such passion for what they do that they want to be better tomorrow than they are today – regardless of any success or awards they may have already achieved (Schempp et al 1998b).

One exemplar of this trait is seen in a study including Bobby Bowden (Smith 2004), the 'most winning' collegiate American football coach in the United States. During an interview, coach Bowden was asked to speculate on how much he knew about coaching American football, he responded with, "Aww, about 60%" (Smith 2004 p 197). What is missing from that comment is the context. Coach Bowden responded with that answer without false modesty and in an instant after it was asked. He did not need to think about it nor was he mindful that he should not 'brag' on his knowledge. It was a completely genuine answer to a question one would suspect would have elicited an answer such as, 'Well, I've been around a long time, I don't think there is anything I haven't seen before...'.

In a recent study, expert coaches reported that they closely and extensively monitor the things they do well and the things that believe they can do better (Schempp et al 2007). These coaches identified both goals and actions in their self-monitoring strategies. Specifically, they monitored their communication skills, personal lifestyle, coaching perspectives, and knowledge. The result of this monitoring led to actions to improve their performance. They reported plans to seek help from others, read, use more technology, and modify coaching practices. Self-monitoring was a skill these experts developed to identify specific areas for improvement, as well as undertaken strategies that would lead to achieving their goals of improving their coaching performance.

Perceptual skills

It would be easy to believe that expert coaches see things the rest of us do not; but it appears that they see the same things we see, but they interpret what they see differently (Woorons 2001). Specifically, they are able to discern the important from the unimportant in what they see while to the rest of us it all looks pretty much the same. Evidence would suggest that with both extensive knowledge and experience, the expert coach detects subtleties in the sport environment that have significant importance to the events taking place. They recognise when something is not working in a player's performance, a practice session or a game.

There are several keys to developing the perceptual skills of an expert coach. First, coaching must be viewed as a dynamic process where many athletes are simultaneously engaged in activities in a practice session or game. Keeping the whole team or other players interested and on task is important, but the challenge comes in focusing on individual performance. It is here the previously discussed skill of 'attending to the atypical' comes into play. The expert coach has the perceptual capacity to attend to individual player performance while monitoring the entire practice or game. Beginners and competent coaches do not seem to have developed this skill (Housner & Griffey 1985). Because they can observe the athletes individually, experts can meet the needs of every player and realise that athletes will be at differing skill levels.

Second, experts are able to sort the important from the unimportant in their observations (Woorons 2001). For example, a beginning coach may notice a player's dress, choice of equipment, or friends, while experts see, but overlook, extraneous factors that don't directly bear on athletes' performance. They thus devote more attention to player performances and lock tightly on the key components that most affect the player's performance. By identifying the critical components in a player's performance they can supply the information and promote activities that will contribute the biggest improvement in the player in the shortest amount of time (Woorons 2001). They are able to

do this because as they observe, they are continually asking themselves the question 'What will increase this player's or team's performance?' Searching for answers to that question helps the expert perceive and recognise the factors most needing her or his attention.

While observing their athletes' performances, less-expert coaches often see the symptoms of mediocre or poor performance (McCullick et al 1999, Bian 2003). The expert, with the advantage of superior knowledge and experience, sees past the symptoms and identifies the cause of errors or inferior player performance. Once the cause has been identified, it is far easier to supply the appropriate cure. Less-expert coaches flounder in futile attempts to cure all the symptoms she or he sees, while the expert efficiently sets about curing the cause, which in turn takes care of the symptoms. This point was made clear in a study of the professional orientations of the *Top 100 Golf Instructors in America* (McCullick et al 1999). One of the experts in the study reported that:

> If someone is slicing the ball because they are swinging over the top, I try to figure out why they are over the top versus just telling them to swing more inside . . . every mistake or swing fault has a reason, when you fix a problem at its cause you can really help someone progress. (1999 p 18)

Coaches can speed the development of their perceptual skills by attempting to identify the environmental cues that are most pertinent to a player's performance. Like any coaching skill, it takes deliberate practice to develop one's perceptual skills. Remember, the simple accumulation of experience will not result in an increase in coaching expertise, it must be thoughtful and consciously done.

Concluding comments

Expert coaches are measured by one standard: a consistent and superior performance in athletic competition. Expert coaches do not necessarily reveal signs of being any more intelligent than other coaches, nor do they necessarily appear to be devoting more effort than others during their performance – at times they even seem surprisingly relaxed. However, appearances can be deceiving. As we have discussed here, the expert coach's skills and knowledge are extensive, complex, and earned in years of experience, deliberate practice, and the drive to always learn more. The path toward coaching expertise is one that anyone can pursue. It is not attained through birthrights, or a product of an innate quality or characteristic. We can say that any coach can become a *more-expert* coach.

Research has consistently revealed that by identifying clear goals, undertaking the practice of important coaching skills, and learning all that can be learned from one's experiences and from others, coaching can and does improve.

References

Baker, K., Schempp, P., Hardin, B., 1998. The rituals and routines of expert golf instruction. Science and golf III: proceedings of the World Scientific Congress of Golf. Human Kinetics, Champaign, IL.

Bell, M., 1997. The development of expertise. Journal of Sport, Recreation and Dance 68 (2), 34–38.

Berliner, D.C., 1994. Expertise: the wonder of exemplary performances. In: Mangieri, J., Block, C. (Eds.), Creating powerful thinking in coaches and athletes: diverse perspectives. Harcourt Brace College, Fort Worth, TX, pp. 161–186.

Bian, W., 2003. Examination of expert and novice volleyball coaches' diagnostic abilities. Unpublished doctoral dissertation, University of Georgia, Athens.

Carter, K., Cushing, K., Sabers, D., et al., 1988. Expert – novice differences in perceiving and processing visual classroom stimuli. Journal of Coach Education 39 (3), 25–31.

Cassidy, T., Jones, R., Potrac, P., 2009. Understanding sports coaching: the social, cultural and pedagogical foundations of coaching practice, second ed. Routledge, London.

Chi, M.T.H., Feltovich, P., Glaser, R., 1981. Categorization and representation of physics problems by experts and novices. Cognitive Science 5, 121–152.

Chi, M., Galser, R., Farr, M. (Eds.), 1988. The nature of expertise. Erlbaum, Hillsdale, NJ.

DeMarco, G., McCullick, B., 1997. Developing coaching expertise: learning from the legends. Journal of Physical Education, Recreation and Dance 68 (3), 37–41.

Dodds, P., 1994. Cognitive and behavioral components of expertise in teaching physical education. Quest 46, 143–163.

Ericsson, K.A., 1998. The road to excellence. Lawrence Erlbaum Associates, New Jersey.

Ericsson, K.A., Charness, N., 1994. Expert performance: its structure and acquisition. Am. Psychol. 49, 725–747.

Ericsson, K.A., Charness, N., Feltovich, P., et al., 2006. The Cambridge handbook of expertise and expert performance. Cambridge University Press, Cambridge.

Fincher, M., 1996. Major league hitting instruction: An expert act. Unpublished doctoral dissertation, University of Georgia, Athens, GA.

Fincher, M., Schempp, P., 1994. Teaching physical education: What do we need to know and how do we find it? GAHPERD Journal 28 (3), 7–10.

Gilbert, W., Cote, J., Mallett, C., 2006. Developmental paths and activities of successful sport coaches. International Journal of Sports Science & Coaching 1, 69–76.

Housner, L.D., Griffey, D., 1985. Teacher cognition: Differences in planning and interactive decision making between experienced and inexperienced teachers. Res. Q. Exerc. Sport 56, 44–53.

Jones, R., 2006. The sports coach as educator: reconceptualising sports coaching. Routledge, London.

Leas, R.R., Chi, T.H.M., 1993. Analyzing diagnostic expertise of competitive swimming coaches. In: Starkes, J.L., Allard, F. (Eds.), Cognitive issues in motor expertise. Elsevier Science Publishers, New York, pp. 75–94.

Martens, R., 2004. Successful coaching. Human Kinetics Publisher, Champaign, IL.

McCullick, B.A., Cumings, R.L., Schempp, P.G., 1999. The professional orientations of expert

golf instructors. International Journal of Physical Education 36, 15–24.

McCullick, B., Schempp, P., Hsu, S., et al., 2006. An analysis of the working memory of expert sport instructors. Journal of Teaching in Physical Education 25, 149–165.

Patel, V.L., Groen, G.J., 1991. The general and specific nature of medical expertise: a critical look. In: Ericsson, K.A., Smith, J. (Eds.), Toward a general theory of expertise. Cambridge University Press, Cambridge, pp. 93–125.

Schempp, P.G., 2003. Teaching sport and physical activity. Human Kinetics, Champaign, IL.

Schempp, P.G., 2006. Where experts find answers. In: American Society for Training and Development Research-to-Practice Conference Proceedings. Alexandria, VA, pp.143–152.

Schempp, P.G., Tan, S., Manross, D., et al., 1998a. Differences in novice and competent coaches' knowledge. Teachers and Teaching: Theory and Practice 4 (1), 9–20.

Schempp, P.G., Manross, D., Tan, S., et al., 1998b. Subject expertise and teachers' knowledge. Journal of Teaching Physical Education 17 (3), 342–356.

Schempp, P.G., Templeton, C., Clark, E., 1999. The knowledge acquisition of expert golf instructors. In: Farrally, M.R., Cochran, A.J. (Eds.), Science and golf III: proceedings of the World Scientific Congress of Golf. Human Kinetics, Champaign, IL, pp. 295–301.

Schempp, P.G., McCullick, B.A., Busch, C.A., et al., 2006a. The self-monitoring of expert sport instructors. International Journal of Sport Science & Coaching 1, 25–36.

Schempp, P.G., McCullick, B.A., Mason, I., 2006b. The development of expert coaching. In: Jones, R.L.

(Ed.), The sports coach as educator: reconceptualising sports coaching. Routledge, London, pp. 145–161.

Schempp, P.G., Webster, C., McCullick, B., et al., 2007. How the best get better: an analysis of the self-monitoring strategies used by expert golf instructors. Sport, Education & Society 12, 175–192.

Shulman, L.S., 1987. Knowledge and teaching: foundations of the new reform. Harvard Educational Review 57 (1), 1–22.

Siedentop, D., Eldar, E., 1989. Expertise, experience, and effectiveness. Journal of Teaching Physical Education 8 (3), 254–260.

Smith, M., 2004. Stories from sidelines past: A story of coach Bobby Bowden. Unpublished doctoral dissertation, The University of Georgia, Athens, GA.

Tan, S., 1997. The elements of expertise. Journal of Physical Education, Recreation, and Dance 68 (2), 30–33.

Vickers, J., 2008. Peer interactions throughout coach development. Paper presented at the American Alliance for Health, Physical Education, Recreation and Dance annual convention, Fort Worth, TX.

Webster, C.A., 2006. A comparison of expert and novice golf instructors' from a communication perspective. Unpublished doctoral dissertation, The University of Georgia, Athens, GA, USA.

Woorons, S., 2001. An analysis of expert and novice tennis instructors' perceptual capacities. Unpublished doctoral dissertation, University of Georgia, Athens, GA, USA.

Coaching philosophy

16

Simon Jenkins

Introduction

All coaches will have developed a personal set of views on coaching, interpersonal relationships, and on issues relevant to their sport. These views will have evolved over time and will be derived from a range of practical and educational experiences. What coaches do in their practice and how they do it will be shaped by these views (Cushion 2006, Cassidy et al 2009). Importantly, these views or personal principles and values are attributes that comprise a coaching philosophy (Cassidy et al 2009). It is widely accepted that the articulation of a coaching philosophy is a means to understanding and developing coaching practice, and this 'reflective' exercise is part of most coach development programmes (Cassidy et al 2009). However, there remains a lack of engagement with this process, and this in part is due to what Cassidy et al (2009 p 56) describe as 'superficial and simplistic assumptions about the value of establishing and locating definitive philosophies'. This situation is aggravated by a lack of detailed research on coaching philosophy.

The purpose of this chapter is to discuss the concept of a coaching philosophy, to review critically the literature in the field, and to make suggestions as to how research and scholarship on coaching philosophy might proceed. Definitions of coaching philosophy are presented from noteworthy texts, such as Lyle (2002), before Milton Rokeach's work on human values is proposed as a framework for clarifying our understanding of beliefs, values and principles. Attention is given to Cassidy et al's (2009) review from a socio-cultural and pedagogical perspective, which

draws particularly from Lyle's (1999) seminal work; while recent studies by Schempp et al (2006), Nash et al (2008) and Denison (2007) are also considered.

In considering future research directions, there are three sections: storytelling, development of coaching philosophy, and coaching philosophy versus coaching behaviour. In the storytelling section, the role of values and storytelling in Kouzes and Posner's (2002) theory is presented, with discussion of points raised about critical incidents and storytelling with reference to Tripp (1993) and Gardner (1995) respectively. The section on the development of coaching philosophy begins by addressing Walton's (1992) notion of the 'great philosopher coach', and then critically examines the development of a coaching philosophy over time. Using the former UCLA basketball coach John Wooden as an exemplar, Martens' (2004) notion that coaches do not begin their careers with the same philosophy that is championed at the end of their careers is examined. The question of how long it takes to develop a coaching philosophy, the influence of background and education, and the issue of self-awareness are also discussed.

In the final section, the attention is on youth sport and a summary is provided of important work associated with the American Sport Education Program, the National Standards for Sports Coaching, and the Positive Coaching Alliance. There is a discussion of the research of McAllister et al (2000), which shows constraints on coaching philosophy, and should be a spur to further research examining inconsistencies between stated coaching philosophy and coaching practice/behaviour.

What is a coaching philosophy?

Definitions of coaching philosophy typically make reference to one or more of the following: beliefs, values and principles. The following example makes reference to all three:

> Your coaching philosophy is a set of *beliefs* and *principles* that guide your behaviour. It helps you remain true to your *values* while handling the hundreds of choices you must make as a coach. (Burton & Raedeke 2008 p 4, emphasis added)

Coaching philosophy is viewed by Lyle (1999) in terms of not only beliefs and values, but also behaviours:

> A coaching philosophy is a comprehensive statement about the *beliefs* and *behaviours* that will characterize the coach's practice. These beliefs and behaviours will either reflect a deeper set of *values* held by the coach, or will be the recognition of a set of externally imposed expectations to which the coach feels the need to adhere. (p 28, emphasis added)

Lyle (1999) is particularly concerned with 'the issue of a potential conflict between stated beliefs, actual practice, and personal values' (p 30). He argues that coaching philosophy should be thought of in terms of 'principles' that guide coaching practice, usually expressed as a list of statements about various aspects of the coach's practice: 'each statement will contain a *declaration of belief* about an aspect of the individual's practice and an indication of the *practical manifestation of this belief* (p 31, emphasis added). From Lyle's experience in coach education, the 'practical manifestation' of the beliefs is not always present and the circumstances in which values will be evident are often not specified (Lyle 1999 p 31–32).

In a subsequent text, Lyle (2002) emphasises values in his discussion of coaching philosophy and states that values underlie opinions and beliefs. He is still interested in the dissociation between a coach's stated philosophy and his or her actual coaching practice, but defined coaching philosophy in terms of a 'set of values or values framework' (p 165) even though a coaching philosophy is 'generally not expressed in the vocabulary of values themselves' but rather 'couched in terms of principles related to behaviour': 'taken as a whole, a coaching philosophy should provide a set of guiding *principles* for coaching practice, and . . . identify those *values* that are felt most strongly' (p 166, emphasis added).

Lyle (2002) draws attention to the fact that there may be dissociations between a coach's personal values and his or her publicly stated values; and between organisational values and coaching values. In their review, Cassidy et al (2009) elaborate on these dissociations to make the point that coaching philosophies are often compromised by constraints such as the desire to meet the needs of the employing organisation (p 56–57).

Beliefs, values and principles

In developing the constructs of beliefs, values and principles more fully, Milton Rokeach in his influential work on human values distinguishes three types of belief: descriptive or existential (i.e. capable of being true or false); evaluative (i.e. judged to be good or bad); and prescriptive or proscriptive (i.e. some means or end of action is judged to be desirable or undesirable) (Rokeach 1973 p 6–7). Values are prescriptive or proscriptive beliefs. Rokeach (1973) makes the following assumptions about the nature of values:

> (1) The total number of values that a person possesses is relatively small; (2) all men everywhere possess the same values to different degrees; (3) values are organized into value systems; (4) the antecedents of human values can be traced to culture, society and its institutions, and personality; (5) the consequences of human values will be manifested in virtually all phenomena that social scientists might consider worth investigating and understanding. (1973 p 3)

Rokeach defines a value as 'an enduring belief that a specific mode of conduct or end-state of existence is personally or socially preferable to an opposite or converse mode of conduct or end-state of existence' (p. 5) and a value system as 'an enduring organization of beliefs concerning preferable modes of conduct or end-states of existence along a continuum of relative importance' (p 5).

Values that refer to a mode of conduct and an end-state are termed by Rokeach instrumental and terminal values, respectively. Examples of instrumental values from Rokeach's (1973) study of values found in American society are ambitious (hard-working, aspiring), courageous (standing up for your beliefs), honest (sincere, truthful) and responsible (dependable, reliable); examples of terminal values are freedom (independence, free choice), happiness (contentedness), self-respect (self-esteem) and social recognition (respect, admiration). Values can be further understood in relation to, and differentiated from, attitudes and norms (Rokeach 1973 p 18). Values are determinants of attitudes and are far fewer in number than attitudes (dozens rather than thousands). Unlike attitudes, values are standards that transcend a specific object or situation. A value is based on a single belief, whereas an attitude refers to several beliefs.

A value may refer to a mode of behaviour or end-state of existence, but a norm refers only to a mode of behaviour. Unlike a value, a norm refers to behaviour in a specific situation and is consensual and external to the person. Values can also be differentiated from principles, which are concerned with implementation of values; i.e. they are guidelines for putting values into practice.

To conclude this section: Lyle (2002) indicates that a coaching philosophy should be couched in terms of values and principles. The work of Rokeach (1973) provides a useful framework that clarifies the relationship between beliefs, values, attitudes and norms. The use of such a framework could be used in framing future studies into coach philosophy. In addition, Rokeach's work offers an analytical or thinking tool that could have practical use for coaches making explicit their coaching philosophies.

Critical review of the literature

Compared to topics such as coaching behaviours, there has been a dearth of research on coaching philosophy (Cushion 2006, Cassidy et al 2009). This is perhaps surprising in light of the importance that understanding a coach's philosophy has on understanding that coach's practice, and given the emphasis that authors of textbooks on coaching have given to coaching philosophy (e.g. Martens 2005 p 4, Vealey 2005 p 21). Indeed, these authors emphasise the pre-eminence of coaching philosophy in informing coaches especially when they are required to make difficult decisions. Much of the research directed at coaching philosophy is anecdotal and found in the numerous books by or about high-profile coaches (e.g. Reynaud 2006), especially in the major American sports, or based on interviews (e.g. Jones et al 2004, Voight & Carroll 2006), again with high-profile coaches.

Cassidy et al (2009) have recently considered coaching philosophy and reviewed the literature from a socio-cultural and pedagogical perspective.

Drawing particularly on the work of Lyle (1999, 2002), these authors argued that coaching philosophies should be regarded as 'flexible guides to action' (p 64), which are based on personal values but account for 'contextual complexity' (p 64) in that they are 'able to adapt to changing circumstances' (p 61). These authors draw on the work of Bourdieu (1977) to argue that coaching can be viewed as 'regulated improvisation'. While a critical discussion of Bourdieu's work and its application to coaching is called for, it is beyond the scope of this chapter. However, the reader is referred to Cushion (2007a, 2007b) as a starting point for exploring the concepts of 'habitus' and 'logic of practice' in Bourdieu's work. Cassidy et al draw on the useful distinction made by Raffel (1998) between 'principled' and 'rule-guided' behaviour. The former refers to practice based on values, while the latter involves a prescriptive approach. The distinction can be summed up with the expression that 'rules are followed by fools but are for the guidance of wise men'.

There has been a distinct lack of studies that examine coaches' personal philosophies in the peer-reviewed literature. Two recent exceptions are Schempp et al (2006) and Nash et al (2008). Schempp et al (2006) found that philosophy (defined as things teachers believe) was one of five themes that emerged from analysis of data collected from 31 coaches listed by *Golf Magazine's* 'Top 100 Golf Instructors in America' as representing the activities and qualities they most often monitored. By self-monitoring is meant 'the reflective practice of tracking and recording one's own performance' (p 26). Within the philosophy theme were four categories centred around beliefs. These were: beliefs about learner needs and characteristics; beliefs about what to teach; beliefs about the purpose and ways of teaching; and beliefs about the structure of teaching (p 32). Schempp et al found that with these coaches there was limited self-monitoring of their philosophy relative to other themes (i.e. skills, knowledge and personal characteristics). This finding was accounted for by the fact that the coaches in their study had on average 17 years of experience, thus it would not be unreasonable to assume perhaps that their beliefs would be relatively stable.

In a study based on semi-structured interviews with 21 coaches of different levels in Scotland, Nash et al (2008) concluded that as coaches gain knowledge and become more experienced, they are able both to articulate a coherent personal philosophy and to contextualise it in their coaching practice. Coaches at the beginning levels of coach education, i.e. Levels 1 and 2, 'generally did not exhibit an obvious awareness of their core values and coaching methods'; whereas more experienced coaches at Level 3 'showed evidence of a more profound consideration of their coaching philosophy and of the recognition the direct impact a coaching philosophy has on their coaching processes and strategies' (p 551). Advanced coaches at Levels 4 and 5, however, 'demonstrated a conceptual awareness of key ideas related both to sport and coaching, as well as appreciation of the social, cultural and political values associated with the practice of coaching' (p 551). Notwithstanding the small sample size, there appeared to be a relationship between not only years of coaching experience but also educational achievements. For example, none of the Level 1 coaches had progressed beyond a high-school education; while all the Level 4 and 5 coaches held university degrees. The type of study carried out by Nash et al (2008) could be enhanced by researchers taking a sociological perspective such as used by Green (2000) in his study of PE teachers' 'everyday philosophies'.

A good example of a study on coaching philosophy from a sociological perspective is Denison's (2007) autobiographical account of his coaching of a male cross-country runner called 'Brian'. In this study Denison presents an alternative analysis to his initial 'psychological' interpretation for Brian's poor performance in a race by utilising Michel Foucault's social theory. Denison argues that Foucault's (1979) theory of disciplinary power provides 'a worthwhile heuristic for coaches to evaluate and enhance their athletes' performance', that is, a theory that can inform a coach's personal philosophy.

Moving the field forward

Storytelling

A number of authors have drawn attention to the role of storytelling in coaching. For example, Thompson (2003) stated that the best coaches are 'master storytellers and story collectors who use stories to develop a culture that helps the team hum' (p 161). Douglas and Carless (2008) suggest that 'most coaches are active storytellers' (p 36).

In Kouzes and Posner's (2002) model of leadership, there are five practices of exemplary leadership: model the way, inspire a shared vision, challenge the process, enable others to act, and encourage the heart. From their research, Kouzes and Posner have found that people look for their leaders to be honest, forward-looking, competent and inspiring. Most importantly, people want their leaders to do what they say they're going to do. They make a number of suggestions for good practice but place a strong emphasis on storytelling. Suggestions include 'collect stories that teach values' and 'put storytelling on your meeting agendas'. The use of critical incidents is paraded as opportunities for communicating key lessons about appropriate behaviour and provides a backdrop for illustrating and reinforcing moral lessons about what should and should not be valued. Critical incidents therefore become stories that are passed from person to person, and generation to generation. Kouzes and Posner point to Gardner's (1995) argument that leaders embody the stories they tell, and also that other rhetorical devices such as analogies and metaphors can be effective means of communication.

Critical incidents

Tripp (1993) defined a critical incident as 'an interpretation of the significance of an event' (p 8). Such an incident appears to be 'typical' at first sight, but is rendered 'critical' through analysis (p 24): 'critical incidents are not simply observed, they are literally created' (p 27). Tripp (1993) uses critical incidents to increase understanding of and control over professional judgements in classroom teaching – 'those expert guesses which result from combining experience with specialist theoretical knowledge' (p 7). The analysis of critical incidents depends on reflection, which is considered essential to the development of professional judgement, requiring 'some from of challenge to and critique of ourselves and our professional values' (p 12) in order to be effective: 'we first must change our awareness through deliberately setting out to view the world of our practice in new ways' (p 12). Tripp argues that critical incidents can help us to do this.

The coaching philosophy of Peter Stanley, one of the coaches featured in Jones et al (2004), is summarised as attaching great value to 'the notions of high-quality instruction, athlete empowerment, the creation of a supportive and challenging training environment and the social well-being of athletes' (p 73). Jones et al report a critical incident that Stanley highlighted when reflecting on his style of giving feedback to an individual athlete:

> It was a freezing cold night and we were working indoors. Anyway, he came down and did his jump and it was bad. It was a bad jump and he landed in the sand and looked up with a look of 'Oh God' and I said, "You ran in well there, you just dropped your hips a bit too early". He said, "Pete, I don't come here to be bullshitted by you. It was crap". He said, "Don't bullshit me. It was crap and I'll go back and I'll do it again". So, I thought, rather than look for positives with everybody, I'm going to base my feedback around what they want to know and what they, as individuals, want to get from each session. (p 79)

It is through reflection on incidents such as these that we can become much more aware of our practice and how we might normally react or respond. This provides the basis for a re-assessment of our underlying beliefs and assumptions about existing practice.

Stories

Gardner (1995) argues that effective communication of a story may be the key to leadership. He delineates stories into three broad categories: stories about the self, stories about the group, and stories about values and meaning. These categories are not to be regarded as mutually exclusive and in fact Gardner invokes Ludwig Wittgenstein's concept to argue that kinds of stories (narratives, myths, fables, dreams, etc.) bear at most a 'family resemblance' to one another. Gardner emphasises the importance of stories of identity:

> Leaders and audiences traffic in many stories, but the most basic story has to do with issues of identity. And so it is the leader who succeeds in conveying a new version of a given group's story who is likely to be effective. Effectiveness here involves fit – the story needs to make sense to audience members at this particular historical moment, in terms of where they have been and where they would like to go. (1995 p 14)

He goes on to emphasise the importance of the leader embodying the message being transmitted. This picture of the visionary and inspirational talk/story given by coaches will resonate with readers, as will the significance of the credibility accorded to the coach.

Gardner describes his approach to studying leadership as 'cognitive in a generic sense' (p 16), but it is also constructivist as it assumes 'an active mind is

comparing stories with one another and highlighting some features, while downplaying others' (p 16). This provides the beginnings of a research agenda. Questions can be asked about the genesis of the stories themselves, the mechanisms for transmitting them, their consonance with previous messages, and their impact on the audience (athletes).

These are questions that Gardner concerns himself with in his study of 11 great leaders such as Martin Luther King and Eleanor Roosevelt, but which can also be applied to a study of great coaches. For example, Percy Cerutty, a renowned athletics coach from Australia, is described by Walton (1992) as 'both a talker and a doer, and his words and exploits released powers in the minds and souls of others' (p 145). Citing Herb Elliott, one of the world's greatest ever middle-distance runners, who was coached by Cerutty, Walton refers to the core of Cerutty's philosophy: the creed of 'Stotan' – a word coined from Stoic and Spartan – that embodies themes of nature and virtues such as self-reliance and determination. For inspirational purposes, Cerutty used not only lectures and demonstrations, but also his poetry and essays. If this seems unlike the majority of coaches, the mythology that has grown around the inspirational 'team talks' of many team sport coach will bear examination from this perspective.

Summary

Kouzes and Posner's (2002) model of leadership shows the role that storytelling can play in clarifying values, articulating a philosophy and aligning actions with values. In considering how practice and philosophy relate, critical incidents can be a useful tool for coaches in their reflective practice and can become stories that impact upon the development of a coaching philosophy. Gardner's (1995) cognitive approach to leadership and his emphasis on storytelling would appear to have currency for investigating coaching philosophy.

Development of coaching philosophy

Philosopher coaches

Himmelfarb (2000), arguing that Nietzsche in the 1880s was instrumental in this process, has discussed how virtues became values in what she refers to as a 'transmutation' that began to associate values with moral virtue. Walton (1992) views coaching philosophy in terms of values or virtues. American football coach Woody Hayes, for example, emphasised independence and self-reliance. In this regard, Hayes was particularly influenced by the philosophy of Ralph Waldo Emerson. So-called 'philosopher coaches' are committed to 'individual integrity, values, and personal growth' (p 162) and are compared by Walton to ancient sages and philosopher kings: 'they are a special brand of leaders, role models for others, coaches and non-coaches alike, to follow' (p 163).

In discussing another great 'philosopher coach', John Wooden, Walton (1992) concludes that Wooden's success derived from building his practice around a framework of values, and embodying those values. However, we should insert a note of caution. Cassidy et al warn that coaches may be aware of the need to evince more socially valued statements than they exhibit in their practice; indeed, 'coaches' notions of their philosophies appear more ideological than philosophical' (2009 p 58). Martens is impressed by Wooden's coaching philosophy, with its emphasis on 'teaching and performing rather than winning', but notes that he 'did not begin with the philosophy he espoused at the end of his career' (Martens 2004 p 7).

The following lengthy quotes describe how those observing John Wooden's career saw the iconic philosophy emerge from more commonplace practice. Halberstam (1981), an American Pulitzer Prize-winning journalist, wrote:

> There were those who coached against Wooden earlier in his career who thought his moral principles fell a little short of the Pyramid's specifications. In those days he was something of a holy terror. He disciplined his own players harshly, he was known to overheat his gym so that opposing teams would wilt in the fourth quarter, and he ragged unmercifully not just refs but opposing players.
>
> But gradually there was a feeling, starting in the mid-fifties, that Wooden was coaching better and attracting better players, and as his teams improved, so finally did his manners. What other coaches resented about UCLA was the surface purity of Wooden and the more complicated morality of its athletic program. For the articles about Wooden that dealt at length with his virtues rarely mentioned the presence of a man named Sam Gilbert, a wealthy Los Angeles builder and fan of UCLA basketball, who helped with some of the more mundane aspects of big-time basketball, such as keeping egocentric superstars happy. (1981 p 315)

Johnson (2004) cites Peter Bjarkman's *The Biographical History of Basketball* (2000):

> Johnny Wooden's success in manufacturing his own mythical persona as coach and inspirational leader was almost as complete as his decade-plus run at manufacturing NCAA championship victories. As other respected historians of the sport have already noted, the methods that coach Wooden piously espoused once he stood atop the sports world were not always exactly those methods that originally had gotten them there. The coach's advocacy of patience, faith and self control always seemed at odds with his own personal impatience with losing, his not-infrequent sideline temper-laced outbursts, and his constant scathing cajoling of officials and opponents during heated game action.

This 'celebrity' example reminds us of the problem identified earlier in the chapter – we may not always 'practise what we preach'. However, it raises two further issues. First, coaches, particularly those in the public gaze, may engage in an element of 'impression management', and second, a coaching philosophy may change over time.

How long does it take to develop a coaching philosophy?

The case of John Wooden would seem to provide evidence that a coaching philosophy evolves (or at least appears to evolve) over time. Indeed, Janssen and Dale (2006) report that many coaches admit that it takes 'a good 10 years of evolution' (p 46) before a coach arrives at a coaching philosophy he or she is comfortable with. There is a good deal of potential for investigations into how the coaching philosophies of successful coaches have developed over time. Two key themes of such investigations – covered briefly in the following two sections – could be the influence of background and education and the level of self awareness.

Influence of background and education

In Jones et al (2004), rugby coach Bob Dwyer spoke of how his coaching philosophy was influenced by his background in engineering and underpinned by 'a belief in organisation, order and precision' (p 98). In the same text, another rugby coach, Ian McGeechan paid homage to his teacher-training background, 'I'm an education man really, and a lot of what I do goes back to Carnegie where I did my teacher training. The preparation that I got there to be a teacher was second to none. They insisted on standards, discipline, it was almost like the army' (p 54). McGeechan was appointed coach for the British & Irish Lions on their 2009 tour to South Africa. He paid homage to former British & Irish Lions coach Syd Millar as one of the most influential people in his career. Millar was coach of the victorious Lions tour to South Africa in 1974 on which McGeechan played: 'He made you feel important and took time with you. I felt I really grew up as a person on that tour because of the way I was handled. As a coach, I try to do the same with my players' (Lloyd 2008).

These short vignettes illustrate that coaches have an awareness that their approaches to coaching, and what they feel to be important, have emerged from their own experiences as performers and from their educational backgrounds.

Self-awareness

Martens (2004) argued that a useful coaching philosophy depends on self-awareness, that is, 'getting to know yourself'. In the words of Pete Carroll, the successful USC Trojans football coach:

> In order to have the opportunity to be authentic as an individual, you have to figure out who you are and what you're all about. Until you know that, you really don't know how to recreate it or replicate it. ... My idea is simply this – "be true to the self you know yourself to be". (Voight & Carroll 2006 p 324–325)

This seems to be particularly important when coaches realise that their practice does not reflect what they truly believe to be the most appropriate approach. Returning to Ian McGeechan, Jones et al (2004) point to an instance recalled by McGeechan in which he demonstrated self-awareness when he veered from his coaching philosophy when he first coached the Scotland B team in the 1980s:

> I coached the way I thought they wanted me to do it, and it was awful. I didn't enjoy it, and I said to a lad who became Scotland coach a few years ago, Ritchie Dixon, who was my assistant coach then, I just said "Ritchie, just remind me, if I ever get the opportunity to coach Scotland B again, Iapos;m going to do it my way" and that's what I have done ever since. (quoted in Jones et al 2004 p 60)

Summary

There is often a need to dig beneath the surface of the idealised and sanitised coaching philosophies espoused by coaches in order to understand how coaching philosophy evolves throughout a coach's career. The influence of background and education can be revealing as shown for example by Jones et al's (2004) study of Ian McGeechan. Self-awareness has been highlighted by Martens (2004) as important in the development of coaching philosophy, and critical incidents and stories of identity – to use Gardner's (1995) term – are likely to have utility in assisting coaches to become more self-aware.

Coaching philosophy versus coaching behaviour

In England, the Football Association (FA) has recently banned teams with players aged under 8 years from publishing the results of their league matches and also from competing in knockout tournaments where trophies and medals are given to the winners (Malvern 2008).

The FA's Director of Football Development, Sir Trevor Brooking, was quoted as saying:

> At the moment we are not at the same level as other countries. In the youngest age groups, there's too much emphasis on winning leagues, often to satisfy parents and coaches. That's what we're looking to change. We need better, more skilful players coming through. (Football Association 2008)

A similar concern for the way youth sport is organised is evident in the USA. In 1976 Rainer Martens founded the Coaching Effectiveness Program (ACEP), which later expanded into the American Sport Education Program (ASEP). In 1981, Martens produced and released the first ASEP course, which included a focus on coaching philosophy. More than a million coaches have participated in ASEP courses since 1976 (American Sport Education Program, n d). The motto of the ASEP, 'Athletes First, Winning Second,' is cited as the cornerstone of its coaching philosophy and the philosophical foundation of the Bill of Rights for Young Athletes: 'Striving to win is proposed as the objective that should be adopted by every athlete and coach' (Human Kinetics, n d).

Martens favours the 'cooperative' style of coaching rather than the 'command' or 'submissive' styles, because it 'shares decision-making with the athletes and fosters the Athletes first, Winning second philosophy' (Martens 2004 p 33) that is the motto of the ASEP. What Martens refers to as cooperative and command styles are often referred to in the literature as democratic and autocratic styles, respectively. Once again we can recognise these distinctions but exercise some caution in their interpretation. Scholars of sports coaching have pointed to the limitations of the democratic–autocratic dichotomy. Cassidy et al (2004), for example, argue that such a dichotomy 'leaves little room for the fact that a coach may be more democratic in one area of practice while being more autocratic in another' (p 57–58). Nevertheless, these notions of sharing decision-making and putting the athletes first are captured in the philosophy of empowerment: 'a philosophy of empowerment also aims to make athletes increasingly responsible for their own performances by giving them a degree of ownership over them (Jones et al 2004 p 159). Related to empowerment is the notion of an athlete-centred approach, which refers to an 'ethos and philosophy whereby the person – and their long-term health and well-being – is seen as central to the coaching process' (Douglas & Carless 2008 p 34).

This athlete-centred approach is embedded in public statements of philosophy in the USA. In the National Standards for Sports Coaching, which were produced in 2006 for the National Association of Sport and Physical Education by the United States Olympic Committee, and the National Federation of State High School Associations (National Association of Sport & Physical Education) there are eight domains; one of which is Philosophy and Ethics. Coaching philosophy is embraced by Standard 1 of Domain 1 – 'Develop and Implement an athlete-centred coaching philosophy':

> A well-developed coaching philosophy provides expectations for behaviours that reflect priorities and values of the coach. An appropriate coaching perspective focuses on maximizing the positive benefits of sport participation for each athlete. (National Association of Sport & Physical Education)

Standard 1 has the following benchmarks; that is, 'performance guides which can be used in developing and assessing coaching competence, and can be applied to any sport or coaching program':

- Identify and communicate reasons for entering the coaching profession
- Develop an athlete-centred coaching philosophy that aligns with the organisational mission and goals

- Communicate the athlete-centred coaching philosophy in verbal and written form to athletes, parents/guardians, and program staff
- Welcome all eligible athletes and implement strategies that encourage the participation of disadvantaged and disabled athletes
- Manage athlete behaviour consistent with an athlete-centred coaching philosophy (National Association of Sport & Physical Education).

These standards are a revision of the 1995 standards for athletic coaches and were intended to be 'more consistent with current sport research and best practice' (National Association of Sport & Physical Education). In 2006, NASPE called on experts from national governing bodies of sport, the United States Olympic Committee, National Federation of State High School Associations, and NASPE leadership to review and revise the popular 1995 standards for athletic coaches to be more consistent with current sport research and best practice.

While coaches may state that their philosophy emphasises development and experience, their behaviour often instead exhibits an emphasis on winning. Vealey (2005) cites three studies illustrative of this lack of alignment between stated philosophy and actual behaviour (Wilcox & Trudel 1998, Gilbert et al 1999, McAllister et al 2000). As an example, in the context of youth-sport softball and baseball programs, designed for ages 7–12, in two communities in the southern region of Illinois, McAllister et al (2000) carried out in-depth interviews with 22 youth-sport baseball and softball coaches (10 women and 12 men) with the purposes being to: 'identify the values and life skills that coaches deem important and the manner in which coaches claim to teach these desired outcomes, and to examine the philosophies of youth sport coaches and the degree to which coaches implement such philosophies (p 35). The authors reported that 'learning skills' and 'having fun' were the two areas discussed most often when coaches were asked about their coaching philosophies. However, the coaches struggled to describe how they taught values and life skills. Many coaches assumed that talking about values or telling their charges how to respond in a particular situation constituted effective teaching:

> 'absent in the remarks of these youth sport coaches were discussions about modifying the environment to facilitate the active learning of values or utilizing developmental teaching progressions to reinforce learning' (p 39)

The authors found inconsistencies between coaches' stated philosophy and their comments about coaching practice/behaviour, particularly about the importance of winning. For example, some coaches believed that having fun was the result of winning, even though they made it clear that having fun was a priority (p 40). While most coaches indicated that their coaching philosophy de-emphasised winning, it was found that team meetings generally took place only after a loss:

> Coaches indicated that this meeting was held with the intent to inform the youngsters that 'winning isn't everything' and 'you tried hard and that's what's important'. Yet it appeared that these meetings were an opportunity for coaches to critique performance with the emphasis being placed on mistakes. As one coach explained, 'they need to know what they did wrong so they won't make that mistake again' (p 41)

In discussing the results, the authors note that all the coaches were volunteers and none were reimbursed for coaching. It also appears that most had at least one child who was participating in the youth-sport program. In attempting to explain the above inconsistencies, the authors point to the fact that 18 of the coaches had participated in youth-sport programmes themselves as a child and 19 had been involved in sport at junior-high or high-school level. Furthermore, many of the coaches appeared to be 'extremely competitive individuals, a quality many cited as having been learned through their own sport participation' (p 41). Expectations and peer pressure from parents also appeared to be a factor in the inconsistencies, as was the influence of professional sport in the USA.

Summary

Research demonstrates inconsistencies between coaches' stated philosophies and their comments about coaching practice/behaviour. Studies like these across a wide variety of sporting contexts and age groups in different countries would surely reveal much about the structure and function of coaching philosophy as well the kind of constraints on behaviour and philosophy that have been indicated by Lyle (2002) and Cassidy et al (2009).

Summary

Overall, there has been a lack of research on coaching philosophy with Lyle (1999, 2002) arguably providing the most useful scholarly coverage over the last decade. In order to develop further Lyle's (2002) notions about coaching philosophies being concerned with values and principles, Rokeach (1973) provides a framework that could be a starting point for future research. Gardner's (1995) work on storytelling in leadership along with the use of critical incidents (Tripp 1993) would also appear to have currency for researchers on coaching philosophy. The development of coaching philosophies over time is an important area for research, including the influence of background and education. There is much that can be learned about the structure and function of coaching philosophies from studies like McAllister et al (2000) that investigate dissociations between what coaches say they do and what they actually do.

Coaches' philosophies or values frameworks provide a potentially fertile ground for research as they constitute a link between the public discourse on coaching, evidenced in 'standards' and social expectations about coaches' behaviours, and the individual coach's belief system and the context in which he or she operates. A greater self-awareness of 'practice values' – but perhaps more importantly how these have been shaped by previous experience, education and influential figures – will be a useful tool for reflecting on and re-assessing coaching behaviour.

It seems incontrovertible that the dissociation of 'practice from preaching' is a function of the coach's impression management, that is, conforming publicly (at least in statements) to expectations in that particular sporting domain. Even this simple awareness of social expectations in relation to personal beliefs is a valuable starting point for coach education.

References

American Sport Education Program, no date. About ASEP. Online. Available: http://www.asep.com/about.cfm.

Bourdieu, P., 1977. Outline of a theory of practice. Cambridge University Press, Cambridge.

Burton, D., Raedeke, T.D., 2008. Sport psychology for coaches. Human Kinetics, Champaign, IL.

Campbell, R., 1977. How to really love your child. Signet, New York.

Cassidy, T., Jones, R.L., Potrac, P., 2009. Understanding sports coaching: the social, cultural and pedagogical foundations of coaching practice, second ed. Routledge, New York.

Cushion, C., 2006. Thinking about coach philosophy. Sports Media. Online. Available: http://sports-media.org/newpedimensionoctober2006.htm.

Cushion, C., 2007a. Modelling the complexity of the coaching process. International Journal of Sports Science and Coaching 2 (4), 395–401.

Denison, J., 2007. Social theory for coaches: a Foucauldian reading of one athlete's poor performance. International Journal of Sports Science and Coaching 2 (4), 369–383.

Douglas, K., Carless, D., 2008. Using stories in coach education. International Journal of Sports Science and Coaching 3 (1), 33–49.

Football Association, 2008. Brooking on development. Online. Available: http://www.thefa.com/TheFA/NewsFromTheFA/Postings/brooking_backs_skills_development.htm.

Foucault, M., 1979. Discipline and punish: the birth of the prison. Vintage Books, New York.

Gardner, H., 1995. Leading minds: an anatomy of leadership. Harper Collins, London.

Gilbert, W.D., Trudel, P., Haughian, L., 1999. Interactive decision making factors considered by coaches of youth ice hockey during games. Journal of Teaching in Physical Education 18, 290–311.

Green, K., 2000. Exploring the everyday 'philosophies' of physical education teachers from a sociological perspective. Sport, Education & Society 5 (2), 109–129.

Halberstam, D., 1981. The breaks of the game. Ballantine Books, New York.

Heywood, M., 2008. Respect the key for McGeechan. The Official Website of the British & Irish Lions Tour to South Africa 2009. Online.

Available: http://www.lionsrugby.com/5366.php.

Human Kinetics, no date. Determining your coaching objectives. Online. Available: http://www.humankinetics.com/SuccessfulCoaching/IG/chp_02.htm.

Janssen, J., Dale, G., 2002. The seven secrets of successful coaches: how to unlock and unleash your team's full potential. Winning the Mental Game, Cary.

Johnson, N., 2003. The John Wooden pyramid of success, second ed. Cool Titles, Los Angeles.

Jones, R., Armour, K., Potrac, P., 2004. Sports coaching cultures: from practice to theory. Routledge, Abingdon.

Kouzes, J.M., Posner, B.Z., 2002. The leadership challenge, third ed. Jossey-Bass, San Francisco.

Lloyd, M., 2008. The Official Website of the British & Irish Lions Tour to South Africa 2009. Online. Available: http://www.lionsrugby.com/5361.php.

Lyle, J., 1999. Coaching philosophy and coaching behaviour. In: Cross, N., Lyle, J. (Eds.), The coaching process: principles and practice for sport. Butterworth-Heinemann, Oxford, pp. 25–46.

Lyle, J., 2002. Sports coaching concepts: a framework for coaches' behaviour. Routledge, London.

Malvern, J., 2008. Football Association bans league tables for under 8s. The Times. Online. Available: http://www.timesonline.co.uk/tol/news/uk/article4222254.ece.

Martens, R., 2004. Successful coaching, third ed. Human Kinetics, Champaign, IL.

McAllister, S.G., Blinde, E.M., Weiss, W.M., 2000. Teaching values and implementing philosophies: dilemmas of the youth sport coach. Physical Educator 57 (1), 35–45.

Nash, C.S., Sproule, J., Horton, P., 2008. Sport coaches' perceived role frames and philosophies. International

Journal of Sports Science and Coaching 3 (4), 539–554.

National Association for Sport & Physical Education, no date. National Standards for Sport Coaches, second ed. Online. Available: http://www.aahperd.org/naspe/template.cfm?template=domainsStandards.html.

Raffel, S., 1998. Revisiting role theory: roles and the problem of the self. Sociological Research Online 4 (3) Online. Available: http://www.socresonline.org.uk/4/2/raffel.html.

Reynaud, C. (Ed.), 2006. She can coach! Tools for success from 20 top women coaches. Human Kinetics, Champaign, IL.

Rokeach, M., 1973. The nature of human values. The Free Press, New York.

Schempp, P.G., McCullick, B.A., Busch, C.A., et al., 2006. The self-monitoring of expert sport instructors. International Journal of Sports Science and Coaching 1 (1), 25–35.

Thompson, J., 2003. The double-goal coach: positive coaching tools for honouring the game and developing winners in sports and life. Collins, New York.

Tripp, D., 1993. Critical incidents in teaching: developing professional judgement. Routledge, London.

Vealey, R.S., 2005. Coaching for the inner edge. Fitness Information Technology, Morgantown.

Voight, M., Carroll, P., 2006. Applying sport psychology philosophies, principles, and practices onto the gridiron: an interview with USC football coach Pete Carroll. International Journal of Sports Science and Coaching 1 (4), 321–331.

Walton, G.M., 1992. Beyond winning: the timeless wisdom of great philosopher coaches. Human Kinetics, Champaign, IL.

Wilcox, S., Trudel, P., 1998. Constructing the coaching principles and beliefs of youth ice hockey coach. Avante 4, 39–66.

Narrowing the field: some key questions about sports coaching

John Lyle and Chris Cushion

Introduction

Our intention for the book was to cover the constituent parts of the coaching process and current themes within the academic study of sports coaching. Our belief is that the book has been effective in providing an updated position statement in a range of topical coaching-related issues. In doing so, the book demonstrates something of the growing interest and research in the many facets of coaching and the coaching process. Importantly, the chapters have attempted, where applicable, to theorise and provide methodological tools for investigating a coaching process within which its operations and functions are shaped by social, cultural, historical and human factors. Indeed, the chapters demonstrate clearly that individual and supra-individual factors lie at the heart of the possibilities for the coaching process. For coaches and scholars alike this perspective provides important tools for the development of an understanding of coaching. Importantly, the book opens up, or rather insists upon, a number of persistent themes that pervade the writing, and an academic imagination that reflects the coaching process as much more than face-to-face interaction, or the unproblematic transmission of prescribed knowledge and skill.

In this final chapter we are exercising our academic imagination and develop a number of themes, perhaps better described as 'conceptual threads' – that require further attention. We have taken the liberty of expanding on these, and we have unashamedly adopted a polemic position on each to suggest possibilities for intervention and change.

It is not our intention to provide a similar position-style account as those in earlier chapters. We have deliberately set out to 'make a statement' about some issues in sports coaching. They are often conceptual in nature, but arise from both research and policy analysis. We believe that they have a very significant role to play in influencing the research agenda in this field.

Coaching domains

In general, and when taken in aggregation, there is a certain untidiness or absence of concerted focus across the chapters. This is not a reflection of the quality of the writing, which was excellent. Rather it is the contextual or 'situationally dependent' caveats that were introduced into that writing. In addition, there were often unspoken or assumed emphases that arose from the use of youth sport or high-performance sport as the exemplar coaching environment. In our discussions this has led to a number of questions or issues that we felt have been inadequately dealt with.

The first of these issues concerns coaching domains. It has become increasingly obvious to us that coaching can only be understood in a particular context or domain. It is not simply that the coaching process (by which we mean the particular mix of behaviours, skills, functional and professional competences, technical demands, interpersonal relationships, intervention styles, and so on) is quite distinct, but that each domain creates a particular set of assumptions and expectations, within which we can understand coaching practice. We believe that it is axiomatic that sports coaching is not a uni-dimensional concept (see our later arguments about the scope of sports coaching), and that any attempt to focus on the generic nature of the coaching process masks the very distinctive and different forms of coaching practice throughout sport. *Coaching domains* is a useful mechanism for conceptualising the aggregation of behaviours and practice that characterise coaching in different sporting environments. Without an adequate recognition of domain-specific coaching practice and motivations we cannot hope to understand accountability and expectations in coaching, coach education and training, arrangements for professional development, research assumptions, or the development of expertise. In particular, any attempt to 'professionalise' must deal with these distinctive domains.

Some authors, however, question the relevance of domains to understanding coaching; asking if, for example, the competitive level of the athlete is a sufficient unit of analysis (Jones 2006). Jones (2006) attempts to reconceptualise the coach as 'educator', to introduce educational theory as a tool to understand better the coaching process. While this is useful to a degree, rhetorical talk about 'educators' carries the danger of fostering the acceptance of a weak definition of the coaching role and of relevant knowledge. This leads to a lack of discrimination about different sorts of knowledge used by coaches. Indeed, knowledge has been demonstrated in the expertise literature to be highly domain specific. By not understanding and differentiating coaching domains, we end up with a spurious equality for coaching and coaching knowledge. This, in turn, leads to an uncritical and undiscriminating way of understanding both coaching and learning, and the interdependencies between coaching and learning in different contexts.

Understanding the issues surrounding domains presents the challenging dichotomy between a desire to simplify sports coaching by stressing the generic components of the coaching process, and acknowledging the potentially context-dependent nature of skills, knowledge, personal relationships, objectives and working practices. Can the 'coaching' relevant to a beginner group of primary school children undertaking a taster programme in tag rugby be meaningfully compared to that of a full-time head coach of a professional rugby club? What is the balance of similarities and differences that might lead us to consider them sufficiently separate to demand individual attention? If the example

given seems too obvious to be helpful, it begs the further question of whether each putative 'domain' is sufficiently homogeneous and how many domains are helpful or defensible.

Understandably, there are some obvious 'drivers' that militate against presenting too fragmented a picture. These might include a desire for employment/deployment mobility, the perceived benefits of a cohesive 'profession', a desire to promote the universality of coach education and training, and a conviction that coaching in one domain, for example, elite sport, should not be perceived to be more valued than in another. Similarly, the extensive range of sports with differentiating characteristics such as team versus individual sports or game versus performance sports, when allied to organisational variety (schools, clubs, local authorities, performance centres), and the 'level' or standard of participation, presents a complex framework that suggests that coaching will be very context-specific. The temptation to find coherence within this occupational diversity is understandable. At the centre of all of this variety is the performer – the youngster, the adult, the employee, the recreationalist, or the professional – each with different ambitions, capacities, and social and sporting capital. The notion of a coaching domain implies that there will be evident distinctions between the performers in these domains.

A coaching domain is 'a distinctive sporting milieu in which the environmental demands lead to a more or less coherent community of practice, with its attendant demands on the coach's expertise and practice'. The environmental demands refer to an accommodation between the performer's aspirations, abilities and developmental stage, the consequent development and preparation provision, and the organisational and socio-cultural context. Remember that coaching domains are a conceptual device; each domain can be thought of as constituted by an aggregation of countless coaching contexts and episodes that exhibit a similar characteristic pattern. It is important to recognise that these domains are not differentiated by a single factor, perhaps the most obvious of which would be the standard of performance of the athlete. Rather, it is a combination of factors. For example, 'community coaching' may indeed deal for the most part with beginners in a sport. However, there are also factors such as the nature of the coach's employment, an after-school context, the extent of the programme, a developmental ethos, and the presence or absence of external competition, perhaps a festival, all of which create a recognisable context or form of coaching.

How are these domains to be recognised? As we have argued, it is the combination of the performers' aspirations and abilities, and their stage of development, along with the 'reward environment' that creates a particular configuration of coaching process. The 'reward environment' is the level of commitment justified by the perceived benefits from participation in that set of circumstances. A young person with aspirations to reach elite status and who is part of an accelerated development programme may commit significantly to preparation, training and competition, and be willing to amend her/his lifestyle to accommodate this. The adult club performer, who is operating within performance sport and organised competition, but who receives modest recognition and may no longer be part of that group of performers from which the elite will develop, is likely to commit to a limited programme of preparation and lifestyle adjustment. The result is a very context-specific coaching process with boundaries that are dictated by the circumstances. Before describing these coaching process boundaries, it is important to acknowledge the place of competition in determining the boundaries. To some extent, there has been an attempt to de-emphasise the place of competition, particularly in children's sport. However, there is no doubt that the nature of the competition is central to both determining and understanding the coaching process. The possibilities range from short programmes without any external competition, 4–6-week programmes with a festival, regular weekly leagues competition, 'circuits' of scheduled competition in athletics, skiing, golf or tennis, and a series of representative matches. When taken with the perceived 'standing' of such competition, it becomes obvious that the nature of the competition programme will influence the coaches' practice.

Coaching domains are likely to differ in a number of ways. These have been elaborated upon elsewhere and we need not expand on the implications of each criterion across domains. A 'starter list' might include: intensity of participation and preparation; complexity of performance components; coach recruitment, deployment and career development; interpersonal skills; value systems; the specificity of competition preparation; and scale and scope of the community of practice and other social networks. The result of these differences is a differential demand on the coach's expertise and the nature of coaching therein. The

coaching process that emerges from each set of circumstances will require different planning skills, tactical preparation, decision making, refining/teaching skills, resource management, interpersonal skills and so on. The knowledge base and associated skills will differ across domains. It is difficult to avoid suggesting that the higher the levels of athlete performance the greater the sophistication of knowledge and skills. However, this should be avoided. The coaching processes in each domain should be thought of as different, and presenting their distinctive challenges. Nevertheless, the arguments for distinctive perspectives on coaching are persuasive. Perhaps most persuasive is the argument that coaches will learn to 'frame' their roles and expectations within a particular set of personal, educational, and experiential circumstances.

Inevitably we attempt to identify a typology of domains. Trudel and Gilbert (2006) argue that a single typology of coaching contexts is required to facilitate research within a meaningful framework, and to assist with the design of coach education. They review a number of classifications, characterised by terms such as community, instruction, competition, professional, volunteer and school. They decide upon a typology of recreational sport, developmental sport, and elite sport. This they acknowledge is most analogous to Lyle's (2002) typology (participation, development and performance domains), which they describe as the most thoroughly described, grounded in concepts of the coaching process, and consistent with empirical research on stages of performance development. Trudel and Gilbert go on to review the evidence (derived from Gilbert & Trudel 2004) on the characteristics of coaches in each domain under the headings of gender, age and experience, sport experience, motives for coaching, education, and stress and burnout.

There seems little doubt that recent developments in coach education have begun to acknowledge these domains. Trudel and Gilbert (2006) describe developments in the USA, in which different curricula for volunteer and professional coaches are proposed. An earlier coaching system in the UK had allowed for specialisms based on coaching children, adults and those with a disability. More recent developments in the UK, with the establishment of the United Kingdom Coaching Certificate endorsement system (sports coach UK 2004), have encouraged the development of 'horizontal' structures; that is, progress through increasing levels of award but within domains. Although this is not yet widespread, there are examples in gymnastics (distinguishing 'general gymnastics' from the competition disciplines), and swimming (distinguishing swimming teaching and competition).

Summary

We would argue that making assumptions about a coherent set of processes and practices across coaching domains is misguided. Indeed, the difficulties occasioned by attempting to sustain this argument have bedevilled professionalisation and coach education and development. Coaching domains must be acknowledged in any academic writing on sports coaching. While coaching is likely to be influenced by themes and principles common to coaching approaches (it is recognisable as coaching), there are significant specific features and contradictory perspectives that define difference in coaching domains. Therefore, we are not convinced by any claims of generalisability or cross-domain expertise. This is not a position that we believe to be particularly contentious. We would not be surprised, for example, that teachers in primary, secondary or tertiary education should be thought of as operating in different domains, nor would we claim that they operated on a continuum of expertise. They may share essential common territory in core educational functions, but they remain different in important ways. In the same way we need to acknowledge distinctive domains in sports coaching.

At the same time, we acknowledge that further work is required to 'piece together' the different domains, and to consider the implications for recruitment, education and development. We have not attempted to be definitive about the domains; we think of this as a lesser-order problem. Indeed, some brief reflection on this raised the possibility that the domains were perhaps culture-specific. The distinctive educational systems and arrangements for community sport (for example, between the USA and the UK), and recent developments in modelling participation (North 2009) may provide us with further work in seeking commonalities.

Definition of sports coaching

Sports coaching is a catch-all and inevitably too imprecise a term; it is assumed to refer to all forms of 'coaching' activity, but the differences outweigh the similarities. Nevertheless, there is a political imperative to delineate an occupational boundary that is sufficiently extensive to justify its professionalisation. This may still be possible. However, sports coaching is not a synonym for all forms of coaching/ leading/teaching/instructing, and this lack of precision is a very serious barrier to research, education/ certification and professionalisation. Sports coaching is a 'family' title; it connotes a family of related roles, roles that are linked but with different degrees of engagement with the coaching process. We suggest that it must not be used as a shorthand term to embrace all of them. There is no one process that we can term 'sports coaching' that adequately covers all of the coaching environments.

Sports coaching is a generic term that implies 'improving sports performance' but its usefulness (other than to assist superficial communication) is limited. There would be little argument that the primary school teacher, the local authority summer programme coach, the community centre leader, the golf club instructor, the national league club coach, and the national representative squad coach are each engaged in different processes. This may seem obvious, but we have come to use the term indiscriminately. More seriously perhaps, our certification structures have uncritically implied, or assumed, that the family of roles are on a continuum, have an interdependent hierarchy of expertise, and have more similarities than differences; we beg to differ.

We have become convinced that the 'concept' of sports coaching has attained such a level of assumed genericism that in many ways it has become an unhelpful term. Throughout the collection of chapters in this book, but also the literature and development policy more generally, an imprecision has emerged about what the term implies. Once again we acknowledge that there are some perceived advantages to a unified concept, but the lack of precision is evident in research populations, and the extent to which generalisations about the findings are possible. This is partly to do with coaching domains, but more importantly about what is assumed about the processes and practices and their impact on knowledge and expertise. In our combined experience of the academic field, but also in coach education and development, there is confusion between role descriptors, levels of certification, the hierarchy of functional demands (the process), and the scope and range of the required coaching competences. We should not mix up role, domain, function, certification and expertise – and, although we tend to shy away from it, the standard of performance of the athlete/participants. This is not because of level per se but because standard of performance, level of reward and commitment, intensity of preparation and lifestyle commitment are linked to each other. More importantly, the family 'groupings' are not on a continuum, but efforts to 'regularise' the whole field may do great disservice to each group.

We question and doubt the education and development continuum implied by the certification structure (North 2009). While acknowledging the work of Erikson et al (2007) and Gilbert et al (2006), our extensive consultation and research experience suggests that much more work is required on career path regularities, recruitment, motives and prior experience in order to inform our conceptual frameworks. Sports that we have worked with are able to draw very clear distinctions between the roles of instructors and coaches, for example. We are also reminded of coach certification structures that imply a functional consequence at each level. The coach's capacity is described in terms of their level of autonomous practice and readiness to operate within programmes that move from the sessional to the multi-year. This continuum will not apply across such populations as children's sport, adult recreation, and even performance development for age groups.

This is not simply a language issue. We cannot accept that terms such as leader, teacher, instructor and coach confer assumed practices that are interchangeable. The verbs 'to coach', 'to teach', 'to instruct' are not interchangeable. We believe that the term 'to coach' may more usefully be employed to describe a relationship, and not a set of behaviours. We should use a vocabulary that is much more precise. If we intend to convey that a coach is delivering and managing a training session, with specific interventions that may include teaching of new skills – then let's say so! By the same token, impoverished notions and assumptions about 'learning' in the coaching process lead to simplistic approaches and attitudes that convey 'learning' as going on in all coaching practice. Clearly, we need to be more discriminating in the way we talk about and understand different types of learning. This may be a matter of language and philosophical approach – certainly many coaches will be engaged in a 'maintenance' and rehearsal programme that might be designed this way, and the athletes' will learn experientially – but the 'young person's skills agenda' should not be associated with all coaching.

Inevitably, this is linked to the development of coaching as a profession. Our most appropriate analogy comes from comparison to other families of occupations. Classroom assistants, nursing assistants, first aiders, and paralegals are not understood to be the first stages of training and preparation to become teachers, doctors, or lawyers. There remains a threshold of competence and certification/qualification, accountability, and regulation of roles that determines the relationship between the family roles. Thus far, either by design or neglect, we have attempted to embrace all roles and levels within the ambit of sports coaching. This is an insurmountable problem if we attempt to embrace an individual with 2 or 3 days' training (and no real vetting of suitability) within the 'profession', when in fact they have a limited degree of attachment and engagement. As the reader might expect, we acknowledge the dictum that each of these roles is simply different and makes an equal contribution, rather than of different status – but we don't entirely believe it! The contribution of the roles is taken for granted. It is vital that we have youth sport 'coaches'; we need to introduce very young people to sport; we need to facilitate the experience of sport for groups of people for whom there may be wider benefits; and there is a role for those who satisfy their clients' wish for technical instruction. However, the expertise required for these roles may not satisfy a threshold of, say, 'chartered' professional status for sports coaching.

What do we suggest? There needs to be function and role clarity, and a clear threshold statement accompanied by regulation. This will lead to more clarity about the development of expertise, and appropriate education and development structures. Note also the importance of distinguishing between the role being exercised, the capacity required to exercise that role, and the coach's expertise. It is common for coaches to 'coach down' (meaning to operate with groups 'below' those for whom they are 'qualified'). Coaches can operate across roles, levels and domains. Researchers cannot assume that coaches' characteristics are only relevant to the context in which they are studied. (There is also the issue of coaches operating in contexts for which they do not have appropriate qualifications or experience.) What is required is a clear understanding of what knowledge and expertise is conferred (assured) by a qualification, and the coaching roles for which this is a prerequisite.

Is there a 'bottom line'? The answer is yes, although we accept that this proposes a narrower view of the role of the sport coach. Our position is that sports coaching is a term for a family of roles and activities that subsume an intention to improve sports performance (an analogy would be the family title 'render medical assistance', this would apply to all practitioners from first aiders to consultant surgeons). It would not make sense to have too many sub-divisions of roles, and we accept that any categorisation will lead to demarcation/boundary issues. We suggest that the key distinctions are between sports teachers, sports instructors, and sports coaches. There may be advantages from aggregating these occupational groupings, but the distinctions should be acknowledged and will impact on professional status.

Sports instructors are a very distinctive grouping; they are characterised by the absence of an extensive intervention programme, normally episodic and infrequent contact, focus on technique, and in general, no accountability for competition involvement. The key distinction is between sports teachers, usually of young people, and sports coaches. We argue that a substantial proportion of the populations being researched and reported in the academic literature is in fact working to a skills framework, without being 'nested' in a longer-term set of competition objectives, which we take to be a distinguishing feature. We believe that there is a threshold of engagement (see Lyle 2002 p 46, for a discussion of boundary criteria) that is expressed best as extended duration. Sports coaches manage (coordinate and/or deliver) a combination of preparation, competition and lifestyle interventions that are marked by longer-term goals, recognisable sport environments, competition, and extended preparation. The demands of such an environment mean that the sports coach needs an extended period of education and training (with implied depth and breadth of knowledge).

We are aware that we have perhaps couched our arguments in a language that is current in the UK. Nevertheless, we believe that the arguments are universal. We are also sensitive to individuals' desires to 'badge' their activities as coaching. The debate is not a sterile one; we have been critical throughout of much of the research being carried out under the banner of sports coaching. The criticism is not of the researchers' expertise and probity. The shortcomings relate much more to the use of opportunity samples from populations that are engaged in 'learning to play sport', and from which authors should be very much more circumspect about generalising beyond their (often unspoken) assumptions about that coaching process. We are also reluctant to couch the argument in terms of 'levels' of coaching award. However, the relevance is the likely use of such 'levels' in setting thresholds for professional recognition (licensing). Using UK terminology (as used in the United Kingdom Coaching Certification endorsement framework), our view (see also Kay et al 2008) is that Level 3 certification (in principle, intended to be an undergraduate degree level) requires the extent of education and experience required to satisfy a threshold for sports coaches. (There may be other thresholds for sports teaching and sports instruction.) It would be inappropriate to 'set the bar lower' if we intend to develop the circumstances that will lead to professionalisation.

Mental models of coaching

The term 'mental model', and other related terms (e.g. schema), has arisen in a number of chapters in this book and is increasingly common in the literature. Our purpose here is to acknowledge this and to identify mental models as a priority research topic. There is no doubt that coaching depends on cognitive capacities and finds expression in the coach's reliance on decision-making. Coaching is also recognised to be a craft activity, but the action behaviour that operationalises coaching practice is clearly reliant on some forms of mental representation. Despite a consensus that this is the case, we do not have a clear picture of how these models work. How are they established, developed, or changed by coach education (a useful agenda item for coach education research)?

The consideration of mental models would also help coaching look at tensions around practice, mind and body dualism, and issues of internalisation and appropriation. These tensions may be resolved; they may not. Indeed, as Lemke (1997) reminds us, the intellectual culture that runs deep through contemporary thinking is that of 'divisions' where perhaps dynamic tensions usefully exist. A better understanding of sports coaching will emerge from the development of theories of mental representation necessary to account for understanding the coaching process. Coaching remains a mediated activity that is social, embodied, and transactional.

It would be interesting to understand the difference between schemata and embodiment, as each demonstrates a multi-level representation of activity between and within persons that are given form at the time of their expression (Daniels 2004). That is, schemata can be used to explore the possibilities for mental representations that are socially formed and modifiable.

When expert coaches attend to features and meaningful patterns of information in the environment, they are using socially acquired, expert schemata developed through participation in particular forms of practice (Glaser 1999). In this case the social nature of coaching consists of a small 'aura' of socialness that provides the input for the process of internalisation and the individual acquisition of the cultural 'given' (Lave & Wenger 1996). What is not clear is the impact of the learning context and the structure of the social world. Mental models should allow culturally shaped cognitive representation, operating within social interchange, and in specific settings, to be better understood.

The concept has had some fertile ground. Côté et al (1995) used the term as a generalised metaphor for coaches' cognitions, although they did not examine this in any detailed way. Lyle (2002) also used the concept of mental models to provide an explanation for coaches' decision making. This owed much to the assumption of mental modelling in Naturalistic Decision Making (Randall et al 1996, Lipshitz et al 2001). What we have termed a 'mental model' is a mechanism for representing the cognitive organisation that underlies the operational craft of the coach. Research into coaching behaviour and practice has worked around this assumption and referred to it in explanations of decision making. This is particularly relevant in coaching, because of its reliance on tacit knowledge and intuition-like practice.

The value of the concept is perhaps limited by our capacity to describe it. The term is intended to convey a capacity to 'hold a mental reference point'. At times this may be a virtual image, but it may also be a more or less-sophisticated network of knowledge structures. The psychological constructs schemata, scripts and frames are often used to describe the organisation of this knowledge and understanding. What is important is that it is sufficiently organised to act as a reference point or guide. Although it is important to appreciate how these 'models' are built, it is equally important to understand how they are accessed and used in practice. We should also distinguish between the use of the term for these mental representations and 'models' as a formula for guiding decision making, although future research may show that their use is similar.

The following comments are intended to be hypotheses. We assume that imaging and building mental representations are learned skills, and that they are domain-specific. Creating these reference points facilitates a further range of cognitive capacities – recognition, matching, identifying discontinuities, making predictions, evaluating progress, and evaluating outcomes. We speculate that these are used in coaching interventions. Indeed the coach seems likely to filter all behaviour through these 'images'. This facilitates the coordination or 'orchestration' (Jones & Wallace 2005) made necessary by the relatively dynamic, complex and highly charged environment in which much of coaching takes place. We further speculate that sophisticated mental models (in breadth and depth) are characteristic of higher-order cognitive abilities and expertise, and should be both a 'marker' for coaching expertise and a central feature of education and training.

We also note that athletes have mental models of performance, game play, training, goals, and so on. There is a further agenda about the complementarily of the mental representation of athlete and coach (and coach and mentor) and their shared understandings. We can also speculate that athletes/players need mental representations as their 'reference points', but how to develop these is rarely a feature of coach education.

It is helpful to think in terms of at least three 'models' – a goal model, a performance model, and various simulation models. The goal model represents planning and intended outcomes. It is used to guide target setting and progression points, and alters as the 'season' progresses. A sophisticated and wide-ranging version of this model may act as a framework for the whole coaching process. The performance model is a 'picture' of what is required in performance terms to achieve the goals that have been identified. This is dependent on 'technical' knowledge and informed by profiling, monitoring, analysis, and so on. The model is used as a reference point for current performance, and has implications for targets, development stages, timescales, progression rates, and is expressed in 'component' (technical, physical, etc.) terms as well as outcome terms. This model tells us 'how we're doing' and 'how we should be doing'. The simulation model helps with day-to-day management of the coaching process. This model provides a representation of what the coach 'expects to happen', and is built on experience, the data available, knowledge of the performers, and cases that the coach has previously experienced. We speculate that coaches use this to 'regulate' (manage progression and expectations) both direct interventions and progress more generally.

The simulation model in particular may hold the clue to coaches' expertise. Novices have a wide set of expectations but expert coaches may be able to 'narrow' these expectations. Experts, through experience (implying that they have incorporated many similar cases), have built in 'inherent variability', which allows them to deal more sanguinely with the 'ups and downs' of coaching. We speculate that the simulation is continuously updated by 'anticipatory reflection' – that is, anticipating the future and already having considered the most appropriate options. Again there are likely to be novice–expert differences. Mental models as a way of helping to explain coaches' behaviour brings with it a new set of skills that are not yet evident in coach education. We also note 'contest management' (match coaching) as a particular coaching environment where mental models of performance and simulation models may be important.

The use of mental models as a mechanism for representing coaches' cognitions, particularly the notion of a 'tacit set of reference points' requires a new vocabulary, better conceptual frameworks for coaching, and appropriate research methods. The anticipated sophistication of the expert coaches' modelling suggests that novice–expert studies will be valuable (but with strong caveats about what the term novice implies, that is, from the same coaching domain). Stimulated recall and other forms of interrogation of practice also need to be used. One particular approach might be to study the impact of critical incidents and crises on routine activity.

Operationalising coaching: models, practice and evidence

We have used the notions of models *of* coaching and models *for* coaching to interrogate and help in classifying coaching models (Lyle 1999, Cushion et al 2006). The distinction is that the former refers to models that are empirically derived, while the latter

are 'idealistic representations that arise from the identification of a set of assumptions about the process' (Cushion et al 2006 p 86). Critiques of existing models and discussions of the issues surrounding modelling per se are well rehearsed elsewhere (e.g. Cushion et al 2006, Cushion 2007a, 2007b). The important point for this discussion is that distinguishing between models *of* and *for* coaching remains a useful tool in developing coaching and understanding practice, as is being clear about a given model's epistemological standpoint.

Currently, different approaches to coaching and coach education offer a range of models and approaches to coaching, with different definitions, different assumptions and placing different emphasis on the directive versus facilitative nature of coaching (Stewart et al 2008). Models such as GROW (Whitmore 1992), principles of Gallwey's 'Inner Game' and so called '360 degree' approaches are increasingly more common in sports coaching as the field is colonised from other domains, such as commercial 'training' and business coaching. (There is a real threat to sports coaching of being overly influenced or colonised from other fields. Of course there is a utility in drawing on relevant theoretical resources from other perhaps 'similar' fields, but also a compelling need to develop *our* own conceptual understanding.)

These approaches are predominantly practitioner-developed and seek to describe and prescribe 'effective' coaching practice. Indeed, while they may incorporate some theoretical aspects, they ultimately remain practitioner reflections of practice (Stewart et al 2008). They are not empirically derived, and, using our typology, are atheoretical models *of* coaching. Indeed, this genre of coaching models has been described as 'proprietary models of coaching with little or no theoretical grounding' (Grant 2007 p 26) that have 'little published research underpinning their efficacy' (Palmer & Whybrow 2007 p 8). Instead of sound empirical support, we are offered considerable amounts of often re-used anecdotal, correlational, cross-sectional and 'opinionnaire' data. As Olson (2008) suggests this type of evidence can become 'circular evidence' with seemingly convincing arguments becoming heavily cited thus reinforcing the circle of believers, without ever leading to any real evidence. Consequently, practitioner beliefs and pre-constructed facts are taken uncritically to create and represent something that is actually far more diffuse and intangible in practice. As a result, limited or decontexualised, models, formula, and schemata dressed loosely in 'theoretical tinsel' (Everett 2002 p 58) can gain a concreteness once framed; and worryingly, can result in dysfunctional changes to coaching practice. Indeed, such models (or prescriptions) run the risk of errors and omissions, and are both limited and limiting if not critically reviewed and empirically grounded.

We need to acknowledge that attempts to model (or perhaps 'represent' would be more accurate) the coaching process (Côté et al 1995, Lyle 2002, Abraham et al 2006) have had limited success if measured by the impact on coach education and research design. Indeed we question whether a model of the coaching process might be inappropriate and/or over-ambitious given our arguments about domain specificity and sports coaching as an aggregation of loosely related roles. Any reduction to the core improvement purpose would be simplistic and unhelpful. On the other hand we have, as yet, been unable to represent the complexity of pedagogy, performance or interpersonal relationships in a way that captures their interrelationships and interdependences. We are not aware that these models have been useful to practitioners, and our view is that existing models lack an 'operational feel'. It is important that we are able to represent the coaching process in a way that identifies its component parts – and processes – rather than provides a prescriptive approach.

The point here is to not be overly critical or negative, but to promote a healthy scepticism to current coaching models and approaches (and those advocating them) that present coaching 'truths', and we suggest a more considered and cautious approach to constructing, developing and re-constructing our understanding and representation of coaching practice. A lack of evidence and theoretical underpinning encourages weak notions of theory–practice relations, and as such has, and will, continue to impoverish practice and develop simplistic attitudes. This, in turn, also helps construct a weak and limited basis for a professional identity that continues to disadvantage both coaching practice and coaching's professional standing (Cushion, 2007a).

Evidence-based approaches will help the field to avoid being dragged into a self-help or 'pop psychology' (Olson 2008) genre. A more holistic approach would ground coaching firmly in the broader 'empirical and theoretical knowledge base' (Grant & Stober 2006 p 5). This, in turn, is a means of integrating theoretical models *for* coaching, with empirical models *of* coaching. A research agenda then suggests an iterative process of refinement simultaneously informed by theory, practice and implementation evidence (Cushion 2007b, Stewart et al 2008). The end result may better represent the dynamic, relational and constructed nature of the coaching process. Coaching and its future development should be informed by a research programme embedded in practice that must be theoretically and empirically sophisticated (Cushion 2007a).

Summary

In the introductory chapter we expressed some disappointment that research into sports coaching had not moved forward as speedily as we might have expected. We are also aware that, despite changes in coach education, we have limited evidence of its effectiveness and impact on practice. There are significant changes foretold in the UK Coaching Framework and in the UK there has been investment in the deployment of coaches; but dispersed coaching populations, the absence of licensing, and the attempt to unify all levels and domains have constrained professionalisation. However, that was the bad news!

The purpose of the academic is to provide critical insight into a specific human endeavour, to ask questions and to provide answers. In aggregation, a body of knowledge and understanding (some of it applied directly to practice) is created that informs the conduct and development of that field. This is not (only) knowledge for knowledge sake, but the basis for education, better practice, and an understanding of how that field contributes to the 'human condition'. As we reflect on this collection of book chapters, we feel more positive about our subject. There is evidence of a more mature body of knowledge. This is demonstrated in its diverse perspectives, more critical questions, and the emergence both of (embryonic) 'schools' of research and common interests. In particular, this emerging maturity is reflected in the level of conceptual debate. We are in no doubt that there is a need for a much better conceptual framework for sports coaching. Nevertheless, it is our perception that this academic field is beginning to look beyond cultural differences, beyond social 'systems', and while relying on theoretical perspectives from many disciplines, the findings are beginning to be aggregated within a set of conceptual understandings that suggests a more cohesive field. We should not exaggerate this progress. The development of 'coaching theory' or 'theories about coaching' is someway off. Yes there are issues to be resolved, but we hope that the reader will accept this collection of academic writing as a marker of this progress and as a stimulus to further study.

References

Abraham, A., Collins, D., Martindale, R., 2006. The coaching schematic: validation through expert coach consensus. J. Sports Sci. 24, 549–564.

Côté, J., Salmela, J.H., Trudel, P., et al., 1995. The coaching model: a grounded assessment of expert gymnastic coaches knowledge. Journal of Sport and Exercise Psychology 17 (1), 1–17.

Cushion, C.J., 2007a. Modelling the complexity of the coaching process. International Journal of Sport Science and Coaching 2 (4), 395–401.

Cushion, C.J., 2007b. Modelling the complexity of the coaching process: a response to commentaries. International Journal of Sport Science and Coaching 2 (4), 427–433.

Cushion, C.J., Armour, K.M., Jones, R.L., 2006. Locating the coaching process in practice models: models 'for' and 'of' coaching. Physical Education and Sport Pedagogy 11, 83–99.

Daniels, H., 2004. Vygotsky and pedagogy. Routledge, London.

Erikson, K., Côté, J., Fraser-Thomas, J., 2007. Sport experiences, milestones, and educational activities associated with high-performance coaches' development. The Sport Psychologist 21, 302–316.

Everett, J., 2002. Organisational research and the praxeology of Pierre Bourdieu. Organisational Research Methods 5 (1), 56–80.

Gilbert, W., Trudel, P., 2004. Analysis of coaching science research published from 1970–2001. Res. Q. Exerc. Sport 75, 388–399.

Gilbert, W., Côté, J., Mallett, C., 2006. The talented coach: developmental paths and activities of successful sport coaches. International Journal

of Sport Science and Coaching 1 (1), 69–76.

Glaser, R., 1999. Expert knowledge and processes of thinking. In: McCormick, C., Paechter, C. (Eds.), Learning and knowledge. Paul Chapman, London, pp. 88–102.

Grant, A.M., 2007. Past, present and future: the evolution of professional coaching and coaching psychology. In: Palmer, S., Whybrow, A. (Eds.), Handbook of coaching psychology: a guide for practitioners. Routledge, London, pp. 25–39.

Grant, A., Stober, D., 2006. Introduction. In: Stober, D., Grant, A. (Eds.), Evidence based coaching: putting best practices to work for your clients. Wiley & Sons, New Jersey, pp. 1–14.

Jones, R.L., Wallace, M., 2005. Another bad day at the training ground: coping with ambiguity in the coaching context. Sport, Education & Society 10, 119–134.

Kay, T., Armour, K.M., Cushion, C.J., et al., 2008. Are we missing the coach for 2012? Report to the Sportnation Panel, Loughborough University, IYS.

Lave, J., Wenger, E., 1996. Practice, person, social world. In: Daniels, H. (Ed.), An introduction to Vygotsky. Routledge, London, pp. 143–150.

Lemke, J., 1997. Cognition, context and learning: a social semiotic perspective. In: Kirshner, D. (Ed.), Situated cognition theory: social neurological and semiotic perspectives. Lawrence Erlbaum, New York.

Lipshitz, R., Klein, G., Orasanu, J., et al., 2001. Taking stock of Naturalistic Decision Making. Journal of Behavioural Decision Making 14, 331–352.

Lyle, J., 1999. The coaching process: an overview. In: Cross, N., Lyle, J.

(Eds.), The coaching process: principles and practice for sport. Butterworth Heinemann, Oxford, pp. 3–24.

Lyle, J., 2002. Sports coaching concepts: a framework for coaches' behaviour. Routledge, London.

North, J., 2009. The coaching workforce 2009–2016. National Coaching Foundation, Leeds.

Olson, P., 2008. A review of assumptions in executive coaching. Coaching Psychologist 4 (3), 151–159.

Palmer, S., Whybrow, A., 2007. Coaching psychology: an introduction. In: Palmer, S., Whybrow, A. (Eds.), Handbook of coaching psychology: a guide for practitioners. Routledge, London, pp. 1–20.

Randel, J.M., Pugh, H.L., Reed, S.K., 1996. Differences in expert and novice situation awareness in naturalistic decision making. International Journal of Human-Computer Studies 45, 579–597.

sports coach UK, 2004. United Kingdom Coaching Certificate: qualification guidance Levels 1 to 3. sports coach UK, Leeds.

Stewart, L.J., O'Riordan, S., Palmer, S., 2008. Before we know how we've done, we need to know what we're doing: operationalising coaching to provide a foundation for coaching evaluation. The Coaching Psychologist 4 (3), 125–133.

Trudel, P., Gilbert, W., 2006. Coaching and coach education. In: Kirk, D., O'Sullivan, M., McDonald, D. (Eds.), Handbook of research in physical education. Sage, London, pp. 516–539.

Whitmore, J., 1992. Coaching for performance. Nicholas Brealey, London.

Note: Page numbers followed by *f* indicate figures; and *t* indicate tables and *b* indicate boxes.

A

Ability, player, 90
Academy coaching, 93
Accountability, 209–210
Action decisions, 27–28, 34
Active coach behaviour, 46, 47
Activity theory, 18–20
Adolescents
  participation coaches for, 71–73
  performance coaches for, 73–75
  see also Young adults
Adults
  feedback, to children, 68
  see also Young adults
Affordances, notion of, 171
Amateur organisations, 200
Anticipatory reflection, 250
Anti-intellectualism, 8
Apprenticeship, 156, 184
Athlete development, 63–84
  athlete-centred approach, 52–53, 240
  athlete-coach relationship, 72
  categories of coaching, 68–78
  coaching frameworks, 64–65
  coaching model (CM), 65–67, 67*f*
  Developmental Model of Sports Participation (DMSP),
    67–68
  mental models of performance, 249
Athlete learning, 184–185
  examples, 178*b*, 179*b*
  see also Practice theories; Theories of practice
Athlete-coach relationship, interaction complexity,
  15–26
Atypical events, 226–227
Audit stage, 89
Authority regulators, 197
Authority (TARGET model), 69
Automatic coach behaviour, 226
Autonomy, 55, 215
Autonomy-supportive environments, 55
Availability, player, 90

B

Basic rules, 38
Behaviour, coach, 43–62
  automatic, 226
  context specific, 52–55
  guidelines for, 50–52
  key behaviours, 46–50
  research, 49–50
  study of, 45–46
  vs philosophy, 239–241
Beliefs, 51, 184, 234–235
  declaration of, 234
  practical manifestation of, 234
Benchmarking, 103
Beneficence, principle of, 214–215
Best practice, 109
Bill of Rights for Young Athletes, 239
Biographies, 121, 147
Body, techniques of, 165–167
Bottom-up approach, 202
Bourdieu, P., 112–113
Burnout, 74

C

Caring, 66–67
  adolescents and, 72–73, 75
  children and, 70
  young adults and, 77
Case studies, 38
Categorical imperatives (Kant), 213
Categories, coaching, 68–78
Certification structure, 247
Character building, 66–67
  adolescents and, 72–73, 75
  children and, 70
  young adults and, 77
Children Act 2004, 210
Children, participation coaches for, 63, 68–71
  implications, 70–71

Classifications, coaching, 5
Client service, 212
Coach education programme (CoDe), theory-based,
    138–139
Coach-athlete relationship, 72
  interaction complexity, 15–26
Coaches' community of practice (CCoP), 129,
    130–132
Coaching Behaviour Assessment System (CBAS), 64,
    136–137, 138, 139
Coaching Behaviour Scale for Sport (CB-S), 64–65
Coaching domains *see* Domains, coaching
Coaching Efficacy Scale (CES) (Canada), 142
Coaching model (CM), 64–67
Coaching process, 8
Code of Ethics and Conduct, 218
Code of Practice for Sports Coaches, 218
Codes of conduct, 210, 211
  professional, 217–219
Codes of Ethics, 210
Cognitive alchemy, 161
Cognitive capacities, 249
Cognitive development, 127
Cognitive dissonance, 51–52
Communication, 226
Communities of practice (CoP), 126–128, 128–129, 156
  coaches' (CCoP), 129, 130–132
  limitations, 129–130
Community coaching, 244–245
Compensation mentality, 218
Competence, 37, 65–66
  adolescents and, 71, 74
  behaviours, features of, 76
  children and, 68–69
  young adults and, 76
Competition, 77
  plans, 120
  programmes, 89, 90
Complexity, 3, 43–44, 182
  coach-athlete interaction, 15–26
  coaching as, 3, 4
Conceptual development, 1–14, 16–18
  coaching domains, 5–6
  features, coaching process, 2–5
  research, 1–2, 6–10
Confidence, 66
  adolescents and, 71, 74
  children and, 69
  young adults and, 76
Confounding factors, 90
Connection, 66
  adolescents and, 71–72, 74–75
  children and, 69–70
  young adults and, 76–77

Consequentialist theory, 213–214
Constructivist theories, 156
Contest management, 250
Context, learning, coaching and subject matter, 169–171
Contingency planning, 94–95
Continuing of experience principle, 161–162
Continuing professional development (CPD), 113, 155,
    157–160, 201
  elements of, 157
  impact evaluation, 160
  key characteristics, 157
  lifelong learning, 146–147, 149–150
Continuity, 96
Course of action, 21–23
  activity theory, 19–20
  analysis, 18–19
  situated action, 20–21
Critical incidents, 236–237
Cultural reproduction, 173–175
Cultural theory of learning, 187, 188

D

Data collection, 198t
Decision making, 27–42, 214
  development implications, 36–39
  intuition, 31–32, 34–36, 225–226
  staged process of, 212–213
  see also Naturalistic Decision Making (NDM)
Decision Skills Training, 37–39
Default role, 53
Deficit model, 102–103
Definitions
  coach philosophy, 234
  high-performance coaches, 119–121
  pedagogy, 167
  practice ethics, 212–214
  professionalism, 100–101, 154–155
  sports coaching, 246–248
Degrees of freedom, 4
Deliberate play, 67, 68, 69, 70, 74
  empathy and, 75
  opportunities for, 75
Deliberate practice, 67, 68, 74, 77, 123
Deliberative decisions, 27–28
Development
  decision making and, 36–39
  sport and, 5
  see also Athlete development; Conceptual development;
      Workforce development
Developmental Model of Sports Participation (DMSP),
    67–68, 75–76, 125
Didactique, 167, 169–170
Disciplinary power, theory of, 236

Distributed cognition, 171, 172
Docile coach, 113–114
Domains, coaching, 5–6, 243–252
    typology, 245
'Drip feed' knowledge, 38
Duty, 211
Dynamic social process, 15–16
    network (DSN), 131

E

Edge of chaos, 15–16
Education, coach, 135–152, 238–239
    examples of, 147–149, 153–154, 162
    formal, 124
    human learning approach, 144–147, 145f
    initiatives, 135–136
    measurement, 149–150
    programme effectiveness, 136–144, 136t, 140t, 143t, 145–146
Ego-orientation, 69, 72–73
Elementary unit of meaning (EUM), 21–23
Elite sport, 5, 77, 106
    athletes, 75–76
    competence in, 76
Empathy, 226
    deliberate play and, 75
Empowerment, 54, 186
'End of season' period, 95
Engagement, clarity of, 217
Environment, learning, task and, 171–172
Episodic concept, 3, 9–10
    learning experience, 144–145
Epistemology, 51
    epistemological gap, 51–52
Ethical pluralist approach, 214
Ethics
    decision-making, 212–213
    service, 109–110
    see also Practice ethics
Evaluation (TARGET model), 69
Evidence-based practice, 210, 216, 250–252
Excellence
    pools of, 105
    standards of, 174
Expectation effects, 48
Experience, 38
    coaches', 221–222
    coaching, 123–124
    pre-mediate experiences, 125
    sport participation, 122–123
Expertise, 221–232
    experience, 221–222
    knowledge, 222–224
    skills, 224–229

F

Fairness, 215
    fair play, 217
Families, 71–72
Feature matching, 31
Feedback, 47, 224
    adult to children, 68
    expectation and, 48
Fixture list, 90
Formal learning, 146
Foucault, M., 236
Frameworks, 64–65
    5Cs, 65, 66t
Friendships, 69, 71
Full-time coaching, 93
Funding, 113, 120, 214

G

Game Sense approach, 185
Goals, 20
    goal model, 249–250
Good practice, 95–96
Governing Bodies of sport, 197, 199, 200, 201–202
    see also National Governing Bodies (NGBs)
Grounded theory, 22
Groupings (TARGET model), 69
Guidelines, 39, 50–52

H

Habitus, 112, 165–167, 169, 235
    concept of, 188
Head Coach position, 95–96
Higher education, 106
High-performance coaches, 119–134
    coaching communities, 126–130
    coaching experience, 123–124
    defined, 119–121
    formal education, 124
    key criteria, 122
    key interrelated tasks, 120
    pathways, 121–122
    pre-mediate experiences, 125
    social learning networks, 130–132
    sport participation experience, 122–123
    stage-based model, 125–126
Home league fixtures, scheduling of, 95

I

Identity, 123
Impression managing, 51–52

Incidental outcomes, 128
In-competition behaviour, 50
Independence, 55
Individual difference, 129–130
Informal knowledge networks (IKN), 130–131
Informal learning, 146
Instruction, 45, 46–47
  feedback, 53–54
Instructors, 44, 248
Intensity, 94
Interpretant, 21
Interpretation, 95–96
Intervention, design of coaching, 89
Introspection, 38
Intuition, 31–32, 34–36
  decision making and, 225–226
  features of, 35
Investment years, 75–76

J

Joint enterprise, 128–129
Judgement, 212, 213, 214, 218
Judgement/Decision Making (J/DM), 27, 29–30
Justice, principle of, 215

K

Kant, I, 213, 215
Key performance indicators (KPIs), 93–94, 96
Knowing, 183
Knowledge, 31–32, 183
  body of, 105–107
  coaches', 222–224
  developing strategic, 224
  gaps in existing, 49–50
  problematising existing, 49–50
  production, 182–184
  'society', 183
  sources of, 223
  structure, 31–32
  types of, 223–224

L

Language, 38, 247
Large-scale education training programmes,
    142–144, 143*t*
Leadership, 121, 237
Leadership Scale for Sport (LSS), 64
Learning
  approach, 160–162
  centrality of, 165–167
  coaching, subject matter and context, 169–171

concept of, 155–157
  lifelong, 146–147
  as participation, 130
  situations, 146
  social networks, 130–132
  task, environment and, 171–172
  see also Athlete learning; Education, coach
Legal redress, 218
Legitimate peripheral participation, 128
Life histories, 121, 147
Lifelong learning, 146–147, 149–150
  see also Continuing professional development (CPD)
Literature review
  coaching philosophy, 235–236
  professionalism, 101–105
Logic of practice, 235

M

Macrocycles, 89–90, 91–92
Management, 121
Managerialism, new, 99
Mastery Approach to Coaching (MAC), 137–138, 139, 144
Mental models, 32, 34, 248–250
'Menus', catalogue of, 86
Mesocycles, 89–90, 91–92, 94
Microcycles, 91, 95
Models, 250–252
  for coaching, 250, 251
  of coaching, 250
  of practice, 85
  for practice, 85
Models-based practice (MBP), 169–170
Monitoring, 91, 120
Moral authority, conditions for, 217
Moral virtue, 237–238
Morality, 209
  development and, 72–73
  responsibility and, 173–175
  see also Ethics; Practice ethics
Multidimensional Model of Leadership, 64
Mutual engagement, 129

N

National Governing Bodies (NGBs), 100, 103–104, 108, 109,
    111, 114, 165, 194
  coach education system, 104, 105–106, 150
  modernisation programme, 104
  see also Scottish Governing Bodies (SGBs)
National sports organisations (NSO), 197–201
  strategic options, 201*t*
National Standards for Sports Coaching, 233
  listed, 240

Naturalistic Decision Making (NDM), 27–42, 249
storytelling, 32–34
Negotiating, 120
Networks of practice (NoP), 130–131
New managerialism, 99
Nietzsche, F.W., 237–238
Non-deliberative decision making, 27–28
Non-formal learning, 146
Non-maleficence, 214–215

O

Object, 21
Obligations, 211
Observation systems, 45–46, 47
Occupational Standards, 194
'Off-task', 47
'One size fits all' approach, 53
'On-task', 47
Opportunities for action, 171
Organisational perspective, 77
Organised knowledge, 31
Outcomes, 52
incidental, 128
predicting, 225
quality of, 90
Outline plans, 92

P

Parents, 70
Participation, 187
coaches, 68–73
sport experience and, 122–123
Part-time coaching, 93, 95
Passive observation, 47
Pathos, 16
Pedagogy
defined, 167
place in coaching practice, 180
practice theories and, 180–181
settings, 172–173
theories of practice and, 181–184
Peer relationships, 69, 71
Perceptual skills, coaches', 229
Performance
analysis, 93
indicators, 93–94, 96
model, 249–250
success, 46–47
Performance coaches, 199
for adolescents, 73–75
for young adults, 75–78
Performer-centred – coach-led principle, 209–210

Periodisation, 86
Peripheral participation, legitimate, 128
Personal-Social Responsibility Model, 66–67, 73
Personnel, 120
Phased skills progression model, 93
Philosophy, coach, 51–52, 233–242
beliefs/values/principles, 234–235
defined, 234
development of, 237–239
literature review, 235–236
vs behaviour, 239–241
Physical conditioning, 94
Physical education teacher education (PETE), 175
Planning, 20, 85–98
expert coaches', 224–225
plan-do-review, 89
procedures, 89–91
process, 87–89, 88f
recipe, 87–88
in rugby union, 91–96
workforce development, 195–197, 196t, 198t
Policy borrowing, 103
Pools of excellence, 105
Positional requirements, 95
Positive reinforcement, 47–48
Positive youth development, 65, 66t
Positivist approach, 7–8, 16, 17
research, 6
Power dynamics, 129–130, 188
Practical issues, 90
Practice ethics, 209–220
codes of professional conduct, 217–219
context, 210–212
defined, 212–214
engagement in, 216–217
justifying/analysing, 215–216
key principles, 214–215
Practice theories, 177–180, 184, 185–186, 250–252
opportunities and limitations, 181, 185–186
pedagogy and, 180–181
see also Theories of practice
Praise, 224
praise and scold, 47–48
Prediction, 225
Pre-mediate experiences, 125
Principles, 234–235
Problem solving, 227–228
Problematised view, 121
Problem-based learning (PBL), 38, 139–141
Process, coaching, 8
Production of knowledge, 183–184
Professional artistry, 35
Professional autonomy, principle of, 215
Professional Codes of Practice, 210

Professional learning communities (PLCs), 157–158
Professionalism, 99–118
   coaching and, 105–107, 110–111
   critical reflections, 111–113
   defined, 100–101, 154–155
   further study, 114–115
   literature review, 101–105
   organisation, 107–109
   relevance, 100
   service ethic, 109–110
Progress markers, 93
Propositional knowledge, 31
Psychological skills, 74, 75

R

Received wisdom, 216–217
Recipe solutions, 30, 31–32, 87–88
Recognition Primed Decision (RPD) model, 27, 30, 36–37
Recognition (TARGET model), 69
Recreational sport, 5
Recreational years, 71
Recruitment targets, factors militating against, 200–201
Reflection, 38, 178–179, 237
   anticipatory, 250
   practices, 224
   'reflection-in-action', 123–124
   'reflection-on-action', 123–124
   techniques, 216
Relational schemas, 18
'Repair people', coaches as, 227
Re-planning, 92
Representamen, 21
Representative team tournaments, 90
Respect, principle of, 215
Responsibility, moral, 173–175
'Retrospective reflection-on-action', 123–124
Reward environment, 245
Risk, 30
Role, of coach, 53–55
Rotation policy, 96, 177
Rules
   basic, 38
   rule-guided behaviour, 218, 235

S

Safeguarding Vulnerable Persons Act 2006, 210
Sampling years, 68, 172–173
'Scaffolding' analogy, 54–55
Scottish Governing Bodies (SGBs), 194–196, 197, 199, 200, 201
Scripts, 31–33
Self-awareness, 239
Self-determination, 215

theory, 55, 65–66
Self-monitoring, 228–229
Self-worth, 69, 224
Semi-structured interviews, 235–236
Service ethic, 109–110
   ideals, 109–110
   priorities, key, 195
Shared repertoire, 129
Silence, 47
Simulation models, 249–250
Situated action, 18–19, 20–21
Situated learning, 130
   theory, 171
Situated training, 38
Situation-action matching, 29–30
Situational assessment, 37
Situational awareness, 30–31
Skills
   analysis, 199
   coaches', 224–229
   framework approach, 199
   gaps, 199
Slow Interactive Script model, 32–33
Small-scale education training programmes, 136–139, 136*t*
Social constructivist theory, 127–128
Social learning
   networks, 130–132
   theory, 72
Social process, 15–16
Social setting, 17–18
Social theory, Foucault's, 236
Socialization, 70, 216–217
Socio-cultural perspectives, 187
Socio-pedagogy, 167–175
Socratic Method, 170
Specialising years, 73–74
Specific Actions, 193–194
Sponsorship, 120
Sport Anxiety Scale (SAS), 137
Sport Competition Anxiety Test (SCAT), 137
Sport Education, 173
   model, 168
Sports coaching, defined, 246–248
Sportsmanship, 217
Stage-based model, high-performance coaching, 125–126
Stakeholder organisations, 120
Standards of excellence, 174
Status, 99, 103
Storytelling, 32 34, 236, 237
Strategic Action Areas, 193–194
Strategic knowledge, 224
Strategic options, 201
Strength and conditioning programme, 96
Structural development, 72

Structured improvisation, 4–5, 85–86
Structured interview, 122
Structured training, 77
Subject matter, coaching, learning and context,
169–171
Success, 46–47
Supply and demand, coaching and, 205–206
Supply planning focus, 197
Symbolic violence, 112
Systematic coaching, 85–86

T

Talent
development, 68
identification programmes, 214
TARGET model, 69, 70–71
Task, learning, environment and, 171–172
Task-orientation, 69, 72–73
Tasks (TARGET model), 69
Teaching Games for Understanding (TGfU), 169–171,
173, 185
Team sports
drills, 90
personnel, 95
see also Planning
Technical development, 92
Technical knowledge, 105
Technical-rational approach, 161
Techniques of the body, 165–167
Technocratic rationality, 7–8, 205
'10-year rule', 123
Terminology, 92
Tertiary education, 125
Theories of practice, 177–180, 184, 186–188
opportunities and limitations, 182–184,
187–188
pedagogy and, 181–184
see also Practice theories
Theory waving, 8–9
Thought-sign model, 21
Threat, 30
Time pressure, 30
Timing (TARGET model), 69
Top-down approach, 202
Tradition, 167–168, 171–172

Training
structured, 77
theory, 86
Transformation, 173–175
cultural, 175
Transformative learning, 156–157, 160
Transmutation, 237–238

U

Uncontrollability, 4
University-based education programmes, 139–142, 140t
Utilitarian theory, 213–214

V

Values, 210–211, 234–235, 237–238
Videos, 96
Violence, symbolic, 112
Virtue ethics, 214
Voluntary ethos, 100
coaches, 104, 110, 113
commitment, 110
Vygotsky, L, 126, 127

W

Waving theory, 8–9
Workforce development, 193–208
national sports organisations and, 197–201, 201t
national vs sports-specific projections, 202–204, 203t
planning, 195–197
wider employment context, 201–202

Y

Young adults, 63
performance coaches for, 75–78
Youth development
literature, 64
programmes, 63

Z

Zone of Proximal Development (ZPD), 54–55

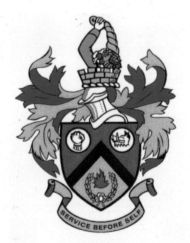